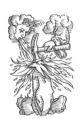

Anna Katharina Münch

Nomadic Women's Health Practice

Islamic Belief and Medical Care among

Kel Alhafra Tuareg in Mali

Schwabe Verlag Basel

Gedruckt mit freundlicher Unterstützung der NCCR North-South, Cogito, Swiss TPH

 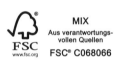

Umschlaggestaltung unter Verwendung einer Fotografie von
Anna Katharina Münch: Thomas Lutz, Schwabe
Gesamtherstellung: Schwabe AG, Druckerei, Muttenz/Basel
Printed in Switzerland
ISBN 978-3-7965-2744-9

www.schwabe.ch

Table of contents

Preface

Mobile pastoralists like the Kel Alhafra Tuareg belong to the most neglected communities in the world. They are devoid of social services for health and education. In addition, they suffer from extreme environmental and climatic hardship. For over fifteen years, through healthcare reform projects in Sahelian countries, the Swiss Tropical and Public Health Institute has engaged in research and development for better social services to mobile pastoral communities. Starting in Chad, the work extended to Mauritania, Mali and Ethiopia.

Initial stakeholder processes brought together national health authorities, the concerned communities and scientists to define agendas for research. Mixed teams of anthropologists, geographers, medical doctors and veterinarians started field work to better understand the context of vulnerability, perceived needs and priorities of the concerned communities. Observational, "etic" perspectives were complemented with "emic" views to assess perceptions by the concerned communities and to analyze the traditional and modern state institutional frameworks. The first results in Chad showed that vaccination coverage was better for cattle than for children and women. This led to the development of joint animal and human preventive health services.

Health perception of mobile pastoralists is divided between traditional care and influences of modern medicine in a syncretistic way. Locally perceived traditional views, while containing numerous misconceptions from a modern western medical perspective, largely determine health behavior and help-seeking attitudes. Attempts to compare results across different countries reveal a very high cultural and ethnic diversity of communities having a seemingly similar mobile lifestyle. Health care provision must be adapted with respect to local geographical, social and cultural contexts. This motivated a partnership with The Institute of Islamic and Middle Eastern Studies at the University of Bern and the medical faculty of the University of Bamako. Close cooperation between cultural and medical sciences was established. It was a bold endeavor as paradigmatic and epistemological differences seem not to converge. With an aim to improve healthcare, however, a pragmatic triangulation of the mobile pastoralists' healthcare determinants by the different involved disciplines was warranted. Particular attention to in-depth understanding of the local language and to representations of perceived illnesses is required.

The present work by Anna Münch is such an in-depth hermeneutic analysis of the perception of illness and health among the Kel Alhafra (a group of the Kel Anṣar Tamasheq confederation in the Republic of Mali, better known as Tuareg). It serves first as a linguistic and cultural science reference with special emphasis on the human body, illness perception and health care. Secondly, it serves as a reference for locally adapted health planning and demonstrates the power and potential of cultural sciences applied to practical problem solving in healthcare. It also serves as a case study for epistemological dialogue between cultural and medical sciences. The advantages of cultural immersion are demonstrated in comparison to cross-sectional epidemiological assessments. The process of information exchange in the studied communities requires the scientist to become part of the community and match its local social and gender standards. For this, Anna Münch has invested heavily in Arabic and Tamasheq language skills and took considerable personal risk, living for months as an accepted family member of the Kel Alhafra more than a hundred kilometers north of Timbuktu. I am convinced that this book will serve as a linguistic and cultural reference and pave the way for effective locally adapted health and social services to the Kel Alhafra. Thus, it provides an important case example for the potential of close cooperation between cultural and health sciences working for the improvement of health in remote communities of sub-Saharan Africa.

Marcel Tanner, Director Swiss Tropical
and Public Health Institute   *Basel, January 2012*

Acknowledgment

The present monograph represents a revised version of my doctoral dissertation, which was accepted on 5 October 2007 by the Faculty of Humanities at the University of Bern (Switzerland).

From 2003–2007, thanks to my advisor Prof. Dr. Reinhard Schulze, the Institute of Islamic and Middle Eastern Studies at the University of Bern provided a quiet environment that allowed me to recuperate from the exhaustion of life in the desert and concentrate on analyzing my data. Professor Schulze showed confidence in my research and gave me intellectual freedom while generously standing as an expert at my side.

Additionally, I feel especially obliged to Prof. Dr. Jakob Zinsstag of the Swiss Tropical and Public Health Institute, who was always there with encouragement and support as a second advisor. Along with Prof. Dr. Bassirou Bonfoh, the Director of the Centre Suisse de Recherches Scientifiques in Abidjan (Côte d'Ivoire), Professor Zinsstag ventured regularly into the innermost corner of the Kel Alhafra transhumance area. With their diplomatic skills, their cautions, their useful advice and their thought provoking inputs, Professor Zinsstag and Professor Bonfoh both provided me with technical and moral support throughout the development of this work. For all of this, I thank them warmly.

This study was made possible principally by the Cogito Foundation, which not only nurtured the beginning of the research project through financial support and unyielding interest but came through once again for its completion. The Commission for Research Partnerships with Developing Countries, KFPE, also made a significant contribution to the project and moreover provided support to Mohamed El Moctar my doctoral partner in Mali.

Of course, this work would not have been possible without the members of the Kel Alhafra families who warmly welcomed me into their circles and answered with patience my many questions. In particular, I would like to express my gratitude to the committed fraction leader Alhassan Ag Alkher. His help facilitated access to many Kel Alhafra tents in remote areas of the Azawad. Furthermore, I feel very thankful to Muhammad Tijani Ag Ousman, the traditional healer and "Agent de Santé". With the vast knowledge he generously shared, he has significantly contributed to the enrichment of this work. With his wit and humor, he made many difficult days of the medical study in the desert bearable. "Achoḍi" and the African "Cousinage" will always be a cheerful reminder.

Dr. Birama Diallo, the physician from Bamako, diligently examined his patients under extreme conditions in the desert. I have great appreciation for his tireless dedication. Dr. Mohamed El Moctar's study on the utilization of health centers has also contributed significantly to the understanding of nomadic healthcare.

Mariamma Wālāt Faṭi was a faithful companion during the ethnographic study. She hiked courageously with me from camp to camp under the scorching sun of the dry season even in times of food shortage and hardship. My thanks go in addition to the interpreter Muhammad Aḥmad, whose work and patience during the clinical study were of great value.

Furthermore, I would like to thank the local Bamako office of the Swiss Direction for Development and Cooperation, SDC, who helped the nomads of the Azawad with food and medical relief during a trying period.

In the realization of this book, I owe particular gratitude to the translator, Dr. Anne Blonstein (1958-2011), who despite serious illness converted the text from German into English. Thanks also goes to Dr. Jan Hattendorf for his invaluable contribution in data analysis and graphics, to Helen Kupferschmied for accounting assistance, and to Toshiaki Ozawa for proofreading the English text.

The book project was generously supported by contributions from the Swiss Tropical and Public Health Institute, the Cogito Foundation, the NCCR North-South and the Berne University Research Foundation. To these organizations and the publisher Schwabe Verlag, I extend heartfelt thanks.

"āfus iyyān wār isirəd iman-ənnes", "one hand cannot wash alone", the Kel Alhafra say. Without the direct and indirect support of many, this work would not have been possible. I am grateful to all my friends, colleagues, relatives and acquaintances, too many to list here by name, who provided me with a nurturing environment throughout the years. Finally, I would like to express my thanks to my parents, Elsbeth Münch-Fiechter and Eric Münch, as well as to my brothers, Christian, Manuel and Matthias, who supported me in so many ways time and time again.

1. Introduction

1.1. General overview

Scarred by years of intense drought that decimated their herds and turned large areas of their habitat into inhospitable desert, marginalized by foreign occupation forces, but also isolated by violent uprisings from their own ranks, the Kel Alhafra in Northern Mali are today once again forced to survive by adapting to the resources within their environment. Sparse rainfall obliges them to be highly mobile and often places them far from urban centers and public services such as schools and health care facilities. Because their lives – unlike those of the men – are largely restricted to the protective shadows of the tent and encampment, sick women and children can rarely avail themselves of outside medical care. Meanwhile, their conceptions of illness, their understanding of the human organism, their ideas about the etiology of diseases and their concomitant responses and behavior remain largely unknown outside the Tamasheq sphere.

In contrast to other Tamasheq groups, among the Kel Alhafra there are no families of traditional healers who pass their knowledge on from generation to generation and who can be approached to treat someone who is sick. Although the Kel Alhafra belong to the social class of the *inaslamān*, the Islamic scholars, among whom there are respected marabouts who can apply the Koranic text to treat sickness, in the female milieu there are no explicitly designated women with traditional healing knowledge. At birth, the umbilical cord is always cut by a relative or neighbor, and when a woman or her children are sick, interventions depend on the type and quality of her own healing knowledge, her social support system and the opportunities she has to use these effectively.

The Kel Alhafra (Arabic *al-ḥufra*) of the Republic of Mali are a branch of the Kel Anṣār Tamasheq who live as nomadic pastoralists in the commune of Ber which is located within the northeastern section of the Timbuktu region. This area covers approximately 72,000 square kilometers and is home to about 25,000 people (70% are Tamasheq *(taneslamt)* speakers and 30% are Arab (Ḥassānīya) speaking "Moors"). As with almost all nomadic communities in the area, camel husbandry, complemented with sheep and goats, comprises the livelihood of the nearly 1,000-member Kel Alhafra group. Only about 194 Kel Alhafra families work cattle. The well Tin Timāɣayān, about 140 km northeast of the desert village Ber, is the geographic center of their transhumance area. Tin Timāɣayān was also the polling station for elections in 2007, where the name "Alhafra" was used as a political entity. Access to water (comprised almost exclusively of groundwater from a depth of 20–110 meters) is critically underdeveloped in the region. In Ber, only half of the major wells are function-

ing. Tin Timāyayān is one of approximately 27 such operational wells. There
are slightly more than 100 other, smaller pits and holes in varying degrees of
dysfunction from which the inhabitants attempt to draw water to supply their
herds (in the municipality: approximately 500 cattle, 7000 sheep and goats,
1,300 camels and 1,300 donkeys). From these animals, milk production yields
about 25–30% of maximum available capacity providing 0.3 liters per capita
based on the population statistics for Ber.

For Kel Alhafra, the nearest health center (CSCOM – Centre de Santé
Communautaire) is in the village of Ber. From the northern transhumance areas of the nomads, this often means a five day camel ride to reach the health
center. There are eleven schools in the settlement of Ber but only four are
open, because the population does not have the means to support them. Only
nine percent of children in the village can attend school.

Studies to date that have dealt with health issues among the Tamasheq in
Mali have been largely undertaken west of Timbuktu and in the Gourma region. However, not only are the Tamasheq groups living in these areas different to those in the far north, since their return from exile and refugee camps,
they have to a large extent become either semi-nomadic or sedentary and have
access to a range of medical systems. The *imɣad* among the Kel Serere in
Gourma, for example, are recognized as experts in a form of traditional medicine, and Kel Serere who fall ill have, quite unlike the Kel Alhafra, recourse to
a variety of healing practitioners within their own group.

What forms of therapy are available to the Kel Alhafra, now that the traditional healer families of neighboring groups have moved into villages and
towns? What medical options for healing can they fall back upon?

Because the national immunization program (PEV, Programme Elargi de
Vaccination) lacks the resources to cover the most remote parts of northern
Mali, neither mothers nor children are sufficiently vaccinated to prevent epidemic outbreaks of whooping cough, measles, meningitis, tuberculosis, or
syphilis, which is endemic. New, previously unknown diseases have also entered the Kel Alhafra tents, especially a severe fever at the end of the rainy
season, which can be fatal and against which they have no remedies. The eating habits of the Kel Alhafra have also shifted significantly since the major
droughts and massive herd losses. Milk and meat are no longer the staples they
once were and are being increasingly replaced by cereals. For the Kel Alhafra
this readjustment disturbs the body's fragile internal equilibrium – maintained
in their view by a balance of cold and hot forces – weakening the individual and
thus rendering him or her susceptible to various diseases. The close physical association of the nomadic groups with their animals exposes them to additional
health risks. Animal slaughter, contact with birth entrails and the consump-

tion of uncooked raw milk are all possible sources of zoonoses. There is a 72% chance that a Kel Alhafra child will survive beyond its fifth birthday, and many women talk about miscarriages, still births, birth complications, the suffering of their children who died, and a general rise in the frequency of several disorders.

Sickness and healing always represent sources for cultural imagination. They are reference points for rituals and coded forms of networks that cannot be measured or appreciated by biomedical rationality alone. Human cultural behavior interprets traditional structures and value systems, and understanding these can yield important insights into options and limitations in health-specific areas. This book is an attempt to describe and present a precise picture of what are considered to be valid representations of sickness, diseases and their dissemination within the cultural context of the Kel Alhafra. The focus is on women and children, the most vulnerable groups in the nomadic society. How, in general, do the Kel Alhafra understand health and sickness? What are the dominant ideas about the human body among the Kel Alhafra? How does a norm-defining value system operate, and in what ways does it determine the scope available to or the restrictions placed on women and children? How do the women take care of their own and their children's health on a daily basis, and what methods do they use to treat and cure their health problems? What are the most frequent women- and child-specific diseases that they identify, and what public health services do they use? Together, these questions and their answers – provided largely by the Kel Alhafra women themselves – form the core of this study. A medical clinical investigation of the health status of the Kel Alhafra women and children was also undertaken. Using a standardized questionnaire, the women were asked about their utilization of external health services, vaccinations, their daily work, food consumption, and the number of their children.

It is in weaving together the two strands of this research into a third approach that the interdisciplinarity of this study becomes most apparent, in the search for correlations between clinically identified diseases and those perceived by the nomads themselves. Where do health-specific statements by the Kel Alhafra and medically ascertained facts drift apart? What are the shortcomings of a standardized questionnaire, and where are complementary cultural studies needed in order to provide a comprehensive picture of the actual, prevailing health status and health needs of the population?[1]

---

1 As Armin Prinz "discovered" among the Azande of Central Africa, the famous example of "hunter disease", *kaza ngua na tuva*, shows the importance of correlation between an interpretation of local perceptions and clinical findings. Because this disease could not be biomedically recognized in 1974, it was classified as a "cultural syndrome". Only in 1983/6, did serological and epidemiological studies show that it was Lyme disease. See here, Armin Prinz,

This is first and foremost a case study in the field of Islamic sciences employing primarily philological and anthropological criteria, in which supplementary empirical epidemiological approaches have also been applied. No claims are made about the general applicability of the research findings to the Tamasheq as a whole: theirs is not a single, homogenous society, and in Mali alone, there are enormous differences in the ways of life and the belief systems among the individual groups. It has not been possible to delve into the descent structures or the Islamization of the Kel Alhafra, and the influences of Greek and Arabic medicine on illness perception by the Kel Alhafra are likewise topics that lie outside the scope of this inquiry.

The Kel Alhafra were chosen as the focus of this study because they are a Tamasheq group that still seeks to live primarily from nomadic pastoralism and moves in a remote area neglected presumably largely for logistic reasons by researchers. Excluded from public health care and education, without proper command of the nation's official language, they feel marginalized and discriminated in the isolated desert of Azawad, where they try to make the most of locally available opportunities and resources. Nevertheless, the Kel Alhafra might be considered as exemplary for other nomadic groups living in inhospitable surroundings and exploring their own way into modernity, far from urban centers, political events and state infrastructures. The inexorable changes to which their society is being exposed are reflected not least in their prevailing medical system. Just as the hierarchic social structures of the past have lost much of their force, likewise, the formerly effective traditional medicine is not able to heal new diseases. Modern drugs circulate that cure symptoms but do not drive the disease in and of itself out of the body. What paths do the Kel Alhafra choose between modern and traditional medicine? How do they perceive themselves surviving in a very uncertain future when they lack state schooling and have been deprived of many of their traditional assets and yet are not sufficiently educated or trained to lead any lives other than those of nomads?

1.2. Methodology

As a Berber language, Tamasheq is one branch of the Afro-Asiatic (Hamito-Semitic) language family. It is subdivided into various dialects, of which the regional languages of the Hoggar in Algeria and the Ajjer in Niger have re-

"Die Lyme-Borreliose als 'Culture-bound syndrome' bei den Azande Zentralafrikas: Beispiel einer ethnozentrischen Fehlinterpretation", Special reproduction *Curare* 14 (1991).

ceived the most attention by scholars.[2] Literature on the Tamasheq dialects in Mali is much sparser, with Heath's *Dictionnaire touareg du Mali* as the only reasonably comprehensive reference work. The book serves as a useful guide to the linguistic structure of Tamasheq but falls short in conveying the richness of the language and its wealth of sayings and idiomatic expressions.[3] The Tamasheq take philology, "love of the word", very seriously, and eloquent speech and poetry are admired and praised. The Kel Alhafra, however, do not use Tamasheq as a written language, and texts are written in the Arabic they learn in the Koranic schools. Because the Kel Alhafra travel across the same regions as the Arabic-speaking Moors, nearly all of them understand and speak the Arabic Ḥassānīya dialect as well.[4]

This study would not have been possible without an active knowledge of Tamasheq: so much of the language is transmitted through proverbs, idioms and metaphors, which often resist an adequate translation. Furthermore, to understand a terminology of illness, as will be shown, knowledge of the source of the words used is critical, i.e. whether it is a Tamasheq word that has always been familiar to the Kel Alhafra, or whether it is a construct or loan word from French or Arabic whose meaning has, therefore, been "imported". The philological approach of this study is one based not on texts but on the (recorded) spoken word, with all the translations attempting to convey as much as possible of the general sense of the Tamasheq.

On the anthropological side, although I apply ethnographic research methods, I have sought wherever possible to give the word to the actors of the "other culture". I follow Geertz's view that an absolutely objective ethnography is impossible, and that a fiction is created whenever an observer describes a – to him or her – foreign world.[5] For this reason, I have taken care to present interpretations only when confirmed by the Kel Alhafra themselves. I hope in this way to have kept the "fictionalization" to a minimum. The intention has

---

2   See Charles de Foucauld, Charles, *Dictionnaire Touareg-Français. Dialecte de l'Ahaggar*, 4 vols. (Paris: Imprimerie nationale, 1951–1952); Karl-G Prasse, *Dictionnaire Touareg-Français (Niger)*, 2 vols. (Copenhagen: Museum Tusculanum Press, 2003); Mohamed Aghali-Zakara, *Psycholinguistique Touarègue. Interférences culturelles* (Paris: Inalco, 1992).

3   Jeffrey Heath, *Dictionnaire touareg du Mali. Tamachek-Anglais-Français* (Paris: Karthala, 2006).

4   All the *inəsləmān* tribes in Mali speak a strongly Arabicized Tamasheq. In contrast to other Tamasheq groups, the Kel Alhafra pronounce the letters ⌐ and ⌐ with an Arabic phonetics. It is for this reason that transcriptions of the Tamasheq alphabet sometimes contain the corresponding ḥ and ç. At the same time, the feminine gender of certain Arabic substantives is retained by the *inəsləmān* in their Tamasheq: *təjmaḍ-t āṣṣahāt* – "he has no force left"– is written by other Tamasheq groups as *ijmaḍ-t āṣṣahāt*, with the noun here considered masculine.

5   See Clifford Geertz, *Works and Lives: The Anthropologist as Author* (Cambridge: Polity Press, 1988).

been to reconstruct the ideational world in which the Kel Alhafra engage with health and sickness, with myself as a scholar of Islamic studies functioning first and foremost as a "cultural translator", someone who, in Good's sense, seeks to convey a social and cultural reality of semantic networks into another language.[6]

Quantitative components from epidemiology supplement the social science methodologies employed in this study, with clinical examinations and a standardized questionnaire providing data about the general health status of the study group.

It is hoped that the cross-disciplinary analysis of all the information obtained by the various approaches will provide not only an accurate picture of the health status of Kel Alhafra women and children, but also of the relationships between culture and illness within this particular nomadic society.

1.3. Data sources and data collection

Between October 2003 and March 2004, I devoted myself to learning the basic essentials of the Tamasheq language in a Tamasheq district of Timbuktu, as well as during shorter stays in Kel Alhafra encampments. Since there are no written records or textbooks for the specific dialect of the Kel Alhafra (taneslɜmt), the language had to be learned directly from members of this group. With basic linguistic knowledge, an ethnographic study was conducted from October 2004 to June 2005 where I stayed in two main camps and fam-

---

6 On the term "semantic networks" see Byron Good: "I introduced the notion 'semantic networks' to indicate that illness has meaning not simply through univocal representations that depict a disease state of the body, but as a 'product of interconnections', in Iser's terms – a 'syndrome' of experiences, words, feelings, and actions that run together for members of a society." Byron J. Good, *Medicine, Rationality and Experience: An Anthropological Perspective* (New York: Cambridge University Press, 1994) 171. The concept of "semantic networks" has been presented in a series of collaborations by Mary-Jo Del Vecchio Good and Byron Good: Byron J. Good, and Mary-Jo Del Vecchio Good, "The Meaning of Symptoms: A Cultural Hermeneutic Model for Clinical Practice", in *The Relevance of Social Science for Medicine* eds. Leon Eisenberg and Arthur Kleinman (Dordrecht: Reidel, 1980) 165–196; Byron J. Good and Mary-Jo Del Vecchio Good, "The Semantics of Medical Discourse", in *Sciences and Cultures,* eds. Everett Mendelsohn, and Yehuda Elkana (Dordrecht: Reidel, 1981) 177–212; Byron J. Good, Byron J. and Mary-Jo Del Vecchio Good, "The Comparative Study of Greco-Islamic Medicine: The Integration of Medical Knowledge into Local Symbolic Contexts", in *Paths to Asian Medical Knowledge,* eds. Charles Leslie and Allan Young (Berkeley: University of California Press, 1992) 257–271; Byron J. Good, Mary-Jo Del Vecchio Good, and Robert Moradi, "The Interpretation of Dysphoric Affect and Depressive Illness in Iranian Culture", in *Culture and Depression: Studies in the Anthropology and Cross-Cultural Psychiatry of Affect and Disorder* eds. Arthur Kleinman and Byron J. Good (Berkeley: University of California Press, 1985) 369–428.

ily associations of the Kel Alhafra within the transhumance area around the wells of In Astilan and In Agozmi. During these stays, I shared tents as an accepted member of a family with at least 7 other persons. I participated in the everyday work of the women, pounded millet with the neighbors, collected firewood, helped to round up sheep and goats, looked for lost animals, gathered wild fruits, visited neighboring camps and shared all aspects of a Kel Alhafra-life in the desert.

Between January and May 2005, Azawad was afflicted by an acute food shortage, during which malnutrition and epidemics claimed a significant number of lives, especially among children. At this time I was living near the well of In Agozmi, 180 km northeast of Timbuktu, without communication media. For weeks I shared with the nomads their highly precarious situation. The food supply was limited to millet, flour and some sunflower oil. Because their animals were emaciated or had died, there was almost no milk or meat, and many Kel Alhafra families were exhausted by the deprivations. After an appeal, Médecins sans Frontières (MSF) finally launched a *"mission explorative"* to evaluate the situation. Their report provoked intervention by the local SDC (Swiss Agency for Development and Cooperation) office in Bamako, which set up an emergency food program and intervened for three months in the area in which I was doing research, until the new rainy season began and the situation gradually became less tense. During this period, the provision of temporary humanitarian aid overrode the claims of research.

I finally returned to this study in October 2005, when two medical surveys were begun. In the first, during seven field missions to 36 encampments around 15 wells in a cross section of the transhumance area of the Kel Alhafra, a Malian doctor examined 177 women and 141 children with the aid of a standardized questionnaire (see chapter 6.1.1.). The data from this clinical study were evaluated later on in collaboration with the Swiss Tropical and Public Health Institute in Basel using the statistics program SAS™ version 9.1 (SAS Institute, Cary, USA). In the second medical study, a trainee doctor investigated the use by the Tamasheq in the commune of Ber of the state health care centers in Ber and Tehārje.[7] I accompanied the Malian doctor of the clinical study on the seven field trips, and in these five months, I conducted 53 unstructured interviews with women participating in the clinical study. Unlike the doctor, I did not use an interpreter, but covered similar themes as those on the ques-

---

7   The results on the use of health care institutions by the nomadic population can be found in Mohamed El Moctar's thesis: *Logiques de production et utilisation des services de santé en milieu nomade au Mali: Cas de la commune de Ber (Tombouctou)* (Doctoral thesis, Faculté de Médecine, de Pharmacie et d'Odonto-Stomatologie, Université du Mali, 2006).

tionnaire, such as their experiences of pregnancy, number of children, mis-carriages, the histories of children who had died, their eating habits, illnesses, treatments they used, their opinions about health care institutions and so on.

During my three-year research stay among the Kel Alhafra, I became im-mersed in the community in order to study local illness hermeneutics from an actor-centered perspective. The objective was to decode and translate local narratives into a broader context of cultural understanding, and integrate them into language where they are comprehensible in terms of concepts of west-ern medicine. By reproducing the Kel Alhafra's worldview, their self-image and their view of illness, insights into their culture should be provided by giv-ing the people unmediated voice. Narratives and spontaneous speech are tran-scribed and translated directly from the original Tamasheq. In fact, I rarely in-terfere in the local hermeneutics of health and illness. Tamasheq statements in the text are either cited as a general synthesis of ideas presented by most of the Kel Alhafra, or they are from a specific person mentioned by name. The clinical investigation of a Malian doctor, in turn, aimed to provide a picture of the momentary health situation of women and children. Using standardized questionnaires with the help of local translators, information was collected about nutrition, number of children, immunization and utilization of health-care institutions.

In weaving together the two strands of this research, and in searching for correlations between clinically identified diseases and those perceived by the nomads themselves, three additional questions emerged: i) Where do health-specific statements by the Tamasheq and medically ascertained facts differ? ii) What are the shortcomings of a standardized questionnaire? iii) Where are complementary cultural studies needed in order to provide a compre-hensive picture of the actual, prevailing health status and health needs of the population?

At the end of the investigations, a feedback process took place during a stakeholder seminar, held over two days in the nomadic environment around the well of Tin Timāγayān on March 11th – 12th, 2006. Eighty-two people were present, comprising 61% of the members (40% women) of the nomadic com-munity under study. In a first step, the investigators of the different fields (clin-ical study of women and children, access to health centers, local illness herme-neutics) presented an outline of their preliminary findings to the Tamasheq community. During an in-depth dialogue, the people were divided into two gender-specific groups in order to allow freer expression in a less hierarchi-cal environment. The in-depth dialogue was recorded. The recorded discourse served the investigators later on recalling the critical points of information that were included in their final narrative analyses.

1.4. Recent trends in research on medical understanding among the Tamasheq

Medical concepts among the Tamasheq in Mali have been the subject of three dissertations: Mohamed Ousmane (1981)[8], Yannick Le Jean (1986)[9] and El-Mehdi Ag Hamahady (1988)[10] have all attempted to identify and classify local diseases according to a western medical typology. Unfortunately, all three theses are limited to descriptive approaches structured around the biomedical system.

Ousmane undertook his study among the Tamasheq in the Gourma region (in the southern bend of the Niger river) and collected interesting statements about the function of various bodily organs as well as traditional medication from plant, organic and mineral sources.

Le Jean's work concentrates on the knowledge and healing practices of a traditional healer and a marabout in Timbuktu. Their clientele are sedentary Tamasheq and Arabs who settled in the city after the 1972–1973 drought. Le Jean interprets their medical systems according to a western perspective, and during this process many important nuances in the Tamasheq conception of illness get lost through a lack of differentiated understanding in the specifics of Tamasheq and Arabic terms.

Ag Hamahady's study of digestive diseases, undertaken in the region of Goundam, Niafunké and Gourma-Rharous, is, however, a veritable treasure trove of information on medicinal plants. Unfortunately his analysis of diseases is limited to a biomedical framework, and Tamasheq terms are constructed based on western concepts of illness that are never used by the Tamasheq themselves. Nevertheless, his plant lists and data about phytotherapy remain invaluable. No other work provides so comprehensively the Latin equivalents for Tamasheq plant names. Although Marceau Gast in his book *Moissons du désert*[11] also analyzes various desert plants, the context for his work is not their use in traditional medicine but as a natural resource of nutritional supplements during food shortages.

Unfortunately in the work of all the above-mentioned authors adequate focus seems to be missing on historical, social and local cultural influences on their research subjects, and they do not analyze critically the boundaries be-

8 Mohamed Ousmane, *La médecine traditionnelle tamachèque en milieu malien* (Doctoral thesis, l'Ecole Nationale de Médecine et de Pharmacie du Mali, 1981).
9 Yannick Le Jean, *Médecine traditionnelle en milieu nomade dans la région de Tombouctou* (Doctoral thesis in medicine, Faculté de Médicine de Paris-Sud, 1986).
10 El-Mehdi Ag Hamahady, *Nosographie tamachèque des gastro-enterites dans la région de Tombouctou* (Doctoral thesis, Ecole Nationale de Médecine et de Pharmacie du Mali, 1988).
11 Marceau Gast, *Moissons du désert* (Paris: Ibis, 2000).

tween mental disorders of supernatural origin and somatic diseases with a natural cause. Ousmane rarely discusses the etiology of his clinically identified
diseases, and in all these dissertations, the classification of foods, symptoms
and diseases into hot and cold categories is contradictory and insufficiently explained.[12]

The book by the traditional healer Fadi Walett Faqqi[13] describes a collec-
tion of diseases which are classified either by their bodily location or on the
basis of various characteristics such as hot, cold, contagious, allergic, hereditary etc. Nevertheless, this compilation lacks a presentation of the context
in which her specific understanding of illness is embedded. Although in the
book's foreword, the editor Barbara Fiore provides some information to assist
the reader in grasping the concept of "hot" and "cold" elements, her accounts
do not explore the topic in greater detail.

In none of the above-mentioned works is any specific consideration given
to the perception of illness during different stages of the life cycle, in particular those of women and children. Jacques Hureiki's study[14] also ignores this
theme. He views the medical system of the Kel Tamasheq as first of all a concept that illustrates the relationship between the human individual and his
or her surroundings. For Hureiki, this relationship is based on a duality between natural and supernatural powers, whose conflicts and outcomes are reflected in the world in the opposition between "hot" and "cold". The interesting dichotomy between "pagan-divine", "cold-hot" and "spirits-God" provides
not only the foundation upon which illness experiences and therapeutic measures are based, but simultaneously reflects, in Hureiki's view, the social hierarchy among the Tamasheq. In his fascination for this idea and the desire to
prove it, however, Hureiki seems to lose a correlation with the Tamasheq nor-
mative reality of illness representation. His study gets caught up in an overem-
phasis of historical belief concepts, which become for him the central axis by
which he analyzes Tamasheq culture and their medical concepts. In my view,
he becomes enmeshed in an imaginative construct. Additionally, various linguistic and Islam-related errors demonstrate limited knowledge of Arabic or
Tamasheq, casting further doubt on the reliability of his claims.

---

12 Le Jean writes: "... the information provided about these concepts in contradictory, and dif-
    fers from healer to healer. It is difficult to gain a precise idea about what is hot and what is
    cold." Yannick Le Jean, *Médecine traditionnelle en milieu nomade dans la région de Tom-
    bouctou* (Doctoral thesis in medicine, Faculté de Médecine de Paris-Sud, 1986) 48.
13 Fadi Walett Faqqi, *Isefran. Maladies et soins en milieu Touareg*, Preface and presentation of
    the scientific edition by Barbara Fiore (Bandiagara (Mali), Perugia (Italy): Editions CRMT/
    PSMTM, 1993).
14 Jacques Hureiki, *Les médecins touarègues traditionelles. Approche ethnologique* (Paris: Kar-
    thala, 2000).

Sara Randall and Susan Rasmussen are among the few scholars whose work engages with the local realities of pastoral women and children. Randall works primarily in the field of medical demography and has published important comparative studies on the Tamasheq of Mali, in which she has shown, for example, how socio-cultural factors influence sickness and child mortality. Her 1984 study established that, unexpectedly, child mortality was higher among the noble Tamasheq than in the dependent, poorer *iklān* class. The social norms condone the lethargy of noble women and their prestige is raised if they do not work. One consequence of this, however, is that they neglect the health of their children who are then more likely than lower-status infants to die of dehydration.[15] With the recent changes in nomadic lifestyle and a shift in thinking about hierarchical structures, these findings are may need further scrutiny vis-à-vis contemporary Tamasheq culture, one in which most women now perform daily tasks and childcare without household assistance.[16] In another interesting case study among the Tamasheq in the Gourma region, Randall identified high maternal mortality as a significant problem following their return from the refugee camps, with one in eight women dying during childbirth.

For Rasmussen, a political and cultural analysis of the dialectic interaction between the female body, power and resistance is essential for understanding medical realities among Tamasheq women. She has focused on the Kel Ewey in Niger where she believes that female sexuality and reproduction are key components in a hegemonic power struggle between western-sponsored state clinics, traditional healers and Islamic scholars.[17] To demonstrate their autonomy, Tamasheq women, according to Rasmussen, are reluctant to admit that they are sick, especially when they have gynecological problems. Although infertile Tamasheq women desire medical treatment, they fear the power of the mostly male health care specialists and mistrust their motives. State-run health care services are often mentioned in connection with the earlier colonial presence of the French, and important interventions like vaccination and oral rehydration are perceived as attempts at political manipulation.[18] Rasmussen pro-

---

15 Sara Randall, "Différences géographiques et sociales dans la mortalité infantile et juvénile au Mali", *Population* 6 (1984): 921–946.

16 Sara Randall, "Demographic consequences of conflict, forced migration and repatriation: a case study of Malian Kel Tamasheq", *European Journal of Population* 21.2-3 (2005): 291–320.

17 "... this power struggle threatens to jeopardize Tuareg women's traditionally high status, prestige, and independence expressed, for example, in ownership of herds and participation in trade, the right to eject husbands from the tent, and self-representation in litigation." Susan J. Rasmussen, "Female Sexuality, Social Reproduction, and the Politics of Medical Intervention in Niger: Kel Ewey Tuareg perspectives", *Culture, Medicine and Psychiatry* 18.4 (1994): 433–462.

18 Ibid.

vides important insights into the local realities and contexts of the Tamasheq in Niger and has given careful consideration to how medical knowledge in African health systems is constructed in a setting of political violence and economic crises.[19]

In general though, much remains to be learned about the perception, attitudes, beliefs, knowledge and understanding of health issues among nomadic women.[20] Information on such topics as child mortality (with the histories of the deceased children), childcare, peri- and postnatal complications, and family planning is sparse. As yet, no interdisciplinary research has been undertaken to identify and analyze current representations of illness among the Tamasheq, especially the women and children; to assess how these representations are distributed among the population and are interrelated; and to ascertain local priorities and problems. Previous studies have been restricted to either biomedical, anthropological or social science approaches, which determine their interpretive scope. Alone these methodologies cannot provide the best possible overall picture of local representations of illness and their distribution in a specific nomadic context.[21]

---

19 See Susan J. Rasmussen, "Parallel and Divergent Landscapes: Cultural Encounters in the Ethnographic Space of Tuareg Medicine", *Medical Anthropology Quarterly* 14 (2000): 242–270.

20 See here: Esther Schelling, *Human and Animal Health in Nomadic Pastoralist Communities of Chad: Zoonoses, Morbidity and Health Services* (Doctoral thesis, University of Basel, 2002); Martin Wiese, *The Context of Vulnerability to Ill-Health as Experienced by Nomadic Pastoralists: A Case Study from Dazagada and Arab Pastoral Communities in Chad* (Freiburg: University of Freiburg and the Swiss Tropical Institute, 2002); Frank Krönke, *Perception of Ill-Health in a FulBe Pastoralist Community and Its Implications on Health Interventions in Chad* (Doctoral thesis, University of Basel, 2001); UNICEF, *Enfants et femmes au Mali. Une analyse de situation* (Paris: L'Harmattan, 1989).

21 In previous research illnesses were mostly analyzed through western categories. To date, the reconstruction of a local hermeneutic background for understanding disease was virtually non-existent in medical and veterinary research of the tropics. In addition, research in so called ethno-medicine (or medical anthropology) deals mostly with healing traditions and healing experiences (in contrast to medical science). Medical anthropology, dedicated to the explicitly local hermeneutics of sickness and health, has existed for almost forty years, but no studies focus on West Africa, much less on nomadic pastoralist native to Mali. See Kathryn Staiano-Ross, *Interpreting signs of illness: a case study in medical semiotics* (Berlin; New York: Mouton de Gruyter 1986) (=Diss. Univ. Kansas 1981); Beatrix Pfleiderer & Wolfgang Bichmann, *Krankheit und Kultur: Eine Einführung in die Ethnomedizin* (Berlin: Reimer 1985); Lars-Christian Koch, *Die ethnischen Varianten des "Krankseins": Krankheitsvorstellungen und Krankheitsverhalten in Stammeskulturen* (Bonn: Holos 1987); Silke von Siebert, *Traditionelle Medizin, Körper- und Krankheitsverständnis in Boca do Acre, Brasilien* (Dissertation der Universität Düsseldorf, 2000); Katarina Greifeld (ed.), *Ritual und Heilung: Eine Einführung in die Ethnomedizin* (Berlin: Dietrich Reimer Verlag 2003); Thomas Lux (ed.), *Kulturelle Dimensionen von Medizin. Ethnomedizin – Medizinethnologie – Medical Anthropology* (Berlin: Reimer 2003); Michael Knipper, *Krankheit, Kultur und medizinische Praxis. Eine medizinethnologische Untersuchung zu "mal aire" im Amazonas-*

1.5. Structure of the study

The study is divided into four main sections framed by a contextual and a concluding chapter. Following this introduction, chapter 2 outlines the geographic, historical, political and economic background to the situation in which the Kel Alhafra live today.

Chapter 3 opens the major part of this work with descriptions the Kel Alhafra themselves give about their way of life, their beliefs, and their image of the world and the body. This framework is then extended by a semantic analysis of the terms used in health and illness and a detailed account of prevailing representations of the human body and its functions. The central section of chapter 3 is devoted to the cultural expression of the female life cycle, with particular attention paid to themes relevant to women's health from childhood to old age. The chapter closes with descriptions of everyday life among the nomads, their general hygiene practices, eating customs, how they process food and how they cope with malnutrition.

The second main section of this study in chapter 4 comprises an analysis of current concepts of illness, and begins with a catalogue of disease categories and applied traditional therapies. This is followed by a discussion of how the Kel Alhafra specifically relate to and understand the various illness classifications. The final part of this chapter deals with the perceived causes of illness and disease, and provides an essential interpretative background for appreciating the illness behavior of the Kel Alhafra.

Chapter 5 provides a classification and description of therapeutic networks, describing the various sectors of the health care system and how Kel Alhafra women seeking help interact with the resources and options available to them.

The results of the medical survey of the health status of the Kel Alhafra women and children are presented and analyzed from an epidemiological perspective in chapter 6.

The final, interpretive chapter compares these clinical results with the illness perceptions of the population, summarizes and critically reflects on the study's findings and poses the questions that still remain open or have been raised by the research.

tiefland von Ecuador (Münster: Lit 2001); Thamar Klein, Globale und lokale Medizinen in Benin (Münster: Lit 2006); Viola Hörbst, *Heilungslandschaften. Umgangsweisen mit Erkrankungen und Heilung bei den Cora in Jesus Maria, Mexiko* (Münster: Lit 2006).

1.6. Notes on style

Those groups that speak Tamasheq in Mali are identified by the French as *Touaregs*, by the Songhai as *Surguboreye*, by the Arabs as *at-tawārik* and by the Peul and Bambara as *Burdame* or *Burdabe*. Their own self-designation is, however, *kel tāmašāyt*, "those of the (language) Tamasheq". I have adopted this designation here, using a transcription that follows the phonetic pronunciation, the feminine ending *-γt* being pronounced in Tamasheq as *-q*.

The major sources for this study are oral statements by the Kel Alhafra, and I have interwoven the original Tamasheq phrases, in italics, throughout the main text. For the transcription of the Tamasheq I have followed the *Guide de Transcription du Tamasheq*, published by the Direction Nationale de l'Alphabétisation Fonctionelle et de la Linguistique Appliquée, DNAFLA, of the Malian Ministry of Education. Where a well-established spelling already exists for a proper name, I have used this; otherwise I have attempted to show stresses and accents using diacritical signs. With the exception of the main map of Mali, I myself have produced all the figures, tables and other maps.

2. The Kel Alhafra in Space and Time

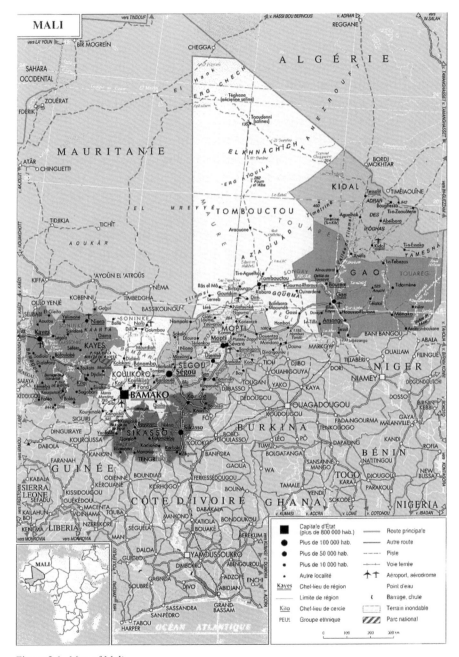

Figure 2.1. *Map of Mali*
Source: Division Géographique de Ministère des Affaires Etrangères, République du Mali.

2.1. Azawad and the commune of Ber

The primary nomadic space for the Kel Alhafra is Azawad, which stretches from 17° N northwards of Timbuktu deep into the Saharan desert. The Kel Alhafra move predominantly within the eastern part of this desert region as well as in the so-called "river zone" around the wells south of In Agozmi (120 km north of Ber). The semi-arid Azawad is divided into two administrative districts, Timbuktu and, further north, Kidal; the Kel Alhafra live in the former, and more precisely in the commune of Ber.

The commune of Ber covers 72,000 km², of which 85% is desert.[22] It is bordered to the north by the commune of Salam and by Algeria. The commune of Bamba in the administrative district of Bourem lies to the east; Hamzakoma (in the district Gourma Rharous) and Bourem Inaly lie to the south. In the west, Ber meets the urban commune of Timbuktu.

The climate is hot and dry, and the commune of Ber is often afflicted by severe droughts. Precipitation is sparse and rare: 136 mm in 2002, 68 mm in 2003, while during 2004–2005, a mere 167 mm fell on eight "rain days". The situation improved again during the rainy season of 2005–2006, with 1,645 mm.[23]

Although the commune of Ber has existed since 1962, it was only officially designated a "Commune Rurale" following decentralization and new subdivision of the country in 1999. At that time, a new communal administration was established for a population of 25,000 covering those living in the main town of Ber and in 35 nomadic fractions.[24]

Of the commune's 25,000 inhabitants, 12,250 are men and 12,750 are women. Seventy percent lead a nomadic or semi-nomadic pastoral existence, while the remaining 30% live from arable farming. The population density is 0.3/km². The village of Ber itself lies 60 km from Timbuktu and about 9 km from the river Niger and today has more than 9,128 inhabitants (ca 75% Tamasheq and 25% Arabs).[25] Ber is growing steadily, and its drinking-water needs are already putting considerable strain on its five existing water pumps. There are four health care centers in the commune of Ber, of which three are

---

22 See Ministère de l'Administration Territoriale et des Collectivités Locales: Commune Rurale de Ber: Présentation générale, 2006.

23 Ibid.

24 In a 1996 census, the commune of Ber had a population of just 7,871. However, with the return of peace, the setting up of a health care center, a school and water pumps, along with investment in gardens, many refugees returned to the area.

25 See "Plan de sécurité alimentaire commune rurale de Ber, 2006–2010", (République du Mali : Commissariat à la Sécurité Alimentaire (CSA), 2006).

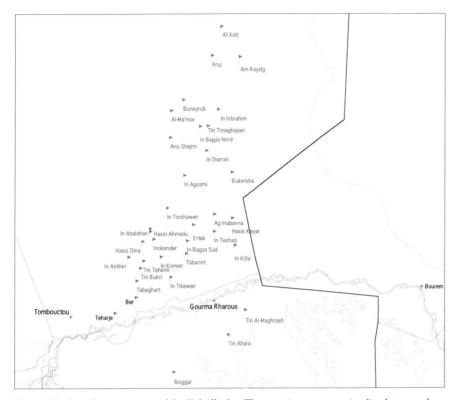

Figure 2.2. *Transhumance area of the Kel Alhafra. The most important region lies between the wells of In Agozmi and Al-Xatt.*

in operation. Although there should be eleven schools (including three Koranic schools) for the children, only four are functioning, because the people cannot provide the funds to maintain them. Only 9% of the children in the commune can attend a school.[26]

Tin Timāyayān, one of the most important wells for the Kel Alhafra, lies 140 km from the commune's main town across rough desert terrain. The Kel Alhafra, comprising 194 families of about 950 individuals, have lived for generations in the dune valleys around these wells, moving across the endless sand plains northwards via Buneyrub to the most northern graze and browse around Aruj and Al-Xatt. The groundwater in this region lies at about 60–110 meters, and the Kel Alhafra bring it to the surface with the aid of draft animals in traditional wells they have built themselves. A treeless desert zone begins at the

---

26 See Ministère de l'Administration Territoriale et des Collectivités Locales: Commune Rurale de Ber: Présentation générale, 2006.

well of Anušejrin, with salt deposits at Al-Ma'mor, Buneyrub, Aruj and Al-Xatt, to which the Kel Alhafra regularly drive their animals for a "salt cure". Three roads cross the area used by the Kel Alhafra. The northernmost route, passing via In Agozmi, Indiārrān and Timətyen (Kidal region), is the most important smuggling route to Algeria. For the Kel Alhafra, this means that an occasional truck will stop at one of the wells, offer goods for sale or take passengers onboard. Young men especially make use of this intermittent travel opportunity, but the usual means of transport for the Kel Alhafra remain the donkey and the camel.

During the drought years of 1972–1973, about fifty Kel Alhafra families fled the northern region and established themselves in the riverine area of Gourma-Rharous 90 km south of the river Niger. Like their kin in Azawad, they lead a primarily nomadic pastoralist life, but while the families in the north raise mainly camels, the Kel Alhafra in Gourma own cattle herds and move with their animals in search of lush pastures around the wells of Tin Ahara, Iboggar and Al Māyraš.

2.2. The basic way of life

As a result of the severe droughts of recent years, the nature of Azawad has changed dramatically. Prior to the droughts, the Kel Alhafra had been able to live solely from the yields of their herds. In the particularly luxuriant pastures of the far north, they had specialized in raising camels but had also owned sheep, goats and donkeys. When food was short, they could supplement their diet with fruits and grains, *ekāde*, and by hunting, *āhoyy*, but the failure of the rains turned vast areas into inhospitable and infertile desert. Trees have died, plant species have disappeared and along with them most of the species of wild animals. Trapping with hand-made traps, *tāṇḍārbaten* (sing. *taṇḍārbatt*), is no longer practiced, and a hare, *temārwālt*, an eagle, *ešeyer,* or a small gazelle, *ašənkaḍ*, is occasionally killed using a shotgun, *ālbārroḍ*. Once basic complements to camel breeding, gathering and hunting are now an activity of the past. Livestock sale, *mamāla*, is likewise no longer an important source of income: the herds are too small, and only when cash is urgently required, is an animal offered for sale at the weekly market in Ber. The Kel Alhafra do in part live from their herds once more, but they own fewer camels and mainly raise goats and sheep, while, as mentioned above, some families in the southern zone of movement have turned to cattle.

The majority of the Kel Alhafra men, however, are obliged to seek additional sources of income. Some work as *imāšrajān* (sing. *amāšraj*), "waterers" at a well, providing water to other people's herds. This arduous and phys-

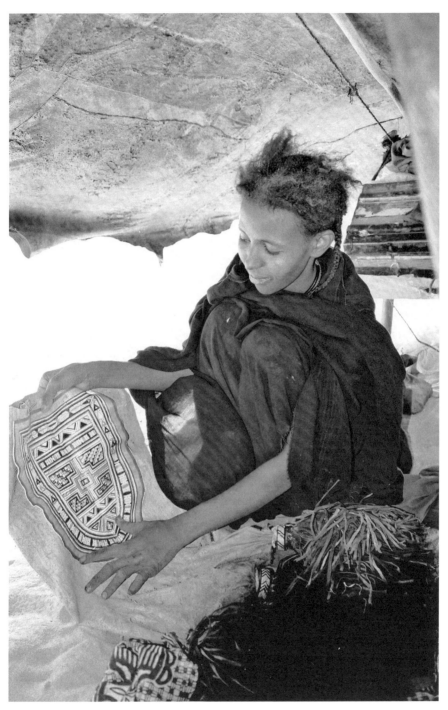

Figure 2.3. *Women prepare leather handicrafts that they sell at local markets to supplement their household income. The picture shows a* tenhāḍt, *a woman from the artisan class, in an encampment near In Teshaq (November 2005).*

ically demanding activity brings them CFA 10,000 a month.[27] Tending others'
herds, *tamāḍent n-irəzzejan*, usually camels belonging to sedentary owners,
provides another source of income. A herder, *amāḍan*, earns the same each
month as an *amāšraj*, but also receives food from the owner and once a year
a new set of clothes and a pair of shoes. A Kel Alhafra man can also act as an
amāsakul, a traveler who drives animals to a market to be sold, receiving in return about CFA 1,000 per animal, or he can take care of animals in a caravan.
He might participate, for example, with ten camels in a salt caravan to Taudenni
and will receive in return the proceeds from the sale of the salt load of one of
those animals. Or, fulfilling a contract to travel with 20 donkeys to sell millet in the south, he will be paid CFA 1,000 per pack animal. As *ināmašālān*
(sing. *anāmašāl*), that is with a "commission" to run an errand for others, the
Kel Alhafra can earn up to CFA 5,000 per job on the market in Ber or in Timbuktu. The Kel Alhafra point out, however, that a man can go at most on three
Saturdays a month to the weekly market in Ber, which will bring him around
CFA 15,000. The taming of camels and bullocks, *assinān n-imənas d-iwdesān*,
provides another income source that garners around CFA 5,000 per animal.
However, *"ma taqālād ad ehāre dāy əššāyāl wadāy"*, the Kel Alhafra sigh, "no
one will make a fortune from that kind of work", and the men are increasingly
traveling abroad in search of more lucrative jobs in Algeria or the Ivory Coast.
The women and children remain in the encampments, the adolescent sons look
after the animals, and after a fashion, life in the desert continues. The women
complain, though, that the men find a better life abroad, marry there and do not
return to the austerities of the desert, abandoning their wives and daughters to
their fate. The Kel Alhafra women say that they are becoming disillusioned
with their economic dependence and would like to establish gardens near a solar pump, to sell vegetables and handicrafts and to break out of their socially an
d economically isolated situation.

2.3. Historical background

In precolonial times, the Tamasheq comprised several tribal groups, *tiwsaten*
(sing. *tawset*),[28] and each individual group was subdivided into several smaller

27 All figures mentioned in CFA refer to the year 2006.
    The officially recommended minimum monthly salary for a non-professional worker is set at
    CFA 22,000 but even that "is insufficient to meet real living costs in Mali". Source: Centre
    National de Promotion des Investissements C.N.P, 2002.
28 Boilley believes that the current translations of *tawset* into the various European languages
    (tribu, tribe, Stamm etc.) are imprecise and he recommends the use of the Tamasheq termi-
    nology for: "the existence of social or political human groups based upon a real or supposed

units under the leadership of a *āmānokal* (pl. *imānokalān*).[29] There was a strong social hierarchy, in which the powerful tribal groups owned enormous herds that were tended by dependents who, in return, received protection from the higher social classes. At the peak of this hierarchical organization were the *əllulātān* (sing. *əllulāt*), the caste of the free (i.e. not enslaved) and nobles, who normally held the status of warriors. However, not all *əllulātān* groups took part in armed raids (Arabic: *ġazawāt*),[30] and following Islamization, a religious class, the *inasləmān* (sing. *anasləm* – Muslim), developed in many *tiwsāten*. They refused to participate in militant activities and devoted themselves to the study of the Koran. The *inasləmān* had their own leaders but their pacifist stance meant that they depended on armed classes among the Tamasheq or Arabs for protection. Thus their status in the general Tamasheq hierarchy oscillated between that of the *əllulātān* and the *imγad* (sing. *amāγid*), the vassals who, although dependent on the *əllulātān*, were free men and women. They took care of the herds, both their own and those of the *əllulātān*. Another vassal group were the *inhāḍān* (sing. *enhāḍ*), the artisans, who made weapons, handicrafts, daily tools and other utensils. They were always tied to a tribal group, *tawset*, for whom they worked and by whom they were paid in kind. Although the origins of the *inhāḍān* have still not been established, they nevertheless form a separate, marginal caste among the Tamasheq and live endogamously. Although their association with the theurgic elements like fire, metal, wood and air meant that they were feared, the *inhāḍān* were also held in contempt due to their specific position within Tamasheq society. The *iklān* (sing. *akli*) formed the lowest social class. They were black slaves from the south who assisted in tending animals, did domestic tasks or raised the children, and lived with their owner's family from whom they could inherit material goods.

kinship. They are connected by numerous blood relationships or shared interests to neighboring groups, from which they consider themselves to be not ethically, but rather socially and indeed geographically distant". Pierre Boilley, *Les Touaregs Kel Adagh. Dépendances et révoltes: du Soudan français au Mali contemporain* (Paris: Karthala, 1999) 624.

In this book, *tawset* is to be understood according to this definition, even when I occasionally use the established translations.

29   In Tamasheq, *āmānokal* (pl. *imānokalān*) is the general term used for a leader, someone who holds a leadership position, *təmənukəla*. In the political context, the *āmānokal*, is always the leader of a political group; earlier, this group was the *tawset*, and the *āmānokal* in this position was the possessor of the *əṭṭəbəl*, the war drum – simultaneously the symbol of power.

30   In precolonial times, *armed raids* (from the Arabic *ġazawāt* (sing. *ġazwa*) – armed campaign, marauding expedition, raid, conquest) served the various Tamasheq groups to increase their resources in the form of stolen cattle, slaves etc. Such raids, though, took various forms and were also used by the Tamasheq as a means of defense. For the significance of these raids among the Tamasheq, see Hélène Claudot-Hawad, *Les Touaregs. Portraits en fragments* (Aix-en-Provence: Edisud, 1993).

The Kel Alhafra form a subgroup of the Kel Anṣār *tawset*, located east of Timbuktu, all of whom belong to the class of the *inəsləmān*.[31] The history and Islamization of the eastern Kel Anṣār are discussed comprehensively in Marty's 1920 study, *Etudes sur l'islam et les tribus du Soudan*, and in Norris' sources,[32] and so here I will simply provide a historical framework highlighting the most important events and issues needed for an understanding of the situation and position of the Kel Alhafra today.

Among the eastern *tawset* of the Kel Anṣār,[33] a leader was selected by the last *amānokāl* and a gathering of the elders, the *ğāma'a* (from the Arabic *ğamā'a* – community), from a single designated family whose descent was distinguished by its close proximity to the prophet's lineage. In this patrilinear succession,[34] they elected a personality they believed to be worthy, upright, as neutral as possible in dealings with other groups of the *tawset*, and knowledgeable and experienced in religious and legal matters. However, in general among the Kel Anṣār, the social borders that were usually clearly demarcated

---

31 As Muslims and promoters of Islam, the Kel Anṣār take their name from the Arabic *al-anṣār*, the Medinan followers of the prophet Muhammad who took him up among their number and supported him after his *ḥiǧra* to Mecca.

   The *inəsləmān* in Mali comprise not only the Kel Anṣār (in the districts of Niafunké, Goundam, Timbuktu, Rharous) but also the Kel Ǝssuk (in the Niger Bend – particularly the districts of Rharous, Bourem, Gao, Ansongo, Ménaka and Kidal) as well as the Iǧəllad (in the district of Bourem).

   Typologically, the *inəsləmān* have a similar function as the Arabic *murābitīn* groups that were disparaged by the French colonial administration as "marabout" (see *Encyclopedia of Islam (2)*, (Leiden: Brill, 2000) X, 379). The *murābitīn* featured in some ways an "elite education", insofar as the privilege of reading and writing (religious texts) was officially acknowledged. Whether the Kel Alhafra – as were often the Arabic *murābitīn* – belonged to a Sufi community, remains undetermined.

32 On the Kel Anṣār, see Paul Marty, *Etudes sur l'islam et les tribus du Soudan*, vol. I (Paris: Leroux 1920); Harry T. Norris, *The Tuaregs: Their Islamic Legacy and Its Diffusion in the Sahel* (Warminster: Aris & Philips, 1975).

33 Once a large *tawset* of *inəsləmān*, all claiming descent from the famous 16th-century ancestor Infa, the Kel Anṣār are today split up into various small groups, although in general reference is made to the eastern Kel Anṣār around Timbuktu and the western Kel Anṣār. On the history and splintering of the Kel Anṣār see Paul Marty, *Etudes sur l'islam et les tribus du Soudan*, vol. I (Paris: Leroux 1920).

   As Arabic sources show, however, not all Kel Anṣār were always peaceful. The Kel Anṣār held protracted disputes, sometimes violent, with the Kunta over the sovereignty of the grasslands in the Azawad. Moreover, the literary production of the Kel Anṣār is considerable, and numerous manuscripts written by Kel Anṣār scholars are kept in the library of Timbuktu. See John O. Hunwick (ed.), *The Writings of Western Sudanic Africa* (Leiden: Brill, 2003) 189–206.

34 In contrast to other Tamasheq groups such as the Kel Ahaggar, in which accession to the position of *āmānokal* is determined matrilinearly, the inheritance system of the Kel Anṣār has been and still is a patrilinear one. Leadership passes through the male line – not from the deceased *āmānokal* to a son but to his brothers. Only when they have died do the sons of the original *āmānokal* and of his brothers gain the right to election.

in other Tamasheq groups appear somewhat blurred. As *inəsləmān*, demonstrated close descent from the prophet's line was certainly recognized and bestowed on some families a degree of prestige, but knowledge of the Koran and piety were also highly valued, and the society was more defined by social relationships, such as the respect shown to elders, sages and marabouts. The *imγad* class seems to be almost non-existent among the Kel Anṣār, and all the individual *inəsləmān* subgroups owned and tended their own animals.[35]

The Kel Alhafra always lived from nomadic pastoralism, which provided them with milk, meat and skins. Every year, some of their camels joined the large salt caravans traveling south to Taudenni, where the rock salt was exchanged for millet. When food was short, the Kel Alhafra gathered wild grasses, hunted and trapped gazelles and other small wild animals. Each subgroup of the tribal fraction or each large family moved within a territory that had grown familiar over generations, in which they had dug wells and which they affectionately referred to as *"ākall-nānāγ"*, "our land".

2.3.1. The French presence

On 12 February 1894, Colonel Joffre leading the French troops stormed Timbuktu and took over the city.[36] Within two years, the French had extended their occupation into the area around Timbuktu. To make contact with groups living in the north, they first sent out two peaceful missions (Toutée: 1895; Hourst: 1896).[37] From 1896, however, their conquest became a violent one, and on 3 November 1898, they subjugated the tribal group of the Kel Anṣār, after they had killed the *āmānokal*, N'Gouna.[38]

In the following years, military units of méhariste camel corps began controlling the desert region of Azawad while the French, from 1903 onward, sought to build up their administrative system. The Kel Alhafra call this decisive year *"awātay wa-dd osān nāsara"* – "the year in which the Christians arrived". The French took pains to respect the traditional lifestyle of the Tamasheq, followed the transhumance of the nomads but, nevertheless, began sewing the seeds for profound changes. Not only were the desert and the wadis reapportioned: tribal associations, *tiwsaten*, were restructured, tradi-

---

35 On the social structure of the Kel Anṣār, see also Jacques Hureiki, *Essais sur les origines des Touaregs* (Paris: Karthala, 2003) 118–119.

36 See General Gaetan Bonnier, *L'occupation de Tombouctou* (Paris: Monde moderne, 1926); Maréchal J. Joffre, "Rapport sur les opérations de la colonne Joffre avant et après l'occupation de Tombouctou", Rapport de M.J. Joffre, lieutenant-colonel du Génie, *Revue du Génie militaire* (Paris: Berger-Levrault, 1895).

37 See Boilley, Les Touaregs Kel Adagh, 62.

38 Ibid.

tional groupings were dissolved and new ones were created, regardless of the customary social structures among the Tamasheq. The French often named these new and smaller fractions according to specifying characteristics, such as the geographical location of a group. In this way the Kel Alhafra received an Arabic name, *al-ḥufra*, from the Arabic for "cavity" or "hole", because the French found the Kel Alhafra hidden in sand hollows and trenches in the dunes [among the Tamasheq, the Kel Alhafra are also called the Kel Abātol – those of an *abātol* (pl. *ibtal*), a sand depression between the dunes].

The leaders of these newly created groups were still chosen by the Tamasheq themselves and usually came from prestigious families, but they were integrated by the French into their system and skillfully used as mediators between the French colonial power and the autochthonous population. The role of these new chiefs was to represent the interests of the French to the nomads and to collect taxes, while at the same time they had continually to justify themselves to the people in order not to be discredited by them. Boilley writes that the Tamasheq leaders were forced to become the "assistants of the colonial power" and were as much bound to the external authority as to their own group.[39] This integration of the Tamasheq leaders into the French administration meant, however, that the French did not need large forces to control the enormous expanses of desert. Until 1948, their administration was placed entirely in the hands of the army, and in Azawad, military posts were set up at the wells of In Agozmi, Inokender, Aruj, In Atlik, In Ibrahim and Al-Ma'mor, which were themselves administered from urban centers such as Rharous and Timbuktu. Boilley writes that, by and large, the French did not interfere with the nomads as long as they remained peaceful: they were not forced into any special activities on behalf of the French, they were not taken into the French army, and they were not obliged to become sedentary.[40]

The Kel Alhafra say that up to this point, they had not perceived the French as wrongdoers, since life in Azawad remained relatively peaceful and the French more or less left them alone. The French not only introduced a taxation and a legal system, they also invested in health care and in pastoral hydraulics. Medical care for the population was provided by the "Assistance Médical Indigène", or AMI, set up in 1926, with 32 medical centers stationed in Bamako, the major towns and each department's administrative center – each one led by a European doctor. These were supplemented by 100 "Dispensaires de Brousse" and

---

39 "… the chiefs became the veritable auxiliaries of the colonization." Boilley, *Les Touaregs Kel Adagh*, 192.
40 See Boilley, *Les Touaregs Kel Adagh*, 195.

30 "Maternités", run by a registered medical assistant.[41] The nearest health care provision for the Kel Alhafra was the military post of Inokender, where a military doctor was responsible for the medical needs of the surrounding population.

However, when attempts were made to introduce a school system, the Tamasheq resisted. They did not want their children to adopt the worldview of the occupying power, to become Christians, Europeans, to become sedentary and to be cut off from their origins. Many Tamasheq groups, including the Kel Alhafra, began to hide themselves in the desert. At this point, a discussion of the so-called "illiteracy of the resistance", an expression introduced by Aghali-Zakara and picked up by others, such as Bernus, Boilley, Clauzel and Triaud, might be expected, but for the Kel Alhafra at least, I find it inappropriate.[42] The *ālfāqqitān*, the Koranic teachers among the *inaslamān*, had always gathered students around them and taught them to read and write the Arabic script. During the colonial period, many Kel Alhafra men had mastered written Arabic without having attended a western-style school. To speak of the refusal of the Tamasheq to send their children to school as part of a general "illiteracy of the resistance" is to suggest that because they were unable to read or write French they were illiterate. I believe this view is misplaced. What the Tamasheq were resisting was not education as such, but the path into a European-molded modernity that they had not elected to take. From this point on, they began to isolate themselves, and today few of the Kel Alhafra belong to the small group of "intellectuals" who attended the French schools in Er Intejeft and Tināwaten during the colonial period.

In his study on the Kel Adagh, Boilley has described clearly the three most important consequences of the 50-year occupation by the French for the nomadic society of the Tamasheq. By restructuring the population, the existing hierarchic system was broken apart, and the large homogenous tribal groups like the *tiwsaten* were divided into smaller, much less stable alliances. To avoid forced schooling, many families fled into and isolated themselves in remote regions of the desert. Finally, a tendency developed to romanticize and idealize the precolonial past. In protest against the colonizers, backs were turned on contemporary events, and the nomads withdrew from the world that was changing around them.[43]

---

41 Georges Spitz, *Le Soudan français* (Paris: Editions Maritimes et Coloniales, 1955).

42 On the expression "analphabetism of the resistance", see Edmond Bernus, Jean Clauzel, Pierre Boilley and Jean-Louis Triaud, *Nomades et commandants. Administration et sociétés nomades dans l'ancienne A.O.F* (Paris: Karthala, 1993) 156.

43 On the consequences of 50-year French presence, see Boilley, *Les Touaregs Kel Adagh*, 259–268.

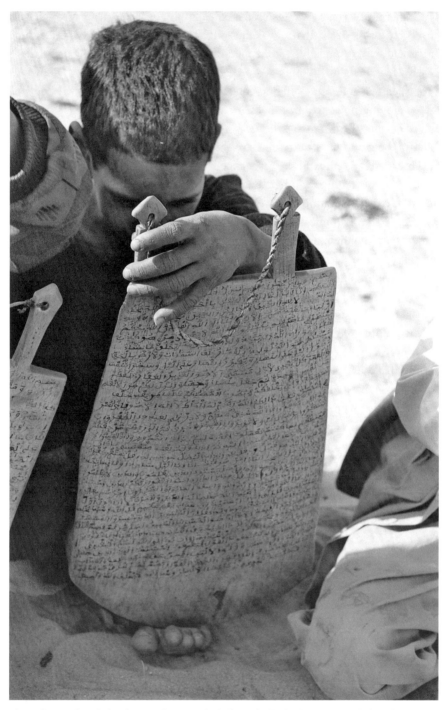

Figure 2.4. *Within the* inəsləmān *class, to which the Kel Alhafra belong, knowledge of the Koran and the Arabic script have always been taught by the* ālfāqqìtān, *the Koranic teachers, to the children (mainly the boys) in the encampments (Inkilla, November 2005).*

2.3.2. From independence to recolonization

In 1944, France had resolved to incorporate the African elite into the administration of its colonies, but because no such elites developed in the most northern parts of Mali, strong imbalances in political participation began to emerge between the north and south. Voting was predominantly reserved for the sedentary population, and only after a legal amendment in 1951 in which the electorate was enlarged were the nomads able to participate actively in elections. Political negotiations, moreover, remained primarily a concern of the south, and the Tamasheq were in fact apprehensive about the approaching withdrawal of the French. Mohammed Ali Ag Attaher, a Kel Anṣār *āmānokal*, campaigned for a separation between the Sahara regions and the rest of (French) Sudan and became the spokesperson for the Tamasheq who did not want to belong to the same territorial unit as the provinces of the south.

The political changes, however, developed rapidly. In 1958, the Sudanese Republic was formed, and an African administration replaced the French system. One year later saw the emergence of the "Fédération Soudano-Sénégalaise du Mali", a political federation with the more developed coastal state of Senegal. This however lasted just nine months. On 22 September 1960, Mali claimed independence under the leadership of Modibo Keïta, oriented itself along the political lines of the Soviet Union and China and established a one-party system.

Between 1958 and 1961, all the French in the administration and army were replaced by Africans, and a new hardline policy began to take shape in northern Mali. The government authorities had no desire to lose the Sahara Provinces whose mineral and oil resources they hoped to exploit. They tightened their control over political expression by the nomads, sought to stifle or monitor mergers and conspiracies and forced charismatic leaders like Mohammed Ali Ag Attaher to flee into exile in Morocco.

Although the Republic of Mali entered full independence in 1961, the Tamasheq still found themselves without political voice and felt themselves to be fully at the mercy of the southern powerbrokers. Two years later in May 1963, the first albeit restricted revolt broke out in Adagh between a few poorly armed individuals and some soldiers.[44] As if they had been waiting for just such an "excuse", the Malian army responded sharply, declaring the entire area between the Algerian border and Kidal as a "zone interdite", in which everyone was regarded as a potential rebel and could be shot.[45] To deprive the rebels of all chances of survival, the state forces systematically poisoned all the

---

44 For a detailed description of the 1963–1964 revolts, see Boilley, *Les Touaregs Kel Adagh*, 317–350.
45 On the "zone interdite", see Boilley, *Les Touaregs Kel Adagh*, 331.

wells in the "forbidden zone" and slaughtered the nomad's animals. Although the 1963–1964 revolt originated primarily among the Kel Adagh, members of other nomadic groups moving with their animals along the transhumance routes were killed in cold blood by the army. Many of the rebels tried to flee to Algeria but the revolt found no support and Algeria extradited the insurrectionists back to Mali. The Malian government now branded all the nomads in the north as "rebels", declared the entire northern region as a "zone d'insécurité" and began to intimidate and traumatize the population with repressions, public executions, prison and torture. Up to 1964, the Mali government used brutal force to impose its authority on the northern part of the country, violently subjecting the Tamasheq to a new form of colonization.[46]

The Malian state imposed an external administration on the area. Azawad, covering the entire north of the country and the northern Niger Bend, was now the sixth and largest region of the country, with Timbuktu as its regional administrative center and the seat of the governor. All the government employees originated from the south, and the political marginalization of the nomads, who after 1964 had representation neither in the administration nor in local institutions or parties, became even more marked. With the introduction of the socialist system at Mali's independence, not only was all wealth declared the property of the state, all the *tiwsaten* were subdivided into 60 equal fractions, *əlqəbīlāten* (sing. *əlqəbīlāt*), whose leaders were used as intermediaries but were placed nevertheless under the control of the local administrative prefect. The former *imānokal*, who had previously held responsibility for several subgroups, were now the representatives of just a single fraction.

Under the rule of Modibo Keïta, schooling again became compulsory and any Tamasheq leader who opposed it was condemned to death. The Kel Alhafra say that at the military post in Inokender where the French school had been taken over by the Malian government, the children were forced with violence to attend classes. It was a period of terror, the army was summoned for the smallest incident, and once more the nomads hid and isolated themselves in an attempt to avoid the repressions exerted by the Malian state.

2.3.3. Drought and rebellion

At the end of the 1960s, large areas of the southern Sahara experienced serious drought. The Kel Alhafra call 1967, the year before the election of Moussa Traoré, *"awātay wa n-tamǝttānt ta n-iwan"* – "the year in which the cows died". In 1968, Modibo Keïta was deposed in a coup, but this was also a year

---

46 On the process of the recolonization of the north, see Boilley, *Les Touaregs Kel Adagh*, 338–348.

marked by the absence of the rains, empty wells, dried-up water pools, over-crowding of nomads around the few remaining water sources, dying animals, starving humans, cholera and other epidemics. The Kel Alhafra say that the Ma-lian government provided no support to the nomads during this difficult period, nor did any international help reach them. They could not know, however, that this first drought year was just the precursor to a whole series of catastrophes. Droughts occurred again in 1972–1973, this time hitting a much wider area ex-tending across the entire Sahara and Sahel in Mauritania, Mali and Niger.[47] 1973 is designated by the Kel Alhafra as *"awātay wa lābasān"* – "the wicked year". Many families lost their entire herds and thus their basic resources. The human death toll was also high. To survive, the nomads had to sell everything they owned – animals, weapons, jewelry, leather wares, saddles etc. – to buy food. A cow fetched just 2,000 Malian francs (CFA 1,000) on the market (the usual price lay around 350,000 Malian francs, equivalent to CFA 175,000), and millet was sold at superinflated prices per tea glass.[48] The fraction chiefs went to the central administration to demand assistance for their people, but they were turned away. Those who still had financial resources left for Algeria, Libya or even the Lebanon; many of the rest, if they had the physical strength, fled to Mauritania and Algeria where they ended up in refugee camps.

Gradually the appalling pictures of emaciated humans and children with bellies bloated by hunger spread around the world, and voices were raised ac-cusing the Malian politicians of purposefully using the drought catastrophe to rid themselves of the nomadic population they found so disagreeable. In an article in *Le Monde*, a French journalist wrote that international aid was not reaching those it was intended for and was being sold at high prices on local markets and that the sedentary population were receiving preferential treat-ment in the distribution of commodities.[49]

There was still no end though to the disasters afflicting northern Mali. 1984–1986 were *"iwatiyān wi n-mānna wa išraynen"* – "the years when the

---

47 On the 1972/1973 droughts in Mali see Mohamed T. Maïga, *Le Mali: De la sècheresse à la rébellion nomade* (Paris: L'Harmattan, 1997).

48 Mali did not convert to CFA until 1984. Instead they were using Malian francs. 2 Malian francs were equivalent to approximately 1 CFA.

49 The accusations by Philippe Decraene stirred up an intense discussion on the international scene. The journalist had visited northern Mali: "At Kabara, where young boys were standing around sacks bearing the label, 'Donation of the European Economic Community,' our guide forbid us to enter the storage area. At Timbuktu, the area commander refused to receive us, 'for lack of time,' and refused us permission to enter the refugee camps because we had 'no legal authorization.' Some of the shops in the town were selling grain that should have been distributed without charge." Philippe Decraene, "Une arme politique contre les Touaregs du Mali", *Le Monde*, 6 February 1974.

drought returned", and the Kel Alhafra joined an even larger wave of migration into settled areas. Those who had survived the 1972/1973 catastrophe now owned too few animals from which to live and fled, mostly illegally, across the border into Algeria. Algeria did not greet this flood across its southern border with open arms. Those without valid papers trying to enter the country and smuggle in their few remaining animals, were arrested, thrown in jail, and had their animals confiscated. In 1986, in the Algerian refugee camp of Borj Mokhtar alone, the Red Cross counted 40,478 people.[50]

Visitors were forbidden to enter the Malian refugee camps around Timbuktu, and only representatives from foreign governments or, on exception, an official from an international organization were allowed in. In 1986, however, the long-awaited assistance finally arrived in Mali in the form of the Red Cross, Médicins sans frontières, UNICEF and other international organizations. The American army distributed aid supplies, and the Malian government eventually also deployed its soldiers for the distribution of food.

It is not known how many Tamasheq lost their lives during these droughts: there are statistics for neither the number who emigrated nor for those who died in the refugee camps. Boilley writes, nevertheless, that there was a significant reduction in the size of the population,[51] and the Kel Alhafra themselves talk of various kinship lineages that were entirely wiped out during these years.

In the 30 years between 1960 and 1990, Tamasheq society was shaken to its very foundations. Not only did they lose a political voice, not only were they forced by repression into increasing isolation, at the same time the new Malian administration that denied the nomads any participation literally took the ground out from under their feet. Affiliation to a *tawset* or a group had no relevance in the new system, with the result that long-standing lines of solidarity fell apart and traditional values were undermined.[52] Many Tamasheq who had lost their herds to the army during the 1963/1964 revolt were unable to return to nomadic pastoralism as their basic way of life, because their already decimated herds had not recovered by the time the devastating droughts set in. The drought years more or less finished off what was left of the nomad's traditional livelihood, and the Tamasheq knew that when they finally returned to their country

---

50 On the Red Cross refugee estimates for 1986, see Boilley, *Les Touaregs Kel Adagh*, 382.
51 See Boilley, *Les Touaregs Kel Adagh*, 375.
52 Ghayshena welet Akedima, a political feminine figure of the Aïr in Niger, expressed this process of transformation from collective Tamasheq identity to an isolated individualistic perspective as follows: "Our space shrank from the 'nation' *(temust)* to the confederation *(taghma)*, then to the tribe *(tawshit)*, then to the encampment *(aghiwen)*, then to the mat tent *(tamankayt)*, and it is now nothing but the space left between the spoon and the mouth." See Hélène Claudot-Hawad, "Neither segmentary, nor centralized: the sociopolitical organization of a nomadic society (Tuaregs) beyond categories", *Orientwissenschaftliche Hefte* 14 (2004): 57–69.

they could expect little support from the Malian government. Meanwhile, however, in the refugee camps, in exile, but also among those who had remained, a new political consciousness began to develop and a new discourse on Tamasheq identity, political rights and autonomy began to take shape and circulate.

Finally, all the anger that had accumulated over the years in the face of suppression, mishandling and marginalization exploded. With an attack on Menaka on 29 June 1990, the Tamasheq began to turn their backs on a story of suffering, resolved to fight for their own identity and win back their decision-making powers. This time, it was much more than the desperate and hopeless revolt of a handful of young men: the rebels had established a dense network of support abroad, both Algeria and Libya tolerated the rebels' use of their countries as bases, and the fighters were armed with modern weapons. The Malian army had trouble suppressing the outbreak of the rebellion and responded to the Tamasheq attacks with ferocious reprisals.

In 1991, power again changed hands in Mali when the Malian army unseated Moussa Traoré and formed the National Reconciliation Council under the leadership of Amadou Toumani Touré, who promised a rapid transition to democracy with the establishment of political parties and free elections. Hopes were raised in the north, only to be quickly shattered by the news of more atrocities. In Gao, members of the Songhai had attacked and destroyed houses whose inhabitants were of nomadic origin, and the conflict in northern Mali gradually took on the contours of an ethnic confrontation. Once more people fled into refugee camps in the surrounding countries, but this time, international human rights organizations were soon involved.

In 1991, the National Conference in Bamako resolved to draft a new constitution and new electoral laws that would serve as the basis for a multiparty system. The first free parliamentary elections were held one year later, in which Alpha Oumar Konaré was elected President of the Republic. Within the context of these political changes, the rebel groups and the Malian government sought a consensus. In 1992, their efforts culminated in the signing of the "National Pact", in which northern Mali, comprising the sixth, seventh and eighth regions of the country, acquired a "special position" with a very large degree of self-determination. The settlement also pledged the belated incorporation of the nomadic groups into the army, administration and economy.[53]

Practically from one day to the next, interregional, regional and local issues were placed in the hands of the population that was supposed to organize itself into assemblies. Suddenly the northern societies were responsible for their own

---

53 For a detailed and critical appraisal of the "National Pact" see Boilley, *Les Touaregs Kel Adagh*, 495–533.

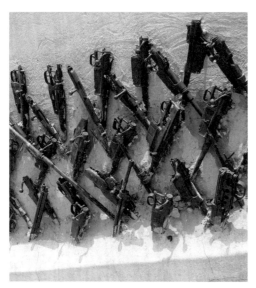

Figure 2.5. *A monument in Timbuktu with Kalashnikovs embedded in its concrete, recalling the weapon burning during the "Flame of Peace" ceremony on 27 March 1996.*

economic, social and cultural development and their own security. It was too much too fast, and overwhelmed by this almost instantaneous autonomy, the situation descended into chaos. There were no regional authorities, bandits roamed the region, and once again terror and uncertainty became the (dis)order of the day.

Feeling themselves abandoned by the Malian state, the settled population built up militant groups for their own self-defense. The Songhai organization "Ganda Koy" ("Masters of the Land"), for example, attacked Tamasheq and Moor encampments, and northern Mali was plunged into conditions resembling those of a civil war, with plundering and the gruesome murder of innocent civilians. Doubts about the "National Pact" were raised among political circles in Bamako, but by 1995, a new functional administration began to take hold, the security situation calmed, and the highly contested decentralization started to take shape. The population of the north longed for security and peace. Finally on 27 March 1996, the various hostile groups came together in Timbuktu and during a "Flame of Peace" ceremony threw down and burned hundreds of their weapons as a symbolic gesture toward the peace and stability they desired for the region.

2.3.4. Return from exile and refugee camps

After 1996, the nomads once more began to return to their homeland from the refugee camps and exile. For three months, the United Nations High Commissioner for Refugees supplied them with tents, food and a small starting credit to rebuild their lives with the animals that had also survived. However, many had lost everything and could not return to their traditional ways. Alternative futures were fostered and encouraged by various international organizations who built villages like Tinjāmbān, Nebket al-Elek, Er Intejeft, Tin Təllun and Tehārje where the returnees could settle, set up gardens, or with the help of microcredit develop a small project.

There was no returning to the past. The tribal associations no longer existed, and every family, whether *inasləmān, inhāḍān* or *iklān*, was on a par with all the others, quasi-autonomous and responsible for their own social and economic relationships. Many Kel Alhafra say that to begin with they had only got by with *aššāyāl wa n-afuss*, temporary jobs, until they could finally afford to purchase a few animals. Some were able to expand their herds in quite a short time, but today the majority of the nomads also tend animals such as camels and sheep whose owners live in the cities.

Furthermore, in exile and in the refugee camps, the nomads had been exposed to a more comfortable way of life that was totally unfamiliar to them. They had running water and access to medical care and educational opportunities. They could send their children to schools that were not kilometers away from their homes and could regularly visit with kin they would not see for months or longer in the vast expanses of the desert. They were also confronted with modern means of communication like television and radio, and saw how their Arab neighbors raised date palms in the desert and vegetables in gardens. For many, the return to the merciless realities of Azawad was hard, and not just a few among the Kel Alhafra complained about their destitute life in the desert. Many of the old people look on all the changes with regret and say that today everyone wants to be an *āmānokal*. They say that the young people no longer show them respect and prefer to move away from the hard nomad life for a more comfortable one in the villages and cities. The changes are not restricted to the social structures that have forfeited their importance. Other traditional values and behaviors have also been lost or modified. The silver jewelry that the women used to wear but had to sell during the drought years has been replaced by plastic beads, and instead of leather sandals, they buy cheap plastic flip-flops from China at the local weekly markets. Metal and plastic utensils have replaced their leather and wood equivalents that were exchanged for food or cash during the droughts. In the towns especially, the traditional indigo-dyed veil, *alāššo*, worn by the women has given way to the colorful variant, *ikāršāyān* (sing. *ekāršāy*), found in Mauritania and Algeria. Many men no longer cover their faces with the distinctive *āγewəd* (pl. *iγiwad*), but are letting their beards grow, as a sign of the piety they wish to declare as a new form of identity.[54]

54 The period of the Tamasheq uprisings between 1990–1996, as well as the resumption and return to pastoral nomadic life, is well described by Georg Klute, "Die Rebellionen der Tuareg

2.3.5. Decentralization begets marginalization

Since the political transformations of 1991, decentralization has been a most important concept for the Malian government. To realize this core program, since 1999, 703 communes have been set up, whose councils are elected by the people. Each commune sends representatives to the "Conseil de Cercle", which in turn sends representatives to a regional assembly that is responsible to the central government. The purpose of this multilayered structure is to ensure that voters can express their political will and participate in political decision-making. Each commune has wide-reaching authority and can raise loans, hire its own personnel and collect taxes. It is also fully responsible for the economic, social and cultural development of its region.

For many of the nomadic Tamasheq groups, however, decentralization has not yet brought the level of meaningful political participation for which they had hoped. The commune administrations are located in settlements, and during elections the nomads believe they are often the victims of electoral fraud practiced by dominant groups among the sedentary population. Corruption and mismanagement hinder important development projects and, together with favoritism, seem to be widespread in bureaucratic institutions. After the election of Amadou Toumani Touré in 2002, the government set up a commission to fight corruption, but it has yet to purge the lowest administrative levels, especially in the northern regions. In a corruption index published by Transparency International in 2006, Mali held the 99th position of the 163 evaluated nations.[55]

The nomads accuse the Malian government of conducting a politics of "laissez-faire" in the north. Alongside the corruption, inadequately controlled northern areas of the desert have developed networks smuggling migrants, weapons, cigarettes, etc. In addition, armed conflicts between individual groups have once again stirred up fear and mistrust among the Tamasheq. Although the weapon-burning ceremony lies only in the recent past, the desert inhabitants have rearmed to defend themselves against resumed assaults because *"wārtilla ālhukuma dāy azāwād"*, "in Azawad there is no government".

in Mali und Niger" (Habil.-Schrift Univ. Siegen 2001/2, Cologne: Köppe Verlag [in print]); Sara Randall, "The demographic consequences of conflict, exile and repatriation: A case study of Malian Tuareg", *European Journal of Population – Revue Européenne de Démographie* 21.2–3 (2005): 291–320; Alessandra Giuffrida, "Clerics, rebels and refugees: Mobility strategies and networks among the Kel Antessar", *The Journal of North African Studies*, 10.3–4 (2005): 529–543; Sara Randall & Alessandra Giuffrida, "Forced migration, sedentarisation and social change: Malian Kel Tamasheq", in *Nomadic Societies in the Middle East and North Africa: Entering the 21st century*, ed. Dawn Chatty (Leiden: Brill, 2005) 431–462.
55 "Corruption Perception Index", *Transparency International*, 6 November 2006, http://www.transparency.org (accessed 11 Nov. 2006).

The Tamasheq say that anarchic conditions prevail in Azawad, and the political situation is tense. For them, politics remains a business of the south – one in which they still play no decisive role.

2.3.6. Resumption of the rebellion and the Agreement of Algiers

In March 2006, Tamasheq fighters, united under the command of Colonel Hassan Ag Fagaga, deserted from the Malian army taking with them vehicles, weapons, and ammunition. Just two months later, the Malian military post in Tinsāwaten near the border with Algeria and Niger became the target of the first attack.[56] Fear of repeated insurgent conflagrations began to wear on the tolerance of the citizenry. On the night of 22nd May 2006, a group of former resistance fighters, including Hassan Ag Fagaga and Ibrahim Ag Bahanga, occupied military installations in Kidal and attacked barracks in Menaka and Tessalit. Calling themselves "Alliance Démocratique du 23 mai 2006 pour le Changement ADC", the rebels accused the Malian government of breaking promises to invest in the north as well as to increase involvement of northern people in the government. Consequently, they demanded autonomy for the city of Kidal.[57] The Malian government immediately dispatched additional soldiers to the north causing the rebels to retreat, for a time, without a fight from Kidal into the mountains of Tiɣārɣār.[58]

On 4 July 2006 in Algiers, a peace agreement, "l'Accord d'Alger", was signed with the help of Algerian mediation. The agreement emphasized the unity of the Republic of Mali and highlighted the "Pacte National" of 1992. It also promised a development program for the region of Kidal, reintegration of rebels and deserters of 22-23 May, as well as employment prospects for young people.[59] In turn, the ADC rebels promised to stop armed attacks and give up their demands for Kidal's autonomy. A splinter group of the ADC led by Ibrahim Ag Bahanga, however, rejected the Algiers Agreement. At the same time, voices in the Malian population accused the government of supporting secessionist movements and rewarding a small group of troublemaker insurgents, who were already involved in the revolt of the nineties, with concessions.[60]

---

56 Cherif Ouazani, "Les dessous d'une attaque", *Jeune Afrique*, 20 May 2007.
57 http://english.aljazeera.net (accessed 6 June 2006).
58 See Wolfgang Schreiber, *Das Kriegsgeschehen 2008* (Wiesbaden: VS Verlag für Sozialwissenschaften, 2010) 191–195.
59 *L'Essor*, No. 15740, 07 October 2006. See also: http://initiatives-mali.info/spip.php?article611 (accessed 12 January 2011).
60 *L'Indépendant*, 13 July, 2006 and 17 July, 2006.

2.3.7. The crisis expands

The supposed peace following the Agreement of Algiers lasted only briefly. In August 2007, insurgents, again lead by Ibrahim Ag Bahanga, attacked the Malian army in the northwest of the country and captured many soldiers. These rebels renamed themselves "Alliance Touareg du Nord-Mali pour le Changement ATNM" and attacked military bases and convoys with some significant losses for the Malian army. Mediators from Algeria, Libya, and even from their own circles continued efforts for peace and the release of prisoners.

In early April 2008, another ceasefire agreement was signed. This document envisaged secession of hostilities, revitalization of the Algiers Agreement, reduction of Malian troops in the north, emancipation of prisoners, as well as financial support for the development of the northern regions. Arguing, however, that the government had not withdrawn soldiers from the north while the rebels complied with their promise to release of prisoners, Ag Bahanga's group continued their violent attacks. Resentment began to grow within the Tamasheq. Many faction leaders sharply condemned the violence of Ag Bahanga's followers, and most rebels continued to support the peace process.

On 6 May 2008, the ATNM attacked barracks near the city of Ségou, a mere 500 km away from the capital Bamako, causing the Malian government to change its course. As Ag Bahanga's assaults spread geographically beyond the confines of the north and military casualties mounted, the Malian army became restless and began to show less and less patience with negotiations. Concerned that the officers' burgeoning discontent might culminate in a coup attempt, President Amadou Toumani Touré began making changes in the highest echelons of the military hierarchy.

Personnel were rotated to positions abroad, and hardliners known for their relentless fight against the rebels took their place. Interestingly enough, many of these new military commanders were from Arab districts north of Mali, thereby adding an ethnic element to the crisis.[61]

While the Malian army ruthlessly countered the violent attacks of the ATNM rebels and other emerging groups, the government appealed to Algeria for mediation in peace negotiations and for better control of the southern Sahara borders. On 21 July 2008, Algeria was able to broker another peace agreement between the Malian government and Amada Ag Bibi, a delegate of the National Assembly, who represented the demands of the rebels. Malian soldiers were released, and the rebels were promised amnesty and reintegration into the Malian army. With the aid of Algeria, the long awaited peace finally appeared to be re-

---

61 Ousmane Daou, "Insécurité au nord: L'Etat entretien le conflit ethnique", *Le Républicain*, 16 January 2009.

alized. Basking in its success as a regional power, Algeria felt it had gained an advantage in its ongoing rivalry with Libya for influence in the Sahara.

There was speculation of another break up in Ibrahim Ag Bahanga's group with many jumping ship to seek a part in the potential peace process. Rumor had it that Ag Bahanga himself had meanwhile withdrawn into exile in Libya, but at the end of the year, he appeared once again in Mali with his men to attack a military base in Nampala, near the Mauritanian border. According to Bamako, nine soldiers died in the fighting – the rebels claimed there were more than twenty. "Trop, c'est trop! Nous ne pouvons pas continuer à subir, à compter nos morts et à chercher la paix", Amadou Toumani Touré declared.[62] According to various press reports, the Malian army reinforced its troops in the north with Arab militias and immediately announced the destruction of Ag Bahanga's base in Tinsālāk. Rebel camps were attacked and the Malian army killed any suspected revolutionaries they found there. On 6 February 2009, the government announced that the Malian army had destroyed the last position of ATNM fighters and that Ag Bahanga had fled with a handful of men to Algeria.[63]

In a public ceremony in Kidal, former ADC rebels and fighters from Ag Bahanga's faction were made to relinquish their weapons, sign a definitive peace accord, and enter temporary military encampments. Meanwhile, the weakened ATNM leader Ag Bahanga signaled his willingness to return to the bargaining table with Algeria and Mali. This time, however, Bamako refused, insisting that the rebels first lay down their weapons. In October 2010, at a ceremony organized by Libya in Oubary, Ag Bahanga finally acquiesced along with the leader of the Tamasheq movement from neighboring Niger.[64]

2.3.8. Trafficking, terrorism and oil

Mali spans over one million square kilometers, an area equivalent to three times the size of France. Additionally, it shares borders with seven neighboring states that have all struggled to control their vast desert regions. The country lacks necessary resources. Moreover, there are simmering conflicts between and within social and ethnic groups. There is poverty, marginality, banditry, the presence of militant Islamists, youth crime and a black market with drugs, alcohol, cigarettes, weapons, and human trafficking.

"Groupe Salafiste pour la Prédication et le Combat GSPC" (the Salafist Group for Preaching and Combat), a radical separatist organization that seeks to

---

62 Christophe Boisbouvier, "ATT entre en guerre", *Jeune Afrique*, 27 January 2009.
63 http://www.temoust.org/mali-les-rebelles-touaregs-fuient,7632 (accessed 12 February 2009).
64 "R.N.", "Ag Bahanga demande à réintégrer l'Accord d'Alger", *El-Watan* (Algeria), 02 April 2009.

overthrow the Algerian government and establish an Islamic state, has wreaked havoc since 1998 along the borders of Mauritania, Mali, Niger, Libya and Chad, with kidnappings, assassinations and smuggling. Since 2003, a splinter group from the GSPC is believed to have withdrawn into the Tamasheq area north of Mali and Niger. In 2007, this group joined al-Qaeda and changed its name to "Al-Qaida au Maghreb islamique AQMI" (Al-Qaeda organization in the Islamic Maghreb). The European Union and the United States consider AQMI and its international network one of the most dangerous terrorist groups in the world.

In its struggle against terrorism, the United States founded the "Pan Sahel Initiative" at the end of 2002. The goal was to destroy the operating base of terrorists in the Sahel countries of Mali, Mauritania, Niger and Chad.[65] In the Malian town of Gao, special units of the U.S. military teach and supply the local troops with necessary equipment and skills to withstand the enemy and fight in the extreme desert conditions. Especially when military maneuvers are conducted in nomadic areas, the people in the tents are insufficiently informed or simply ignored, and the U.S. presence is not fully comprehended. There are voices in northern Mali whispering that the U.S. would like to buy the Kidal region from the Malian government since the region is of strategic military importance. With its anti-terrorist presence, the U.S. military is in fact already "occupying" Malian military institutions throughout the north.

However, the interest of the U.S. seems to focus not only on counterterrorism but also in particular on the region's potential oil reserves. Rebellions, banditry, terrorism and organized crime could jeopardize unhindered access to those precious resources. In early 2004, the Pan Sahel Initiative was renamed "Trans-Sahara Counter Terrorism Initiative TSCTI" and expanded to include the countries of Algeria, Morocco, Tunisia, Senegal, Ghana and Nigeria.[66] Since Africa has the potential to be the most important oil and natural gas supplier to the U.S. after the Middle East, protection of these transport routes is of central strategic importance.

As for the current peace between Tamasheq rebels and the Malian government, the future remains uncertain. The northern regions of Timbuktu, Gao and Kidal were promised large investments that might lead to equally large disappointments. The donors who have pledged help are reluctant to invest while the area remains insecure. The units of the "Al-Qaida au Maghreb islamique AQMI" are more active than ever, and without international involvement, Mali alone does not have the resources necessary to manage its vast desert regions and control the issues presented by Islamist groups within its borders.

3. Local Frameworks for Health and Sickness

3.1. Lifeworlds as symbolic constructions

3.1.1. Complementary dualities in a holistic worldview

At first sight, the world of the Kel Alhafra appears to be a dualistic one, divided into seemingly oppositional pairs that constitute the entire universe: day and night *ašāl d-ehāḍ*, sun and moon *tāfukk d-iyor,* heaven and earth *išǝnnawān d-ākall*, fire and water *efew d-aman,* heat and cold *tākusse d-tǝssǝmḍe,* rainy season and dry season *akāsa d-ewelān*, light and darkness *ǝnnor d-tihāy*, north and south *afālla d-ajuss*, feminine and masculine *eyy d-tunte*, body and spirit *tayǝssa d-unfas*, life and death *tāmudre d-tamǝttānt*, this life and the hereafter, *āddunya d-ālaxirāt*, paradise and hell *ālžānnāt d-ālžāhānnām*. Together, however, these pairs form a mythical living space, *āddunya*[67], in which all directions and positions are directed toward an affective focus, namely Mecca, *mākkāt*, the center of the Islamic world.

In this way, the mythical[68] comprehension of the Islamic world achieves an identificatory purpose, because it constitutes an explanation of the world in which every element stands in meaningful relationship to every other element. Potential oppositions are tempered by a holistic world view,[69] and emphasis is placed on the complementarity of all phenomena: day can only be classified as such if I know what night is; I can only comprehend what life is when I am able to conceive its end and thus death – *wār tǝzzayād tāmudre a-fāl wār tǝssanād ā-wa aqqālān tamǝttant,* the Kel Alhafra say, "you do not know life if you are not aware of the significance of death". Every conceivable being is essentially monistic, and anything that one tries to place outside this mythological

---

67 The Kel Alhafra apply the term *āddunya* not only as the opposite of *ālaxirāt*, but also in their cosmological understanding as a designation for the entire universe. This illustrates that the bipolar world construed by the Kel Alhafra is not an absolute self-contained system but one that reflects the occasional incoherence of the lifeworld.

68 Myth is to be understood here in the original sense given to it by the Greeks and not as the purely material explanation of the world envisaged by Auguste Comte. For Plato, μῦθος is a creation of humans that unlike λόγος is transmitted not by constructive education but in suggestive narration. Aristotle describes μῦθος as a symbolic emulation of action, a construction of the elements of the act, the soul of a drama, always subjective, a projection and expression of human skills. (On the Greek use of the term myth, see Heinz-Günther Nesselrath, "Mythos-Logos – Mytho-Logos: Zum Mythos-Begriff der Griechen und ihrem Umgang mit ihm", in *Form und Funktion des Mythos in archaischen und modernen Gesellschaften*, eds. Peter Rusterholz and Ruppert Moser (Bern: Paul Haupt, 1999) 1–26.

69 On the holistic worldview of Islam, see Edith Jachimowicz, "Islamic Cosmology", in *Ancient Cosmologies*, eds. Carmen Blacker and Michael Loewe (London: George Allen & Unwin, 1975) 143–171.

space must, ultimately, be situated in reference to it and thus encompassed by it. Meaning for the Kel Alhafra resides in the relationship between complementary elements, and each individual is held answerable for his or her life before a unique power on the judgment day, *ašāl wa n-tebādde*. Each person seeks unity, *taməddāwt*,[70] in the irreducible diversity of the physical world by following a righteous path, *tābarāt ta tāhuskāt*, toward God, so that spirit and body, *ənniyāt d-tayəssa*, this life and the next life, *āddunya d-ālaxirāt*, substance and meaning, *eyās d-ālmāyna*, will be united when he or she leaves the existential lifeworld.

For the Kel Alhafra, the condition or status of things in their world is first made possible by the Islamic creation myth. This constructs a clearly demarcated basis for perception, determining the position of things and the activities of daily life while also establishing a coexistence between the human body and its surroundings – one in which the human is always understood as dominant to nature. God created existentiality by naming it, and he taught Adam[71] and no other living being (the angels included) the names of things.[72] Humans were accorded certain cognitive faculties that place them above all other living beings: they have the "knowledge of the visible", *tāmusne ta ti-tənhəy*, but its complementary pole, "the knowledge of the invisible", *tāmusne ta wār ti-tənhəy*, remains withheld.

Instead of the Arabic term, *āddunya*, older people among the Kel Alhafra often use a Tamasheq word-image: *tesāyt n-ākall fuk*. In Tamasheq, *tesāyt* is a woven dish used in preparing millet to separate the grain from the chaff. Viewed metaphorically, the world in this sense comprises "the sieve of the entire earth", whereby the millet stands for everything that exists. The conceptual meaning of this term is constituted in a gestural signification – that of tossing the pounded millet. In this act of tossing, grain and its complementary coat are separated: the naturally visible things of the world, *āẓẓahir n-ākall*, remain in the *tesāyt*, while the chaff falls through it, disappears from the human visual field, and from that moment on is understood as the invisible and inapprehensible, *ider n-tesāyt*, under the *tesāyt*.

---

70 *taməddāwt* is the verbal noun from the Tamasheq verb *imda* and literally means "finished, complete, total being", "being realized in every aspect", but also "end" and "death".

71 In Tamasheq the human is also called *āwadəm: āw*, descended from, *adəm*, Adam.

72 In Koranic teaching, the human is "created with My own hands", *ḫalaqtu bi-yadayya* (38/75), "and [I] breathed My spirit in him", *wa nafaḫtu fīhi min rūḥī* (38/72), and God created Adam after his image, *lataqabbahu-l-waǧh fa'inna-llāhu ḫalaqa ādam 'ala ṣūratihi*, as expressed by a *ḥadīṯ* from the *Ṣaḥīḥ al-Buḫārī* (see *Buḫārī: istiḏān* 1; and *Muslim: birr* 115, *Ǧannah*: 28, *Ibn Hanbal: musnād* Vol. II, 244, 251, 315, 323). Adam was characterized by the special gift of knowledge, because God taught him the name of all things: *wa 'allama Adama –l-asmā'a kullahā ...* (2/31).

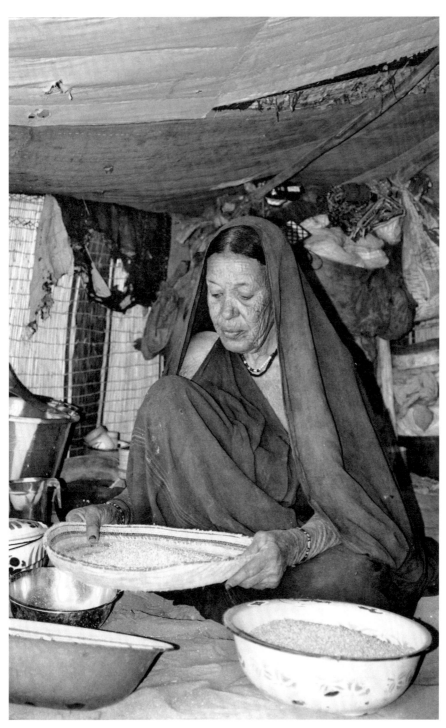

Figure 3.1. *Tossing the pounded millet in a* tesāyt *separates the grain from the chaff (In Astilan, February 2005).*

On the *tesāyt n-ākall* as lifeworld, the Kel Alhafra are engaged with the physical space of the here and now, with its concrete, variably characterized regions that are always directed toward the *qiblāt*, the sanctified direction of prayer, eastward toward Mecca. Nevertheless, aware of the complementaries, of the invisible above and beneath the earth, the lifespace with its interchangeable dimensions always forms a homogenous and indivisible whole.[73]

In Tamasheq, the word-images *āddunya* and *tesāyt n-ākall fuk* already incorporate the complementary polarities of the visible and invisible, this life and the afterlife, light and shadow. In contrast to the Arabic, in the Tamasheq of the Kel Alhafra, the word *āddunya* stands not only for the immanent world but also designates the entire universe in analogy to the Arabic *'ālam* (while *ākall* refers explicitly to the physical, immanent lifespace). *'ālam aš-šahāda* (or *'ālam aẓ-ẓāhir*), the Koranic world of the visible, becomes in Tamasheq *āẓẓahir n-ākall*, the world of the inapparent, while *'ālam al-ġayb* becomes *ider n-ākall*. In this monistic worldview, the bipolar is resolved as a synthesis in the divine unity, *touḥid* (Arabic *tawḥīd*) – unification, the one, unique, transcendent God.

3.1.2. Symbolic use of the tent space

It is through the Islamic creation myth, then, that the Kel Alhafra strive to integrate their world into a universal order. The myth establishes a living space, a unity, in which every element has a meaningful relationship to every other element. It is a cognitive and perceptual foundation that provides the nomads with a certain orientation and sense of stability in the vast expanses of the desert. In analogy to the macrocosm, *āddunya*, the tent forms a microcosm constructed according to the same oppositions and homologies that regulate the entire universe.

The tent *ihānan* (sing. *ehān*) is oriented by the *qiblāt* toward the east *s-emāināj*, such that its entrance is always on the western, *s-ātārām*, side.[74] In this way, anyone entering the tent does so with his or her face toward the east, thus bringing the divine auspiciousness, *ālbarāka*, of the holy city into the mi-

---

73 Hureiki's three-part representation of the Tuareg world into *"eder n amadal"* (foundation of the earth*), "aẓẓahir n amadal"* (surface of the earth) and "the divine or celestial world" must be questioned because this division is not made in the Tamasheq language usage. See Jacques Hureiki, *Essai sur les origines des Touaregs* (Paris: Karthala, 2003) 140–141.

74 In contrast to the Kel Alhafra, according to Pandolfi and Foucauld, the tents of the Kel Ahaggar are oriented toward the south: "For the Kel Alhaggar, east is the direction of Mecca. The opening of their tents is always on their right side, that is to the south, when they are praying." Charles de Foucauld and Adolphe de Calassanti-Motylinski, *Textes Touaregs en prose (dialecte de l'Ahaggar),* Critical edition by Salem Chaker, Hélène Claudot and Marceau Gast (Aix-en-Provence: Edisud, 1984) 359; Paul Pandolfi, *Les Touaregs de l'Ahaggar, Sahara algérien. Parenté et résidence chez les Dag-Ghâli,* (Paris: Editions Karthala, 1998) 147.

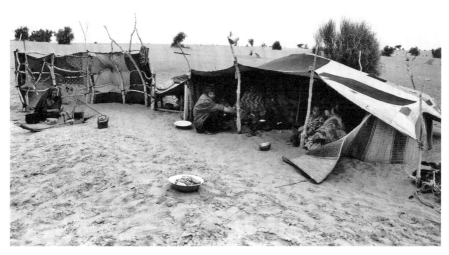

Figure 3.2. *Tent,* ehān, *with its opening toward the west, a cooking area,* edāgg wa n-əsink, *and windbreak,* eff, *in the north (In Astilan, February 2005).*

crocosm. At the same time, because the tents are low structures, it is necessary to bend down to enter the tent, and thus one bows symbolically in the cardinal direction that is connotated as holy.

Correspondingly, the Kel Alhafra always sleep with the head in the west and the feet to the east. In this way, the lower, sensitive and subjective part of the body is symbolically anchored in the mythical perceptual ground *(tāmusne-ta wār ti-tənhəy),* while the objective part of the visual field observes the empirical world *(tāmusne-ta ti-tənhəy).* The head and gaze are, once again, directed toward Mecca.[75] The perception of Mecca as the mythical center is synonymous for the Kel Alhafra with sharing in a common origin and beholding from this center the side of all things that are turned toward it. At least five times a day, this consummate center is bathed in the gaze of an uncountable number of

75 The Kel Ahaggar, in contrast, apparently never sleep with their head to the west: "A Kel Ahaggar always sleeps with his head toward the east or the south, but never toward the west let alone the north." The Kel Ahaggar fear being attacked by evil spirits, which usually come from the north, if they sleep with their heads in that direction. They also believe that anyone who falls ill while sleeping with his or her head toward the north will henceforth be chronically and incurably sick. Paul Pandolfi, *Les Touaregs de l'Ahaggar, Sahara algérien. Parenté et résidence chez les Dag-Ghâli* (Paris: Editions Karthala, 1998) 147.
According to Casajus, the Kel Ferwan sleep like the Kel Alhafra in the east-west orientation in the tent. Dominique Casajus, *La tente dans la solitude: La société et les morts chez les Touaregs Kel Ferwan* (Paris: Fondation de la Maison des Sciences de l'Homme, 1987) 236.

believers, which endows it with something eternal, incomprehensively transparent, and at the same time, magically attractive.

The Kel Alhafra explained to me that the head of a believer must never lie
in the east, either in sleep or in the grave, because it will not have the holy center of the world within its visual field and can lose the connection to Mecca. The
dead are therefore always placed in the grave in a precisely prescribed position, *asətāqbil*, with the feet to the north, head to the south and lying on the right
shoulder turned toward the east. In this way, by always being oriented toward the
mythical center, the objective world of the visual gaze preserves its meaning.[76]

The east, *emāināj*, is symbolic for Mecca and the shared origin and genealogical linking of each individual believer with this center. As the sacred cardinal direction, the east is always positively connotated. The believer prays in
the direction of the *qiblāt*, and the Kel Alhafra take care that no impurities are
found in the eastern part of the tent and that no unclean acts take place there.
Defecation and urination toward the east are frowned upon, as is throwing any
form of refuse in this direction.

At the same time, the sun rises in the east, bringing light and life after the
dark night with its unpredictable dangers from the desert. The Kel Alhafra pur-
sue their early morning activities in the shadow of the western opening of the
tent. The shadow, though, soon moves to the other side, and during the day
the eastern side of the tent is opened. It is on this side, therefore, that millet is
pounded, tea is brewed, small-scale craftwork is undertaken, food is eaten and
guests are received, until shortly before dusk. It is only during the early evening, *takāst tārnašet*, before the fourth prayer, *amud n-ālmaẓ,* at sunset, *almāẓ,*
that the tent inhabitants return to its western side.

The east-west opposition that represents holy and profane, sunrise and
sunset, light and dark, day and night, pure and impure, is mirrored by an analogous contrast between the north, *afālla*, and the south, *ajuss*.

Among the Kel Alhafra, the north of the tent is the woman's side, the south
is assigned to the man.[77] The two sections are separated inside the tent by two
central, vertical wooden poles, *timānkayen* (sing. *temānkayt*), connected by
two horizontal wooden beams, *iloban n-ehān*, thus forming a framework that
supports the roof of the tent.[78]

---

76 The Kel Ferwan in Niger, however, bury their dead with the head in the north and the feet in
   the south. See Dominique Casajus, *La tente dans la solitude: La société et les morts chez les
   Touaregs Kel Ferwan* (Paris: Fondation de la Maison des Sciences de l'Homme, 1987) 236.
77 This division appears to be reversed among the Kel Ferwan in Niger, i.e. north is the masculine and south is the feminine side. See Casajus, *La tente dans la solitude*, 56–57.
78 Surprisingly, among the Kel Ahaggar, Pandolfi identified no symbolic element that divides
   the north and south into sex-specific areas: "The interior of a tent is divided into two halves,

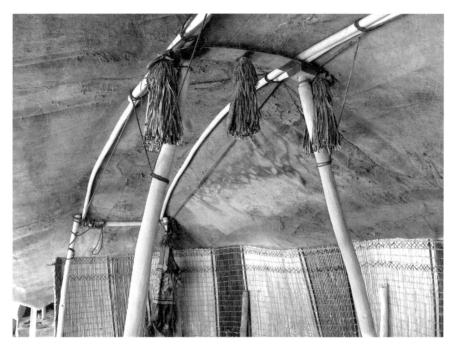

Figure 3.3. *Symbolic division of the tent into female and male sections by vertical poles,* timānkayen, *connected by two horizontal poles,* iloban n-ehān, *that together support the tent roof* (*Tin Timāɣayān*, *March 2006*).

Standing in front of the western tent entrance with the face toward Mecca, the male southern side of the tent is on the right, and the female northern side is on the left. Two wooden stakes, *tijəttawen n-ilalān* (sing. *tajəttawt*), are placed in each side of the tent on which the property of the husband and wife are hung out of the reach of rodents and scorpions. Every Kel Alhafra tent is constructed and organized in this specific manner, and every tent pole, every utensil, every small item has its assigned place in the tent (see table 3.1).

The cooking area, *edāgg wa n-əsink*, is always constructed outside, north of the tent, and all refuse is also deposited in this direction. The south is for the water store, *tijəttwen n-iddidān*, and for the animals (although camels, the "holy animals", are bedded down in the east). Goats spend the night in a pen constructed from thorn branches, *afāraj n-tisādwa*, which is divided into two sections, *afāraj wa n-ulli d-afāraj n-eɣāydān* – one for the adults and a smaller one for the kids. Cattle, donkey and sheep are stabled in the south or west of the tent. The lambs are tied together at night by a cord, *asəddi n-ikrāwatān*.

although no fixed or moveable element marks this separation symbolically." Pandolfi, *Les Touaregs de l'Ahaggar,* 149.

Table 3.1. *Assignment of objects to the female and male sides of the tent*

Woman's side – *teje ta n-tamāḍt* left – *tesālje*	Man's side – *teje ta n-āhalis* right – *āɣəll*
Personal objects	**Personal objects**
tābawānt – leather bag to store the woman's personal property *iməlsan n-tiḍeḍen* – the woman's clothes *tāsāgāmmut (pl. tisəgomma)* – woven rug/blanket *adāfor (pl. idfar)* – cushion *tawset (pl. tiwsaten)* – mat for sitting on *āsadd (pl. isaddān)* – cosmetic stick *tiset, (pl. tiseten)* – mirror *oɣnawān* – jewelry *āṣṣabu, (pl. āṣṣabutān)* – soap	*taɣrək/āššākwa* – leather bag to store the man's personal property *iməlsan n-meddan* – the man's clothes *tabārde (pl. tibardāwen)* – blanket *eben (pl. ibenān)* – tobacco pipe *taba* – tobacco *iɣəmdan* – tweezers for removing thorns *ālkitab* – Koran *asəllum, (pl. isəllumān)* – Koran boards
Food	**Food**
tafārkit – dried meat *bidon n-udi (n-esem)* – pitcher for butter (fat) *dilwil* – oil *tesəmt* – salt	*āllon n-tafāɣāt d-enāle* – millet and rice store *āla* – tea *əssukar* – sugar
Utensils for processing milk	**Equipment for collecting wellwater**
tazāwāt ta n-axx – large wooden bowl for milk *taɣəšut (pl. tiɣəšuten)* – small wooden container for milk *āsilkā (pl. isilkāwān)* – wooden milk ladle *afāranfār (pl. ifāranfārān)* – wooden "whisk" *ākāləkkol* – leather tube-bag to churn butter *asəggəfi* – wooden funnel *eləffi (pl. ilāffān)* – woven lid to close open vessels	*iddid (pl. iddidān)* – goatskin waterbag *terewit* – ropes for the waterbag *tekerkert n-anu* – wooden winch for the well rope *asāqqārqānna* – pole for the winch *āja* – general term for vessels to raise water from a well *aɣān (pl. iaɣnān)* – rope in general *taɣānt (pl. teɣunen)* – rope for tethering animals
Utensils to prepare millet and for cooking	**Utensils to prepare tea**
tesāyt – woven dish for tossing pounded millet *temey ta n-ejel* – sieve to prepare millet *eɣer (pl. iɣerān)* – iron cooking vessel *teɣert (pl. teɣerin)* – metal vessel *asərwi* – large wooden scoop *so (pl. sotān)* – plastic vessel *telāɣt* – small knife *ākoss (pl. ikassān)* – any kind of container *tasəlkot n-aman* – small vessel to scoop water *tāsokālt (pl. tisokālen)* – spoon *ajədod n-tisokalen* – small leather sack to store the wooden spoon *azāwa (pl. azāwatān)* – large, wide vessel	*āfus n-efew d-tizuẓam* – iron tea ladle *ālbārrad* – tea pot *ālkas (pl. ālkisān)* – tea glass *āttabla n-ālkisan* – metal tray for serving tea *ašākwa n-ātay* – leather sack for storing tea utensils *tādara* – small wooden box for holding tea utensils *ālmāɣraš* – water jug *ālfārna n-ātay* – tea warmer
Craft utensils and medicaments	**Weapons and hunting tools**
tistant (pl. tistanen) – needle, awl *lam (pl. lamtān)* – razorblade *elām (pl. ilāmawān)* – tanned skin to be worked *asāfar (pl. isəfrān)* – medicaments (traditional and modern)	*tutāla* – axe *ālbarroḍ (pl. ālbarroḍān)* – gun *absār (pl. ibsārān)* – large knife *ajor* – lance *goẓma* – dagger *tākoba* – sword *tāndərbat (pl. tāndərbaten)* – animal skin

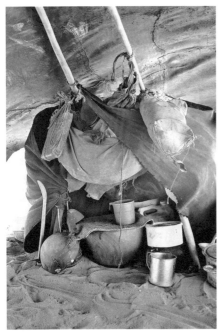 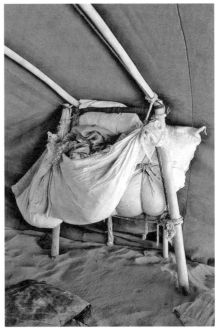

Figure 3.4. *Woman's side* – teje ta n-tamāḍt
(Tin Timāɣayān, October 2005).

Figure 3.5. *Man's side* – teje ta n-āhalis
(Buneyrub, October 2005).

Table 3.2. *Distribution of objects north and south of the tent*

North of the tent – *s-afálla n-ehān*	South of the tent – *s-ajuss n-ehān*
Kitchen – *edāgg wa n-əsink*	Water store – *tijəttwen n-iddidān*
Windbreak for the kitchen – *eff n-əsink*	Camel saddles – *tiriken (sing. tārik)*
Mortar – *tende*	Goatpen – *afāraj wa n-ulli d-eɣāydān*
Pestle – *ešāɣān (pl. išəɣnan)*	Cord for tethering lambs – *asəddi n-ikrāwatān*
Iron tripod for hanging the cooking vessel over	Container for milk – *akābar*
the fire – *ilānkāɣād n-əsink*	Rope to tether donkeys – *tefrānen n-išādān*
Wood – *isāɣerān*	
Wooden tripod for food provisions – *ijettān n-āllon*	
Wooden shovel to remove refuse – *āsaltəf*	
Leather bag to collect refuse – *ejābeš*	
Sieve to clean the sand – *temey ta n-eɣāssiwān/āsaltāf*	
broom – *asəfrāḍ (pl. isəfrāḍ)*	

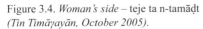

   While the objects in the north on the woman's side testify to a life within,
dāɣ-āmmas n-ehān, and near the tent, *ɣor ehān* (i.e. the pounding of millet,
processing of milk, cooking, handwork, as well as taking care of children, the
sick and the aging), the implements on the southern male side reflect a world

that is directed toward the outside, *s-ajāma/tenere*.[79] The men are witnesses to a life of work with animals, fetching water from the well, hunting, travel, the dangers and challenges of the external environment that the male Kel Alhafra must face. Their realm also includes hospitality (guests are always received on the southern side of the tent), exchange of news, preparation of tea, and engagement with the holy book, *ālkitab*, the Koran.

For a man, the tent is rarely a space that he enters except to sleep or if he is sick. It is rather something from which he originates, *ifal ehān-ənnet*, leaves, *izjar*, or departs early in the morning for a journey, *inšay*. It is the place from where he goes to the market, *ikka ewet*, to fetch water, *israj*, or to take the animals to their pasture, *iḍan irəzzejān-ənnet*. In contrast, the woman puts up the tent, *təday ehān*, an act equivalent to founding a family, and spends the day in the encampment, *təkall yor āmazzoy*. There, she pounds millet, *taddāh enāle*, tidies up, *təsədəw*, cleans the tent and the area around it, *təšašdəj ehān d-āyālād*, cooks, *saŋŋā*, and keeps an eye on the children, *ijəmmiyāt i-išākkātewān*.

The tent belongs to the woman, and while a husband and wife are living together in it, a balance is maintained between the activities of the man in the outside world and those of the woman who takes care of the inner world of the tent – the world of intimacy, privacy and mysteries. In Tamasheq, *ehān n-tamāḍt* signifies not only tent/house but also uterus and is used generally as the term for the inner female genital area. This double meaning reflects the receptivity, passivity, protectiveness and continuity associated with the feminine, while for the Kel Alhafra, the masculine is procreative, active and outwardly directed. The *ehān* as uterus and protective housing represents a life of security within the society, an antithesis to the *tenere*, the vast, lonely and capricious desert.

The "mythical-ritual system" in Bourdieu's sense, in which the tent and everyday life of the Kel Alhafra are integrated, cannot function contrastively without simultaneously unifying. Everything is subsumed into an order, and if the north stands for the feminine, damp, cold, impure, weak, left, and tempting spirits, the complementarity of the south as masculine, warm, pure, right, strong and steadfast is not conceivable without its opposite. Significantly, the fire on the northern side warms the "damp-cold", *immihād d-sāmmeḍ*, associ-

---

79 *ajāma* and *tenere* convey the meanings of "wilderness, desert, uninhabited and empty territory". The Kel Alhafra who lead a nomadic life in Azawad feel themselves to be members of the *kel ajāma*, those who belong to the *ajāma*, in contrast to the *kel āyram* or *kel tāyrəmt*, the settled and "cultivated" population living in cities and villages. See section 3.4. "The body in time and space".

ated with the female, while in the south, the "hot-dry", *ikuus d-əquur*, is symbolically cooled and offset by the water store.[80]

Nevertheless, *"ālbarāka iha s-afălla"* – "God's blessing is in the north" – the Kel Alhafra say, "because there lies fertility and health" – *"iha akāsa d-āṣṣahāt"*.[81] Only the strongest plants can survive the extreme climatic conditions in the treeless zone of Azawad, but they often contain remarkably more nutrients than those of the south. Analogously, God's blessing, *ālbarāka*,[82] is symbolically found in the microcosm in the northern half of the tent. It is where the union of oppositions bears fruit: where children are delivered, milk is processed, food is cooked, and provisions are produced. Quite significantly, it is also where healing takes place, often using medicinal plants from the north that are considered to be especially effective.

Both in the macrocosm and in the tent interior as microcosm, orientation imbues the Kel Alhafra with a sense of identity. Sedentarized Kel Alhafra sym-

---

80 See here Bourdieu's similar observations on the Kabyle house: "L'opposition qui s'établit entre le monde extérieur et la maison ne prend son sens complet que si l'on aperçoit que l'un des termes de cette relation, c'est-à-dire la maison, est lui-même divisé selon les mêmes principes qui l'opposent à l'autre terme. Il est donc à la fois vrai et faux de dire que le monde extérieur s'oppose à la maison comme le masculin au féminin, le jour à la nuit, le feu à l'eau, etc., puisque le deuxième terme de ces oppositions se divise chaque fois en lui-même et son opposé... ce système mythico-rituel ne peut opposer sans unir simultanément, tout en étant capable d'intégrer dans un ordre unique un nombre infini de données, par la simple application indéfiniment réitérée du même principe de division." Pierre Bourdieu, "Trois études d'ethnologie Kabyle", in *Esquisse d'une théorie de la pratique* (Paris: Seuil, 2000) 70–71.

81 For the Kel Ahaggar, according to Foucauld and Pandolfi, and also for the Kel Ferwan in Niger, according to Casajus, *ālbarāka* is always attributed to the south, while the north is always and only negatively connoted. See Charles de Foucauld, *Dictionnaire Touareg-Français: Dialecte de l'Ahaggar* (Paris: Imprimerie nationale, 1951) 570; Pandolfi, *Les Touaregs de l'Ahaggar*, 148; Casajus, *La Tente dans la Solitude*, 56.

82 *ālbarāka* derives from the Arabic root *baraka* and literally means "to kneel down". Chelhod writes that in the Semitic, this "kneeling down" is always associated with sexual union, with the fertilizing power of the man, and that it was only later, after Islamization, that this male "vital force" acquired its signification as the divine "benediction".
For the Kel Alhafra today, *ālbarāka* embodies in its Islamic sense the divine power of blessing, an arbitrary gift of God that manifests itself in the world when it adheres to objects and people. It is still associated with fertility, generative, procreative, creative, and especially healing powers. Marabouts and healers possess *ālbarāka*, but medicinal plants, valuable food sources such as camel's milk or fertile pastures have also internalized this divine power. On *ālbarāka* see: Joseph Chelhod, "La baraka chez les Arabes ou l'influence bienfaisante du sacré", *Revue de l'histoire des religions,* 148 (1955): 68–88; Edward Westermarck, *Ritual and Belief in Morocco*, vol. 1 (London: Mcmillan and Co., 1926): 35–261; Clifford Geertz, *Observer l'Islam. Changement religieux au Maroc et en Indonésie* (Paris: la Découverte, 1992) 58–59; Susan J. Rasmussen, "Accounting for Belief: Causation, Misfortune and Evil in Tuareg Systems of Thought", *Man* 24.1 (1989): 124–144; Johannes Nicolaisen, "Essais sur la religion et la magie touarègues", *Folk* 3 (1961): 118–119; Rudolf Kriss and Hubert Kriss-Heinrich, *Volksglaube im Bereich des Islam*, vol. 1 (Wiesbaden: Harrassowitz, 1960–1962) 4–5.

bolically divide their living space and arrange their belongings as in the tent. Moreover, they undertake their activities in the same cardinal directions as described above. Corresponding to this human orientation, the material objects that belong to the Kel Alhafra, their "l'entourage matériel" as Comte describes it, are also accorded a specific spatial disposition that is socially determined and offers "an image of permanence and stability".[83] As a group, the Kel Alhafra with their appurtenant space assume a "symbolic social entity", to use Assmann's term,[84] to which they cleave, even when they are separated from their nomadic environment, "by symbolically reproducing the holy city" and representing their genealogical descent by directing their entire lifeworld toward Mecca.

3.1.3. From world-image to body-image

The Kel Alhafra represent the human body according to the same structural principles that apply to the spatial partition of the world as macrocosm and the tent as microcosm.[85] The body is described with such oppositions as inner and outer, *āmmās d-afālla*, upper part and lower part, *s-afālla n-tāsa d-ider n-tāsa*, front and back, *s-dat d-s-ḍarāt*, right and left, *aɣəl d-tasālje*, contributing to an overall design homologous to that of the tent or the world. God created the human in his image, *"'ala ṣūratihī"*, the Kel Alhafra say citing an Islamic tradition,[86] and it is assumed that in essence the human body is complete and pure, while impurity is to be ascribed merely to each human's personal comportment with his or her body.

From the head to the navel, *s-eɣāf i-tābutāt*, the body, *taɣəssa*, belongs to the objective world, *s-afālla n-tāsa* (above/north of the stomach). It can always be named or talked about and, following certain rules, exposed. The upper part of the body includes the breast in which the heart, *ulh*, resides as the lifesource and seat of the divinely inspired soul, *iman* (that is, by *unfas*, the divine spirit).[87] As its crowning glory, the creator formed on the shoulders the

---

83 See Auguste Comte, *Cours de philosophie positive* (Paris: Hermann, 1975).

84 Jan Assmann, *Das kulturelle Gedächtnis. Schrift, Erinnerung und politische Identität in frühen Hochkulturen* (Munich: Beck, 2002) 39.

85 See here, Bourdieu: "On observe à peu près universellement que la plupart des distinctions spatiales sont établies par analogie avec le corps humain qui constitue le schème de référence par rapport auquel le monde peut s'ordonner, ..." Bourdieu, "Trois études d'ethnologie Kabyle", 289–290.

86 *lataqabbahu-l-waġh fa'inna-llāhu ḫalaqa ādam'ala ṣūratihi,* as a *ḥadīṯ* from the *ṣaḥīḥ al-buḫārī* says. See *Buḫārī: istiḍān* 1; see also: Muslim: *birr* 115, Ǧannah: 28, Ibn Hanbal: *musnād* vol. II, 244, 251, 315, 323.

87 In the understanding of the Kel Alhafra, the *iman* together with the *unfas* comprise the divine life principle as such. *iman* is considered the bearer of life, an independent being that can be separated from the body, that is molded by individual characteristics, and is the Self

head, with its visual, auditory and other senses, through which the human is in-formed of the activities and state of the outer world. For the Kel Alhafra, the upper part of the body, as active, courageous and communicative, is always oriented out toward an other, be it a living being or the divine power.

In contrast, the lower body from the navel to the feet, *ider n-tāsa*, is as-signed to the subjective world of intimacy – to the invisible and inner-directed receptive processes and powers strongly connected with the natural world and constant re-creation. Parts of this corporeal zone belong to the private, inti-mate area of the protective tent. They are mentioned at most in whispers be-hind raised hands and only then to trusted members of one's peer group.

As discussed above, it is the men who move in the outside world, who go to the market and the well, participate in religious and political discussions, brave the desert and expose themselves to its dangers, while the women re-main in the protective environment of the tent and the encampment.[88] The ob-jects in the southern half of the tent reflect the externally directed and active male principle, while the northern side attests to intimacy, familiarity, nutri-tion, sexuality, process and creative powers. Likewise, the upper body incar-nates the active male principle, while the lower body represents the receptive, modest area of the naturally feminine inner world.

The Kel Alhafra balance these two aspects in symbolic ways. Outside the protective embrace of the tent, the men veil themselves as a defense against temptations and harmful influences, while the women can move around inside their divinely blessed and familiar tents unveiled. Nevertheless, if a foreigner penetrates into the world of feminine intimacy, the Kel Alhafra women cover their faces with the indigo-dyed veil, *alāššo* (pl. *ilāššan*), and never offer, for example, their naked hand to an unknown guest. In this way, symbolically, their nakedness and vulnerability do not draw the attention of strange eyes, and they remain protected against exposure to possibly malign influences.

---

of an individual human. In Tamasheq, *ənta iman-ənnes* means "he himself", *fāll iman-ənnes* implies "of his own account", "for himself alone", "left to his own resources". Nevertheless, *iman* always exists in close relation with *unfas*, the creator's spirit that exceeds the soul and, as divine breath, is shared by all living beings. *unfas* and *iman* should always exist in a con-stant communicative bond with one another so that through wisdom, *zārho*, and faith in God, *tafləst dāɣ māssināɣ*, *iman* can, in an active process, build a bridge to *unfas*. Should, however, the soul, *iman*, abandon itself purely to reason, *tayətte*, and neglect its bond to *unfas*, it will find itself on false paths, *terk tibarāten*. It will become *nafs*, the "carnal soul" described by the Islamic mystics, and on the Day of Resurrection, *ašāl wa n-tebādde*, will stand in judg-ment before God.

88 The women of the Kel Alhafra usually spend the entire day in the encampment, only occa-sionally visiting a neighboring one. In contrast to their Arab neighbors, they do not go to the wells or tend animals. At most, they milk the goats or sheep and take on the men's tasks only when they are absent.

The left side of the body stands for the natural, the earthly, that has developed from its own innate powers and laws, and in analogy to the tent, it also represents the northern side when facing Mecca. Left, *tasālje*, in Tamasheq is thus synonymous with north, while right, *ayəl*, is used as a term for the south.

Because the left hand, *āfus wa n-tasālje*, always performs functions related to bodily excreta and contact with hidden, intimate zones of the body, it is viewed as unclean, *innokāl*, and may not be used for eating, to greet someone or for any action that might expose the body to external damage. The right hand, *āfus wa n-āyəl*, is thus the stronger, steadier, cleaner hand that when washed, is used to eat food, *itatt*, greet, *isikārdut*, congratulate, *itajj tābušer*, and give gifts, *ihak hārāt bānnan*, and alms, *ihak tilāqqiwen*.

The right side of the body is associated with those who visibly and courageously push forward, outward and upward, those who are active and communicative, while the left side is aligned with inside, behind and below, and is linked with the personal and intimate. The Kel Alhafra always arrange the dead so that they lie on their right side in the grave: the dark powers under the earth are unable to penetrate this resistant side of the human body and thus cannot interfere with its natural decay.

3.1.4. Spirits, devils and *təšoṭṭ*, the evil eye

The world of the invisible and intangible, *tāmusne ta wār ti-tənhəy*, that for the Kel Alhafra symbolically lies under the *tesāyt n-ākall*, the visible lifeworld, *ider n-tesāyt*, is inhabited by spirits and demons that sometimes intervene in the events, *fāll tesāyt*, of the naturally visible world, *āẓẓahir n-ākall*.

The common designation used by the Kel Alhafra for these spirits is *kel tenere*,[89] "those of the desert, the vastness, the emptiness, desire and loneliness". However, among the Kel Alhafra the term *kel esuf* is also used as a synonym for *kel tenere*, and one sometimes also hears *kel ākall* ("those of the earth/the elements") and *kel ehāḍ*, ("those of the night") or *ğinn*.[90]

As the invisible doubles of human beings, the *kel tenere*, according to the Kel Alhfra, live as humans do and tend their own herds. As with the Arabic *ğinn*, the *kel tenere* are always designated as a collective and possess no indi-

---

89 For the Kel Alhafra, the meaning of *kel tenere* is highly metaphorical: as "those of the desert, the emptiness, desire and loneliness", they prey upon individuals in a certain emotional state and can possess them. This will be discussed in more detail when I consider the causes of mental diseases.

90 *ğinn* derives from the Arabic root *ğannana* and thus implies something concealed or hidden. The verb stems *istağanna* and *ağanna* are identical to *saḥara*, "to hide", while *ağanna* can also be translated as "to become dark". Additionally, *al-ğanīn* is the term for the human embryo concealed in the mother's body. See Ernst Zbinden, *Die Djinn des Islam und der altorientalische Geisterglaube,* (Bern: Haupt 1953) 75.

viduality. They can take on either human or animal form, and their character may be good or evil. For the Kel Alhafra, they are creatures created by God,[91] just as he created all other living beings, to praise and to serve him.[92] Their deeds will also be weighed on the judgment day, and if the bad outweigh the good, they will roast in hell, *dāɣ temse*, alongside the disobedient humans.[93] Because the *kel tenere* inhabit a world that is not visible to humans, these beings possess knowledge to which humans have no access (*tāmusne ta wār titənhəy*). Just a few humans are endowed with the rare, innate and inheritable gift of being able to see and to contact the *kel tenere*, to engage, and to make deals with them. Nevertheless, as will be discussed later, there are also humans who can use supernatural powers and occult energies to acquire these abilities.

In contrast to humans whose active life is concentrated during the daytime and who favor a life in the sociality of the tent and encampment, the *kel tenere,* as invisible beings of the underworld, prefer the night and darkness – lonely areas and places imbued with natural forces, – to enact their deeds. Sand and dust columns, which occur frequently in the desert, are attributed to the *kel tenere*. They lurk at the bottom of wells, in heavy rain showers, in pools that remain at the end of the rainy season, and in the floodwaters of the Niger River. Although particularly energetic during the sand and dust storms of the hot and dry season, *s-ewelān*, the *kel tenere* are also active at the real and symbolic thresholds between life and death, between the natural and the supernatural. They gather at places where animals are slaughtered, *idāggān wi n-aɣārras*, at places where people have died, *idāggān wi n-nānāmetān*, at sites inhabited by past cultures, *tezəmbaẓ*, near cemeteries, *tifəska* (sing. *tafāskot*), as well as during sexual intercourse, *tenāsse*, at births, *tiwiten* (sing. *tiwit*), by the childbed, *amẓor*, near the newborn, *itiwātān*, at a boy's circumcision, *illuy*, and at wedding celebrations, *āddāl wa n-āẓli*. Two trees whose roots and leaves are used medicinally, *Balanites aegyptiaca*, *tāboraɣt*, and *Maeura crassifolia*, *ājār*, are also said to be sites favored by the *kel tenere*.

The *kel tenere* are magically attracted to places where bodily excreta and blood are mixed on the ground, uncleanliness prevails and the smells are bad. Their preferred cardinal direction is north, where energies immanent to nature

---

91 The Kel Alhafra do not accept the thesis made by Casajus that the *kel esuf* or *kel tenere* represent the world of the dead. The dead will live in paradise or hell, no longer in direct contact with the visible or invisible life on earth. The *ǧinn* are God's creatures, albeit another category than humans in that they are made from fire not from earth, but like humans they live a limited life on earth and will stand before God on the judgment day (as is the view of the Koran).

92 See surah 51/56: *"wa mā ḥalaqtu -l-ǧinna wa-l-insa illā li-ya ʿbudūni;"* see also 6/100.

93 The Koran states that on judgment day, the deceased *ǧinn* will also stand before God (6/130) and will be sent to paradise or to hell (7/38, 7/179).

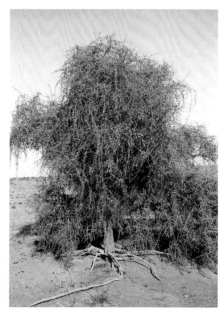

Figure 3.6. *Balanites aegyptiaca* – tāboraɣt
(In Killa, November 2005).

Figure 3.7. *Maerua crassifolia* – ājār
(In Killa, November 2005).

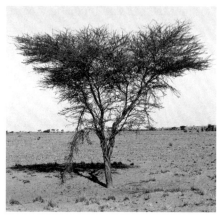

Medicinal properties are ascribed to both trees that are also considered to be haunts favored by the kel tenere.

dominate (such as the northern half of the tent), where covert and intimate acts take place, and where the woman lives and, through her menstrual cycle, is irreversibly affiliated with these invisible energies. The Kel Alhafra believe that women and young children are much weaker and more easily influenced by the *kel tenere* than adult men whose procreative, active, pure and outwardly directed nature empowers them to defend and protect themselves.

By and large, the Kel Alhafra view the *kel tenere* negatively, as irritant beings who attempt to interfere with the natural course of events, who take pleasure in frightening humans and animals, who enjoy misleading them and making life in general difficult by means of their cruel tricks. Particularly crafty and pernicious *kel tenere* are known as *šāyaṭin* (sing. *šāyṭan), ifritan* (sing. *āfrit*) or *tināriwen* (sing. *tenere*), little demons/devils. They are responsible for all the things the Kel Alhafra cannot explain: they can penetrate people and make them mad, or by possessing them, they can cause epileptic fits, sudden death, epidemics, unaccountable sicknesses, acute pain and high fever. They are responsible for excessive emotional outbursts of anger, jealousy, hate, fear, sexual passion and deep mourning. They can interfere in reproductive processes, making men impotent, women infertile and provoking abortions. The *kel tenere* seem to have particular fun encroaching into the intimate sphere between a man and a woman, and the Kel Alhafra never undress fully without first having drawn an imaginary circle around themselves while uttering the basmala[94] under their breath. Sexual intercourse may never take place in the open, because the *kel tenere* might intrude to make the child that is conceived deaf or blind, and a pregnant woman should never move outside alone or sleep outside the tent, because the *kel tenere* might cripple her unborn child or exchange it for one of their own.

The *kel tenere* are also co-responsible for *təšoṭṭ*,[95] "the evil eye", that can provoke an unexpected misfortune, but in this case, the causal agent is a human. An *enāmenšāɣ*,[96] who from birth is of poor character, is able to communicate with the *kel tenere* and sends these in bad faith against his or her victims, an act called *āsəbdar* in Tamasheq, which means literally "to lead someone astray". Here, the *kel tenere* become an instrument of the *enāmenšāɣ*, often taking on human form and causing all kinds of problems (often illnesses) that may even lead to death. There are families of *ināmenšāɣān* among the Kel Alhafra, the gift of communication with the *kel tenere* being hereditary. However, these individuals are never identified aloud, and in order not to provoke their displeasure, they are generously entertained should they visit the tent, or in their presence, one protects oneself against their influence by very quietly pronouncing the basmala.

The concept of *təšoṭṭ*, the evil eye, is closely connected with *terk mājārād*, "bad speech", that, in the form of burning passion or impetuous emotions magically attracts and activates the *kel tenere*. The Kel Alhafra take great care not to mention foul or pernicious objects or acts by name, in order not to invoke the *kel tenere*. *terk mājārād* is primarily associated, however, with jealousy, an emotion the Kel Alhafra frown upon and which is considered the main catalyst for *terk mājārād*. *terk mājārād* can have particularly unfortunate consequences for a pregnant woman. As I will examine later in more detail, "bad speech" is identified by the Kel Alhafra as one of the most common causes of miscarriage.

In contrast to the *ināmenšāɣān*, who pass on their shamanic abilities from generation to generation, the *kel toxni* and the *imāssāḥārān* (sing. *emāssāḥār*)

---

94 The Kel Alhafra introduce all acts of significance with the phrase *bi-smi-llaāhi-r-raḥmāni-r-raḥīm* ("In the name of God, Most Gracious, Most Merciful") and also use it as protection against the *kel tenere* and *təšoṭṭ*. On the use of the basmala see also Kriss and Kriss-Heinrich, *Volksglaube im Bereich des Islam*; Ignaz Goldziher, "Bismillah" in *Gesammelte Schriften*, vol. 5 (Hildesheim: Olms, 1970) 167–169.

95 *šāṭṭ, pl. šiṭṭawen* is a Tamasheq term for the eye.

96 *enāmenšāɣ* (pl. *ināmenšāɣān*) derives from the Tamasheq verb *nemenšāɣ* which literally means "reciprocal inhalation of another's exhalation". A human can merge with a *ǧinn* in this way to acquire supernatural knowledge, obtained through this direct communication with the *kel tenere*. But because the *enāmenšāɣ* has a perverse character, he or she will nearly always apply this shamanic power for bad ends.

This possible act of "mutual inhalation" can provide one explanation for face veiling by the Kel Alhafra men who, unlike the women, travel through open spaces and by covering their nose can avoid the undesired inhalation of a *ǧinn* that might take possession of them.

learn their *métier*. They too are specialized in magic and occult powers and can, thanks to demonic inspiration, see into *tāmusne-ta wār ti-tənhəy*, the world of the invisible, but they utilize these powers professionally and require payment for their services.

The *kel toxni*, "those with black magic", are particularly sought after for their divinatory powers. They are consulted when a camel goes missing, when a valuable object is lost, to predict the future outcome of an event, or to interpret strange visions or dreams. Unlike the *ināmenšāyān*, however, the *kel toxni* do not possess the power to kill someone. An *emāssāḥār*, is therefore much more dangerous, because as a master sorcerer, he can metamorphose into an animal and devour another human being.

Because they can make the impossible possible, *itajjān a-wa wār imukān mušam ad ajjān a-s-imukan,* these three groups of humans who collaborate with the *kel tenere* and use them to execute their will are profoundly despised by the Kel Alhafra but at the same time deeply feared.

To protect themselves from the noxious influences of the *kel tenere*, the Kel Alhafra take pains to avoid them, and when they travel, the men always carry a weapon either wholly or in part made of metal (today often a shotgun, *ālbārroḍ*, or a rifle, *kālaš*; in the past, a lance, *ājor*, a sword, *tākoba*, or a large knife, *absār*), because the *kel tenere* dread all forms of metal, *iqsoodān taẓoli*. Essential oils, *aḍutān*, that release aromatic fumes when poured on glowing coals can also frighten off the *kel tenere*, and hennaed feet and hands are also believed to provide effective protection. Most effective, however, is the *ālkitab*, the Koran, and many Kel Alhafra wear leather amulets, *tikarḍiwen* (sing. *tākarḍe*) around their waist, neck or upper arm that contain Koranic verses to protect the individual's weak points.[97]

Although, in general, the *tināriwen* seek to mislead humans and are perceived as servants of Iblis,[98] it is always the individual who lets him- or herself be misled, gives into these spirits, strays from the righteous path, *tābarat-ta tāhuskāt*, and performs pernicious deeds, *terk timašālen* (sing. *terk tāmašālt*). *tāllābāst*, evil, which as a verbal noun derived from *ilbas* incorporates "bad, hard, strict and dangerous being", is always associated with a course of action,

---

97 The Kel Alhafra employ many other symbols in amulets, objects or in nature as protection against evil powers, and the reader is referred to Nicolaisen's essay on Tuareg religion and magic in which the most important Tamasheq rituals and protective customs are described: Nicolaisen, "Essais sur la religion et la magie touarègues", 113–162.

98 The Kel Alhafra will often use Iblis as a synonym for strong emotions like anger and jealousy: *"ǝlyǝn Iblis!"* – "calm down", ("subdue Iblis!") they will say to someone who gets into a rage. See here also David Sudlow, *The Tamasheq of North-East Burkina Faso*, vol. 1 (Cologne: Rüdiger Köppe, 2001) 310.

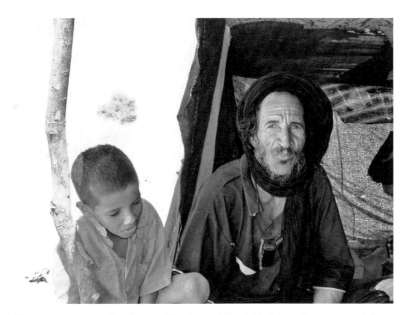

Figure 3.8. *Koranic verses sewn into leather,* tikārḍiwen *(sing.* takārḍe)*, and worn around the neck protect the wearer from corruptive powers (In Agozmi, March 2005).*

with an individual's conduct, rather than being an abstract category contrasted with divine omnipotence. And just as a human being can only understand life in its finiteness by being aware of death, so too, the good and the beautiful can only be appreciated if one knows about evil and ugliness, *wār təzzayād ālxer d-tihussay a-fāl wār təssanād ā-wa aqqālān tāllābāst d-iləššān.* It is for this reason that evil appears in the world in the form of *šāyaṭin, ifritān, tināriwen* and *ǧinn* – to test one's piety, to punish if necessary, or through torments, to lead one back onto the righteous path and to the all-powerful mercy of God.

3.2. The language and semantics of health, sickness and pain

3.2.1. Health – the terms *āṣṣexāt, āṣṣahāt* and *ālxer*

Both the Tamasheq term for health, *āṣṣexāt*[99], and that for strength, *āṣṣahāt,* imply an origin from the Arabic root *ṣaḥḥa,* which on the one hand means "healthy and strong" in terms of the absence of physical or psychic suffering, but with a religious connotation is also understood as "fautless", "true", "authentic" and "genuine" with respect to God's word and the utterances of the Prophet. *āṣṣexāt* denotes not only physical and psychic health as a situation free of illness, *iba n-torhənna,* but at the same time the flawless and con-

---

99 *āṣṣexāt* is the verbal noun from the Tamasheq verb, *ṣoxət* – "to be healthy".

summate state of a healthy individual who has devoted him- or herself fully to God, the ultimate source of human existence.

"tāɣlassed?"[100] – "Are you saved and redeemed?" – is the opening question of every Tamasheq greeting. When asked, *"ma tāxlaqād?"* – "How are you?" or, literally, "How are you created (by God)", from the Koranic perspective, only one answer is possible: *"ālxer ɣās, təbarāk allah!"* – "Only the good, the best, the most excellent, God be praised!" To respond to the question negatively would be to attribute defectiveness to God the creator who is responsible for all human life. At the same time, the expression *təbarāk allah* embodies a person's gratitude for the grace, *ālbarāka,* and the benevolence of God.

In Tamasheq a healthy person is called *āwadəm āṣṣohen,* someone who is strong and energetic, whose spirit is at peace, *tosja tayətte-ənnet,*[101] and whose soul enjoys lightness and contentment, *fāssus iman-ənnet,*[102] because there is a strong connection through belief to the creator of all being.

The Tamasheq adjective *āṣṣohen,* healthy, strong, unshakeable, is contained in the concept of *āṣṣahāt,*[103] which implies not only strength, energy, impetus, but also power, *tādabit* or *təmmənəya,* hardness and steadfastness (in religious conviction). Through meekness, a healthy person, *āwadəm āṣṣohen,* has control over his well-developed senses, sound bodily functions, and inherent physical and psychic powers: *ihannāy ihusken,* he sees well; *anāšaj-ənnet ihusken,* he has a fine sense of smell; *isall hullen,* he hears well; *itatt šik,* he eats quickly; *itak tenere d-itajj āwas ihusken,* he defecates and urinates without any problems; *ikann əššāɣāl-ənnet s-tihussay d-šik,* he completes his tasks well and quickly; *itišəl azāl ihusken,* he runs well; *āṣṣahāt illee,* he is powerful and strong.

---

100 The meaning of the Tamasheq greeting, *tāɣlassed,* seems to be derived from the Arabic root *ḥalaṣa,* even though the Arabic consonant ﺥ has been replaced in *tāmašeq* by a ɣ/ɣ̣ and the Arabic ص by s/ﺱ. Nevertheless the meanings "to be pure, genuine, unadulterated; to be saved, redeemed and blessed" are retained in the Tamasheq.

101 *tayətte* in Tamasheq signifies "intelligence, consciousness, reason, wisdom and spirit".

102 In contrast to the Kel Alhafra for whom a "light soul", *"iman fāssus",* is associated with vitality and carefreeness, according to Walentowitz, for the Kel Eghlal and Ayttawari Seslem in Niger a "light soul", *"iman ifasusnen",* is viewed negatively: "To have a light and open soul provokes distraction and lapses in memory *(iba n təlla n eɣaf)*; it is said that the person forgets things easily. Someone with a light soul frequently 'makes mistakes' *(izulelan)* and slips of the tongue *(šimədəgga)*". Saskia Walentowitz, "Enfant de soi, enfant de l'autre. La construction symbolique et sociale des identités à travers une étude anthropologique de la naissance chez les Touaregs (Kel Eghlal et Ayttawari de l'Azawagh, Niger)," (Paris : Thèse de doctorat, Ecole des Hautes Etudes en Sciences Sociales, 2003) 13.

103 *āṣṣahāt* is the verbal noun from the Tamasheq verb *ṣohət,* "to be strong, forceful, powerful, tough".

In the Kel Alhafra understanding of health, the term *ālxer*[104] is perhaps best translated as "well-being". It conveys the idea not only of spiritual wellness but also of bodily and material well-being including contentment and resources, that can nevertheless only bring the individual happiness through generosity and social undertakings on the behalf of others. *āṣṣexāt āšəkrəš n-ālxer*, as the Kel Alhafra saying goes, "health is a garden of good fortune", a god-given state of bodily, spiritual and social well-being for which the healthy individual must show his or her gratitude through religious faith and acts.

3.2.2. Sickness, ill health and healing – *torhənna, irhan d-tāməzzuyt*

For the Kel Alhafra, *torhənna* (pl. *torhənnawen*) signifies general physical and psychic disturbances that they classify and to which they ascribe defined symptoms (more detail in chapter 4.1).

By an observer, a sick person, *āmarhin,* is described by the Kel Alhafra as follows: he cannot walk around with an erect body, *wār ādoobed tekāle*; he cannot eat, *wār ādoobed tetāte*; he does not drink very much, *wār isəss ajen*; he has joint pains, *ikma tafəkka-ənnet*; he has no appetite, *wār irha imənsiwān*; he cannot sleep, *wār ija edes ihuskən*; he is weak, *ārəkkəm*; he is gradually losing his vitality, *iba n-āṣṣahāt-ənnāt*.

The term *torhənna*, however, is drawn from the Arabic root *rahana* meaning "putting down a deposit" or "to be encumbered with a mortgage". If the behavior of a healthy person, *āwadəm āṣṣohen*, is all too independent and self-satisfactory, the Kel Alhafra feel his pomposity and ingratitude distance him from God, *wār ināqsood māssinay*. God then places a mortgage (a sickness) on him so that he becomes *āwadəm irhiin*, subjugated, someone who has been provided with a certificate of debt – the sickness. *ijrāw-t hārāt* – "he has received (earned) something" – the Kel Alhafra say of a sick person; *torhənna t-təjrawāt* – "a sickness has been placed upon him". In Tamasheq, the sick person, *āmarhin,* is metaphorically placed in debt, so that he becomes conscious again of his weakness and helplessness vis-à-vis the divine power, and he pays off this debt through suffering that will finally, through trust in God, *tafləst dāɣ-māssinay* (Arabic *tawakkul*), bring him back to awareness of the divine presence.[105]

In this scenario, sickness, *torhənna*, is a divine burden whose purpose serves to strengthen the individual's orientation toward God as he follows the

---

104 *ālxer* is derived from the Arabic root, *khāra*, which literally means "to elect" or "to privilege". *al-khayr* (pl. *khuyur*) signifies "goods, property, possessions, welfare, charity and charitable act".

105 In this situation, the Kel Alhafra often cite a well-known hadith from *Ṣaḥīḥ al-Buḥārī*: "God placed no disease on the earth without also providing the appropriate cure" (34/1).

specific path to becoming cured. As he undertakes this process of purification, the sick person, *āmarhin*, experiences an inner agitation, *āyrəswəl*, provoked by the sickness, *torhənna*, that weakens him, *ārəkkəm-t*, and harms his mental state, *ənniyāt wār ihusket*, so that his soul weighs heavily on him, *aẓẓayān fāll-as iman-ənnet*.

torhənna tojarāt āṣṣexāt-nanāy – "sickness is stronger than our health" – the Kel Alhafra say, and God alone decides when the process of purification is complete. The sick person can certainly negotiate with God through prayer,[106] but in the end, it is God who decides about the existence and fate of all things including the healing, *tāməzzuyt,* of a sick person.

In Tamasheq, *izzāy* simultaneously means, "he is healed", "he has recovered", and "he is aware (again)". However, *wār tāsmātāllāt taməzzuyt n-hārāt d-taməzzuyt dāy torhənna* – "do not confuse the awareness of something with the healing of a sickness" – the Kel Alhafra say, because only God knows about the unseen (*innamā-l-ġaybu li-llahi*, surah 10/20) and thus the timing of a cure. At the same time, the term *tāməzzuyt* suggests a reacknowledgement of one's gratitude toward the merciful, divine power, a drawing near again by the human to his creator who must metaphorically speaking, from time to time, place a mortgage (sickness) on his most important creation.

3.2.3. Concepts of pain: *teẓẓort, tākmo* and *tedeje*

The Kel Alhafra use three concepts of pain to describe bodily and emotional suffering. In the first concept, pain, *teẓẓort,* is a general description for severe physical or psychic suffering that brings the sick person to the limits of his or her strength and may even be life-threatening. The Arabic root *waẓara* is contained in the term *teẓẓort* and means "to take upon oneself", "to bear a burden" or "to commit a sin". If one asks of a sick person, *"ma t-ijrawān?"* – "what has he (harvested from God)?" – the answer often refers to a precise part of the body that is tormenting him: *"oẓar eyāf-ənnāt"* – "his head hurts"; *"oẓar ārori-ənnet"* – "the pain in his back is excrutiating" or *"oẓar tāsa-ənnet"* – "he has violent stomach pains".

teẓẓort implies a strong, uninterrupted pain that is so agonizing that the sick person suffers, *āmarhin oẓar*, can no longer concentrate, *wār ənniyāt ihusket*, works poorly, *itaj terk əššāyāl*, and may even be driven mad by the constant pain, *ija dāy teẓẓort as oyšad n-eyāf* (*oyšad n-eyāf* means literally: "the head is 'destroyed'").

Another pain concept is represented by *tākmo* (pl. *tākmotān*), which draws on the Tamasheq verb *əkmu*, meaning "to cause pain, to be painful". *tākmo* is

---

106 See here, the Koranic account of the prophet Job (21/83–84).

used to describe both physical as well as emotional pain.[107] This ambiguity is graphically depicted in the term *tākmo n-ulh*, which on the one hand is understood as emotional pain such as grief or anxiety (literally, "pain of the heart"), but also designates such bodily ailments as nausea, hypotonia (low blood pressure), hypertonia (high blood pressure), bradycardia (slow heart rate), tachycardia (high pulse rate) and so on, and their associated symptoms (see *tākmo n-ulh* chapter 4.1.1.).

One can inflict pain, *tākmo*, on someone or experience it oneself: *"ija-hi āwadəm tākmo"*, "someone injured (upset) me", *"ikma-hi hārāt"*, "something has annoyed me", *"ikma-hi isənnan"*, "I was hurt by a thorn", *"ikma-hi tāsanin"*, "my stomach hurts". Combined with a term for a part of the body, *tākmo* is also used to designate an illness *per se*, for example *tākmo n-timāẓẓujen* for an ear infection, and *tākmo n-tioṭṭāwen* for an eye infection.

The third term for pain, *tedeje*,[108] is the verbal noun from the Tamasheq verb *ədəj* meaning "to sting/prick/bite", and describes a physical, stabbing pain at a specific location inside the body. Kel Alhafra use *tedeje* for a sharp pain whose cause is always a sickness. *tedeje ta n-idmārān*, for example, describes a "sharp pain in the breast", often accompanying bronchitis or pneumonia; *tejede ta n-aḍu* is the "sharp pain of the wind/air" that circulates through the organism, mostly in the stomach, knee or thorax.

In general, pain is understood by the Kel Alhafra as *ašāmol n-torhənna*, a "sign (symptom) of a sickness", as suffering, *teẓẓort*, inflicted by God as a test and that must be born with patience, *tāẓidert n-hārātān wi kāy as tārmās-t māssināγ*.

3.3. Representations of the human body

3.3.1. Bodily balance – the concepts of *tākusse* and *təssəmḍe*

The Kel Alhafra conceive of the human body as a mixture of the various forces that comprise the entire universe. The interactions between such contrasts as day and night, sun and moon, heaven and earth, fire and water, heat and cold generate a dynamic whole whose balance depends on a harmony among these interdependent energies. In the human body too, every single organ exists in

---

107 The Kel Alhafra use both *tākmo n-iman* and *tākmo n-ulh* to describe emotional pain. The terms are used synonymously, the soul, *iman*, in the Kel Alhafra view, being seated in the heart.

108 The term *aslim* as a synonym for *tedeje* is rarely used by the Kel Alhafra.

relation to all other organs, and should even the tiniest part of the balanced wholeness of the body change, the entire organism responds.[109]

Components of the oppositional partners in the universe are assigned by the Kel Alhafra to the categories "hot", *wa n-tākusse,* and "cold", *wa n-təssəmḍe:*[110]

In an analogy to these categorized energies that govern the universe, the human body is also comprised of a cold and a hot life principle, *tākusse*

Table 3.3. *Composition of the universe from oppositional pairs*

Universe - *āddunya*	
wa n-tākusse ← ———————— →	*wa n-təssəmḍe*
Day – *ašāl*	Night – *ehāḍ*
Sun – *tāfukk*	Moon – *iyor*
Life – *tāmudre*	Death – *taməttant*
Fire – *efew*	Water – *aman*
Heat – *tākusse*	Cold – *təssəmḍe*
This world – *āddunya*	The next world – *ālaxirāt*
Light – *ənnor*	Darkness – *tihāy*
South – *ājuss*	North – *afālla*
Masculine – *eyy*	Feminine – *tunte*
Dry – *əquur*	Wet – *immihāḍ*
Visible – *āẓẓahir*	Concealed – *ider*

109 Concepts of a cosmological balance reflected in the microcosm of the body are also found in other cultures, as described, for example, by the following authors: Keith H. Basso, "Western Apache Witchcraft", *Anthropological Papers of the University of Arizona*, No. 15. (Tucson: University of Arizona Press, 1969); Joseph W. Bastien, "Qollahuaya-Andean Body Concepts: A Topographical-Hydraulic Model of Physiology", *American Anthropologist* 87.3 (1985): 595–611; Pierre Bourdieu, *Esquisse d'une théorie de la pratique* (Paris: Editions du Seuil, 2000); Clark Cunningham, "Order in the Atoni House", in *Right and Left: Essays on Dual Symbolic Classification*, ed. Rodney Needham (Chicago: Chicago University Press, 1973) 204–238; Victoria Ebin, "Interpretations of Infertility: the Aowin People of Southeast Ghana", in *Ethnography of Fertility and Birth*, ed. Carol McCormack (London: Academic Press, 1982) 131–149; Gabriella Ferro-Luzzi, "Women's Pollution Periods in Tamilnadu (India)", *Anthropos* 69 (1974): 113–161; Marcel Griaule, *Conversations with Ogotemmeli* (Oxford: Oxford University Press, 1965); Alan Harwood, "The Hot-Cold Theory of Disease: Implications for Treatment of Puerto Rican Patients", *JAMA* 216.7 (1971): 1153–1158; Christine Hugh-Jones, *From the Milk River* (Cambridge: Cambridge University Press, 1979); Charles Leslie (ed.), *Asian Medical Systems: A Comparative Study* (Berkley: University of California Press, 1977); Dennis McGilvray, *Symbolic Heat: Gender, Health & Worship among the Tamils of South India and Sri Lanka* (Ahmedabad: Mapin, 1995); Gerardo Reichel-Dolmatoff, *Amazonian Cosmos: The Sexual and Religious Symbolism of the Tukanao Indians* (Chicago: Chicago University Press, 1971); Evon Vogt, *The Zinacantecos of Mexico: A Modern Mayan Way of Life* (Belmont: Wadsworth/Thomson Learning, 2002); Dominique Zahan, *The Religion, Spirituality and Thought of Traditional Africa* (Chicago: University of Chicago Press, 1979).

110 The polarized assignment of elements into "hot" and "cold" categories that are responsible for certain events through the immanent tension between their opposing forces was a popular explanatory model among the pre-Socratic natural philosophers. Anaxagoras, for example, opposed a cold, wet, dense and dark category (earth) to a hot, dry and tenuous one (ether). Parmenides associated hot and light with the element fire, cold, dark and heavy with night/darkness. See Geoffrey Lloyd, *Polarity and Analogy: Two Types of Argumentation in Early Greek Thought* (Bristol: Bristol Classical Press, 1987) 57.

d-təssəmḍe, whose equilibrium is dependent on its balance in the natural world. The natural environment, foods and illnesses are classified into hot and cold categories and they can influence the corporeal balance between *tākusse* and *təssəmḍe*. In a healthy individual, *tākusse* and *təssəmḍe* are well adjusted, but if this equilibrium is disturbed and a large discrepancy develops between the two categories, the organism is weakened and will fall sick.

Humans can, however, develop an affinity – a temperament – for one or other direction that may shift[111] according to context and that he or she will spend a lifetime trying to counterbalance. The Kel Alhafra divide these individuals into *kel tākusse*, people of the warmth/heat, and *kel təssəmḍe*, people of the cold.

In the understanding of the Kel Alhafra, heat, *tākusse*, is a living heat, a driving force based in the heart from where it stimulates the living processes in the body via the blood.[112] *"təlla tākusse jer-elām d-iγāssān"*, the Kel Alhafra say, "heat exists between the skin and the bones", meaning, "he is full of vitality and his body is equilibrated". As will be seen, the inner workings of the body are perceived as a kind of "cooking", and attention must always be paid to ensuring that an optimal temperature is maintained so that the body neither overheats nor cools down too much.

To begin with, newborn babies have a warm character, *n-tākusse*, but may soon adopt the mother's temperament through her milk. Not until the infant begins to eat solid foods is it possible to assess the digestibility of various foods and thus establish the body's affinity or to assign the child to the category of hot or cold.

Such classificatory systems whose corresponding pairs are bound to one another by an inner correlation that often reflects a deeper-lying one can also be found, however, in earlier cultures. See here, William K.C. Guthrie, *A History of Greek Philosophy*, vol. 1 (Cambridge: University Press, 1962–1965) 251–256; Robert Hertz, "La prééminence de la main droite: étude sur la polarité religieuse", *Revue philosophique de la France et de l'étranger* 11 (1909): 553-580; Symon Byl, *Le dualisme ou les couples d'opposées. Recherches sur les grands traités biologiques d'Aristote: sources écrites et préjugés* (Brussels: Académie Royale Belgique, 1980) 210–237.

111 Menstruating and pregnant women, for example, regardless of their usual bodily affinity, are always in a "hot" state, *n-tākusse*, while older people have a tendency to show a "cold" character, *n-təssəmḍe*. This association is closely connected to the concept of innate warmth as a life energy that is responsible for the stimulation of inner bodily processes (especially reproduction) and progressively cools down during a human life until the individual dies.

112 The idea of an "implanted heat" is well attested in antiquity and in the medieval Arabic-Islamic literature as *al-ḥarāra al-ġarīzīya*, and is responsible for the organism's entire metabolism. According to both Aristotle and the author of the hippocratic texts this "inborn" heat has a particularly important function during reproduction. See Karl Deichgräber (ed.), *Hippokrates: Über Entstehung und Aufbau des menschlichen Körpers. Περί σαρκών* (Leipzig/Berlin: 1935); see chapter 'Die Entstehung der Körperteile und Organe nach 'De carnibus' und Aristoteles', 28–30; M. Roussel, "Ether et chaleur dans l'embryologie aristotélicienne: influences archaïques", *Mélanges d'études anciennes offerts à Maurice Lebel* (Quebec: 1980) 157–180.

kel tākusse have a tendency to retain too much heat in their bodies. This renders them nervous, impatient and irascible, *wār ti təha taẓidert d-tārma tāllābāst-ənnes*. They sweat easily and heavily, *təhe tide tajjet*, try to avoid the sun and hot places, *wār ərhen tāfukk d-tākusse*, and suffer from frequent headaches, *tākmo n-eyāf*, and nosebleeds, *ahunšar*, when the internal heat begins to accumulate in the head. The *kel tākusse* have a tendency to eat too much, *itattān ajjen*, and to drink too little, *wār isəssen ajjen*, which means that they do not urinate very often, *wār itajjan āwas ajjen*, and their excreta are hot and have a bad smell.

In contrast, *kel təssəmḍe* tend toward too little heat in their bodies because the "cooking processes" in their organs are functioning on a low flame. Individuals in this category demonstrate a passive, if not apathetic character, always have cold hands and feet, *iḍārān d-ifassān-nāsān sammeḍān*, and generally suffer from a poor digestion, with the result that their excreta are odorless because they do not absorb nutrients adequately, and food often passes undigested through their gut. *kel təssəmḍe* tend to drink a lot, *isəssān ajjen*, but suffer from a lack of appetite, *wār irhan imənsiwān*, and they prefer warm and sunny to cold and damp places, *irhan idāggān wi ikussnen d-tāfukk*.

kel tākusse among the Kel Alhafra compensate for their hot temperament through a diet rich in foods of the "cold" category, *isəssmaḍ*, while the *kel təssəmḍe* attempt to counteract their overcool temperament with foods that are classified as "hot", *issukās*. At the same time, both *kel tākusse* and *kel təssəmḍe* have a low tolerance for foods and illnesses of their own category.

Depending on their affinity to one or other character, "cold" or "hot", individuals can react totally differently to the same foodstuffs or illnesses. In the traditional medicine, therefore, it is crucial to first identify the patient's temperament and the character of the illness in order to prescribe a therapy that will be effective (see chapter 4.1.). In general it is said of the *kel tākusse* that they often have a shorter lifespan than the *kel təssəmḍe* but that they are also less susceptible to disease. If they fall sick, the illness is usually severe and serious, but in general they respond rapidly to appropriate treatment. With their cold bodies, the *kel təssəmḍe*, on the other hand, are susceptible to chronic diseases that are difficult to cure and, though they do not necessarily shorten the life of the *kel təssəmḍe*, may condemn them to a life of permanent suffering. The Tamasheq say, *"wa n-tākusse enematin, wa n-təssəmḍe āmarhin"*, "those of a hot character are the ones who die, those of a cold character are the invalids".[113]

---

113 Although Le Jean writes, "The terms hot (takusse) and cold (tessemde) convey no notion of good or evil. They simply express a dualistic organization of the elements without reference to an ethic that privileges one of the two aspects" (Le Jean, *Médecine traditionelle*, 49),

3.3.2. Structure of the inner and outer body

The outer body

When the Kel Alhafra describe their outer body, they can do so in detail for every area of the body above the navel, *afalla n-tābutut*, and below the knee, *ider n-afud,* using precise names that often have a metaphoric content.

From the armpit, literally translated, "that which is tickled to make someone laugh", *tidāydāyen n-ifāssan*, to the middle finger, described as "the gratuitously long one", *tassəkāḍt ta təzjərət bānnan*, and the index finger, "the one that licks out the bowl", *tassəkāḍt ta tətoɣ ikassān,* every part of the body receives a specific illustrative terminology. For the description of rounded elevations like the finger tip, *abārkot n-tassəkāḍt*, body-related metaphors are used: *abārkot n-tassəkāḍt* means literally "stomach of the finger", while the back of the hand and the instep are correspondingly described as "back of the hand surface", *ārori n-edekel*, and "back of the sole of the foot", *ārori n-etāfar*. For openings of the body, the word *em* (pl. *imawān*) (mouth, opening, door, gate) is linked to the specific body part: *em n-tinšar* describes the lower part of the nasal cavity (vestibulum nasi), *em n-timāẓẓuj*, the external auditory canal (meatus acusticus externus), *em n-uzəf*, the vaginal canal (introitus vaginae) and *em n-tezz*, the anus.[114]

The entire outer body below the navel, *ider n- tābutut*, and especially between the navel and the knee, *jer tābutut d-afuḍ,* is regarded as a private and intimate zone whose parts are not mentioned in public, except to be extremely disrespectful and to revile or to shame another person. It was only among women of my own age that, with the help of drawings, I was able to learn the names used by the Kel Alhafra for the individual parts of pubic area, which in Tamasheq are usually referred to with such vague expressions as *jer iḍāran*, between the legs, *ider n-tāsa*, under the belly, or *ider n-tābutut*, under the navel.

---

the Kel Alhafra would disagree and would invite her to refine her distinctions. "Cold" and "hot" foods are certainly not positively or negatively connotated, nor are natural elements endowed with explicit values based on their "warmth" or "coldness", nevertheless, as will be shown later, the geoclimatically "hot" zone of the south is perceived as unhealthy, while the "cold" areas of the north are viewed much more favorably. In contrast, a "hot" character, at the individual level, is definitely preferred to a "cold" one and this has consequences not only with respect to disease, but becomes particularly apparent in the choice of a partner, with men showing a definite preference for a wife with a "hot" character, *tamāḍt ta n-tākusse*, to one with a cold temperament, *tamāḍt ta n-təssəmḍe*.

114 In Tamasheq, *em* (pl. *imawān*) means both "mouth" but also "entrance, door, opening" – as in for example, *em n-anu*, "wellshaft" – or "border, bank" – as in *em n-ejreu*, "river bank". The Kel Alhafra attitude to such body "openings" is one of control, caution and discretion. The outside with its harmful influences can enter the body through such openings to disrupt the organism's delicate balance, and excreta leave the body through certain openings, exposing it to the *kel tenere*, who are attracted by bad smells and impurities.

In general, Kel Alhafra women call their female genital area either *uzəf* (pl. *uzāfen*), which translates literally as "the exposed being", and stems from the verb *ezzef*, "to expose oneself, to be naked", but they also use a more specific term, *akədil* (pl. *ikədal*) for the vulva. Many Kel Alhafra women however also employ the name for the birth canal of female animals *tasāssarut* (pl. *tisəssiraw*). The term for the clitoris, *eẓerjəj* (pl. *iẓerjəjān)*, is a verbal noun from *ẓerəjjət*, meaning "to penetrate", "to arise" and "to enter the day". The labia are referred to as *timāsṭaren* (sing. *timāsṭar*) from the verb *əsṭər*, "to cover over", "to protect with chasteness", "to hide".[115] No woman of the Kel Alhafra ever mentioned the hymen in this context, possibly due to the fact that they have no rituals for young women focussing on virginity.

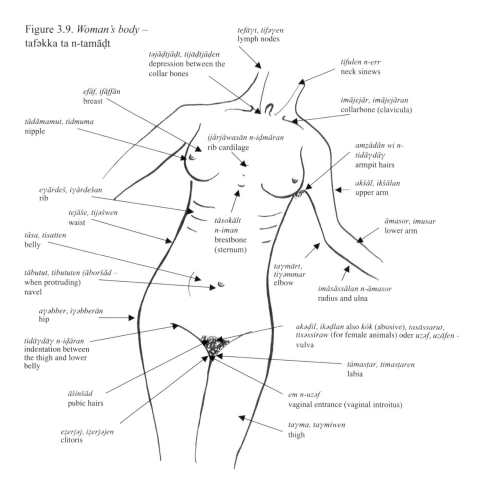

Figure 3.9. *Woman's body –* tafəkka ta n-tamāḍt

tefāɣt, tifəɣen lymph nodes

təjāḍtjāḍt, tijāḍtjāḍen depression between the collar bones

tifulen n-err neck sinews

efāf, ifāffān breast

imājejār, imājejāran collarbone (clavicula)

tādāmamut, tidmuma nipple

ijārjāwasān n-iḍmāran rib cardilage

amẓādān wi n-tidāɣdāɣ armpit hairs

akšāl, ikšālan upper arm

eɣārdeš, iɣārdešan rib

tejāše, tijəšwen waist

tāsokālt n-iman brestbone (sternum)

āmasor, imusar lower arm

tāsa, tisatten belly

tābutut, tibututen (āboršād – when protruding) navel

taɣmārt, tiɣəmmar elbow

imāsāssālan n-āmasor radius and ulna

ayəbber, iɣəbberān hip

akədil, ikədlan also *kôk* (abusive), *tasāssarut, tisəssiraw* (for female animals) oder *uzəf, uzāfen* - vulva

tidāɣdāɣ n-iḍaran indentation between the thigh and lower belly

tāmasṭar, timasṭaren labia

āšinšād pubic hairs

em n-uzəf vaginal entrance (vaginal introitus)

ezerjəj, iẓerjəjen clitoris

taɣma, taɣmiwen thigh

115 There is no tradition of clitoridectomy among the Tamasheq.

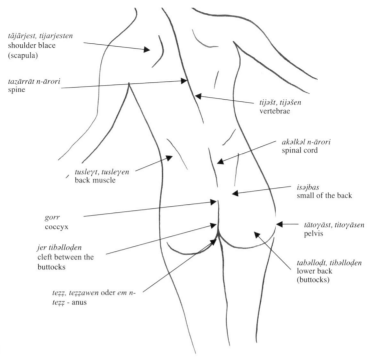

tājārjest, tijarjesten
shoulder blace
(scapula)

tazārrāt n-ārori
spine

tijəšt, tijəšen
vertebrae

akəlkəl n-ārori
spinal cord

tusleγt, tusleγen
back muscle

isəjbas
small of the back

gorr
coccyx

tātoγāst, titoγāsen
pelvis

jer tibəlloḍen
cleft between the
buttocks

tabəlloḍt, tibəlloḍen
lower back
(buttocks)

teẓẓ, teẓẓawen oder *em n-
teẓẓ* - anus

Figure 3.10.
The back –
ārori, irorəyawān

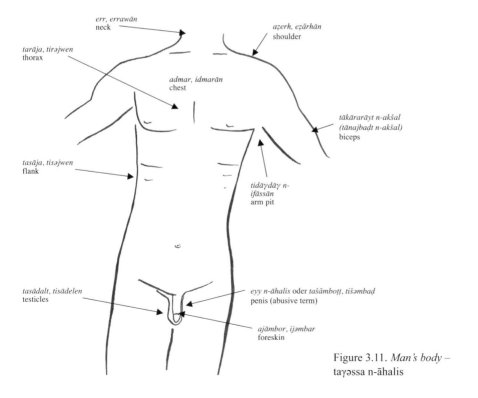

err, errawān
neck

aẓerh, eẓārhān
shoulder

tarāja, tirəjwen
thorax

admar, idmarān
chest

tākārarāyt n-akšal
(tānajbaḍt n-akšal)
biceps

tasāja, tisəjwen
flank

*tidāγdāγ n-
ifāssān*
arm pit

tasādalt, tisādelen
testicles

eyy n-āhalis oder *tašāmboṭṭ, tišəmbaḍ*
penis (abusive term)

ajāmbor, ijəmbar
foreskin

Figure 3.11. *Man's body –*
taγəssa n-āhalis

Figure 3.12. *Woman's head* – eɣāf n-tamāḏt   *Man's head* – eɣāf n-āhalis

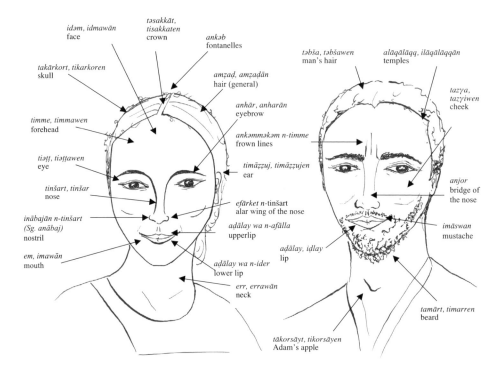

idəm, idmawān
face

təsakkāt, tisakkaten
crown

ankəb
fontanelles

takārkort, tikarkoren
skull

amẓaḏ, amẓaḏān
hair (general)

anhār, anharān
eyebrow

timme, timmawen
forehead

ankəmmkəm n-timme
frown lines

tiəṭṭ, tiəṭṭawen
eye

timāẓẓuj, timāẓẓujen
ear

tinšart, tinšar
nose

efārket n-tinšart
alar wing of the nose

inābajān n-tinšart
(Sg. anābaj)
nostril

aḏālay wa n-afālla
upperlip

em, imawān
mouth

aḏālay wa n-ider
lower lip

err, errawān
neck

təbša, təbšawen
man's hair

alāqālāqq, ilāqālāqqān
temples

tazɣa, tazɣiwen
cheek

anjor
bridge of the nose

imāswan
mustache

aḏālay, iḏlay
lip

tamārt, timarren
beard

tākorsāyt, tikorsāyen
Adam's apple

Figure 3.13. *Hand* – āfus, ifassān

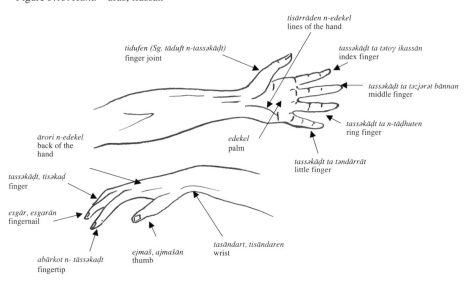

tisārrāden n-edekel
lines of the hand

tidufen (Sg. tāduft n-tassəkāḏt)
finger joint

tassəkāḏt ta tətoɣ ikassān
index finger

tassəkāḏt ta təzjərət bānnan
middle finger

tassəkāḏt ta n-tāḏhuten
ring finger

ārori n-edekel
back of the hand

edekel
palm

tassəkāḏt ta təndārrāt
little finger

tassəkāḏt, tisəkaḏ
finger

esgār, esgarān
fingernail

abārkot n- tāssəkaḏt
fingertip

ejmaš, ajmašān
thumb

tasāndart, tisāndaren
wrist

Figure 3.14. *Leg* – aḍār, iḍarān

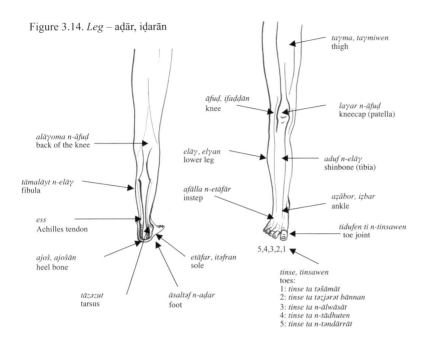

tayma, taymiwen
thigh

āfuḍ, ifaḍḍān
knee

layar n-āfuḍ
kneecap (patella)

alāyoma n-āfuḍ
back of the knee

elāy, elyan
lower leg

aduf n-elāy
shinbone (tibia)

tāmalāyt n-elāy
fibula

afālla n-etāfār
instep

azābor, izbar
ankle

ess
Achilles tendon

tidufen ti n-tinsawen
toe joint

5,4,3,2,1

ajoš, ajošān
heel bone

etāfar, itəfran
sole

tāzəzut
tarsus

āsaltəf n-aḍar
foot

tinse, tinsawen
toes:
1: *tinse ta təšāmāt*
2: *tinse ta təzjərət bānnan*
3: *tinse ta n-ālwāsāt*
4: *tinse ta n-tādhuten*
5: *tinse ta n-təndārrāt*

Figure 3.15.
Mouth – em, imawān

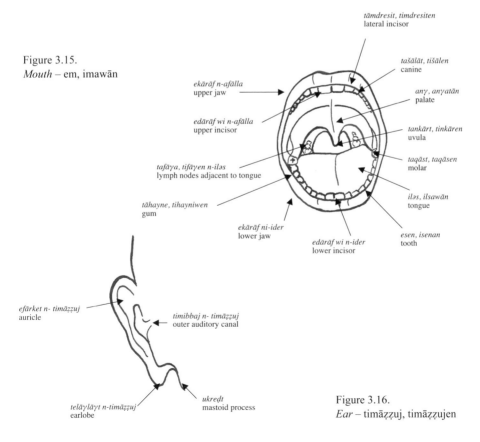

tāmdresit, timdresiten
lateral incisor

tašālāt, tišālen
canine

ekārāf n-afālla
upper jaw

any, anyatān
palate

edārāf wi n-afālla
upper incisor

tankārt, tinkāren
uvula

taqāst, taqāsen
molar

tafāya, tifāyen n-iləs
lymph nodes adjacent to tongue

iləs, ilsawān
tongue

tāhayne, tihayniwen
gum

ekārāf ni-ider
lower jaw

esen, isenan
tooth

edārāf wi n-ider
lower incisor

efārket n- timāẓẓuj
auricle

timibbaj n- timāẓẓuj
outer auditory canal

telāylāyt n-timāẓẓuj
earlobe

ukreḍt
mastoid process

Figure 3.16.
Ear – timāẓẓuj, timāẓẓujen

Figure 3.17. *Eye – tǝṭṭ, tǝṭṭāwen*

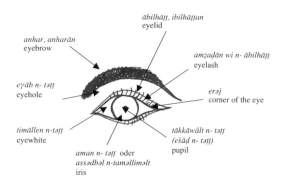

ābilhāṭṭ, ibilhāṭṭan
eyelid

anhar, anharān
eyebrow

amẓaḍān wi n- ābilhāṭṭ
eyelash

eɣāb n- tǝṭṭ
eyehole

erǝj
corner of the eye

timāllen n-tǝṭṭ
eyewhite

tākkāwālt n- tǝṭṭ
(ešāḍ n- tǝṭṭ)
pupil

aman n- tǝṭṭ oder
assǝdbǝl n-tamǝllimǝlt
iris

Beauty of body and character

The Kel Alhafra distinguish between outer and inner beauty, between physical attractiveness, *tihussay n-taɣǝssa,* and grace of character, *tihussay n-tašni.* Here again though, perfection is viewed as the harmonious union between inside and outside, between an inner ethical and an outer esthetic ideal that gives pleasure to the observer and stimulates his desire, *tihussay ijraẓ-ǝnnāt i-āwadǝm wa tāt ihannāyan d-wa tā n-t-irhan.* Beauty is a gift of God, *tihussay ihukkam n-māssināɣ,* and more important for a woman than a man, the Kel Alhafra women explain, because it insures that she will always be desired and will constantly have a male admirer at her side who pampers and looks after her.

The ideal of beauty among the Kel Alhafra, though, appears to have changed quite dramatically during the recent past. Before their experiences of war and flight during the years of the rebellion (1990–1996), the ideal was a well-fed, curvaceous woman. A woman with a large body was synonymous with wealth, *tihussay n-tamāḍt ta māqqārāt ehāre aqqālnāt.* In other words, it demonstrated that she had access to adequate reserves of milk and butter, *axx d-udi inuflayān daɣ amǝzzāɣ,* which in turn indicated that the herds were both extensive and healthy, *irǝzzejān yāẓiḍnān.* It would also mean that the mistress of the tent had a sufficient number of assistants, *iklān meɣ taklaten n-ehān,*[116] to relieve

---

116 *akli* (pl. *iklān*) is the Tamasheq term for former slaves (in Songhai also known as *bella*), captured by the Tuareg during the 19th century during raids on sedentary populations in the south [see here Michael Winter, "Slavery and the Pastoral Tuareg of Mali", *Cambridge Anthropology* 9 (1984): 4–30]. *taklaten n-ehān* (sing. *taklit*) were female slaves who performed the general daily chores and childcare for the mistress of the tent. From the colonial period on, the *iklān* gradually obtained their freedom, but many stayed with their owners and continued to undertake wage labor for them. During the droughts, however, and the rebellion, they were dismissed because there were no longer means to remunerate them. Today, many *bella* in Mali live as sedentary arable farmers or traders, although some manage herds and live a nomadic life or are sedentary agro-pastoralists. Only a few *iklān* remain as free workers with their former owners among the Kel Alhafra.

her of daily tasks so that she herself did not have to undertake any physically arduous activities, *kāla wār təššāγāl*. From their seventh year, girls were fed a diet rich in fats, *ādanda n-amaqqos*, to hasten the development of puberty and a woman's rounded form (i.e. the indices of reproductive maturity and fertility signaling readiness for marriage.)

During the severe droughts of 1972–1973 and 1984–1986 and the years of instability that followed, many Kel Alhafra lost virtually everything and fled, before the outbreak of war in 1991, to neighboring Algeria or Mauritania. There, they often spent years in refugee camps. The overweight beauties suffered during the physically exhausting flight and the subsequent deprivations, *ənhāynāt aγāna*. In the same period, the traditional lifestyle as well as basic concepts and values began to change substantially.[117] Following repatriation, which began in 1996, many Kel Alhafra had to rebuild their lives from scratch. They could no longer afford to pay for domestic labor, and the women had to do their share of the work, take care of their children, pound millet, and when the encampment moved, pack the household goods and load up the donkeys themselves. With the herds so depleted, there were no surpluses of butter and milk, and indeed, families were content simply not to suffer from hunger. Significantly, young women no longer yearned to be fat. Under these impoverished conditions, the opportunity to develop the formerly desired corpulent bodily ideal had in any case evaporated, and such a body type would only have been a hindrance to performing the necessary daily work.

The ideal body for a contemporary Kel Alhafra woman as described by Mariamma and Zainabu[118] is neither too fat nor too thin, but *ālwāsāt,* the "golden mean". A beautiful Kel Alhafra woman should have a "medium-sized" back, *ārori edāgg-γās a-iha,* and "medium-sized" hips, *iγəbberān edāgg-γās*

---

117 In the refugee camps, the Kel Alhafra had access to sufficient clean water and basic medical care. There were vaccination programs, the children could attend school, and training courses were offered to the women so that they might achieve a degree of financial independence after repatriation. Ideas began to change, and after the return to Mali, there was a vociferous demand for educational opportunities for the children, for adequate water supplies and basic health care provision. The women discussed planting and tending the kind of gardens they had seen in their guest countries, while the models of beauty for the young women had become the Arab film stars they had admired on television in the refugee camps. See here also McLuhan's discussion of the symbolic extension of the body through the media: Marshall McLuhan, *Understanding Media: The Extensions of Man* (Corte Madra: Gingko, 2003); as well as Randall's observations for the Tamasheq of the Mema and Goundam region: Sara Randall, "Demographic consequences of conflict, forced migration and repatriation: a case study of Malian Kel Tamasheq", *European Journal of Population* 21.2–3 (2005): 291–320.
118 Interview with Zainabu Wālāt Muḥammad and Mariamma Wālāt Alfaqqi, Indiarran, October 2005.

a-āhan, so that the thorax, waist and hips create a gracefully curving line. The tummy should be small and round, *tāsa təndārrāt d-tajāllālāt,* with a navel, *tābutut,* that disappears inside: this is very important because a protruding navel, *āboršād,* is considered to be particularly ugly, *iləšš.* The breasts should also be well proportioned, not to big and not too small, and the thorax so structured that jewelry placed around a long, slender neck does not "fall into the breasts", *wār tiwār dāɣ ifāffān.* A beautiful face has regular, harmonious features – large shining eyes outlined in black, *tiəṭṭāwen ti māqqoornen a-ti-imāɣmarnen attayen-nāsnāt ikkāwālnen,* and a fine well-formed nose, *tinšar sədudnen.* The lips should also be set off by a barely visible black line, *aḍālay ḍāmḍām (təbibbālāt s-tazolt),* and regular, white teeth, *isenan imāllan,* should gleam in the woman's mouth when she speaks and laughs. Gaps, *timāzzayen* (sing. *tamāzzai),* between the teeth are acceptable, while the gums should be blackish, *tāhayne ikkāwāl.* Hair ought to be artfully braided, black, long, and lie smoothly on the head, *amzāḍān tišləkitnān, ikkāwālān, išəjudnān, sədudnān.* Two skin types are recognized as beautiful: *tāroye,* in which the skin tone is somewhat yellowish, and *tāyole,* a blue tint (also known as "skin in the shadow"). A beautiful woman moves gracefully with a measured step, *tajjet tikle tāhusket wār-ta tarmāḍāt* – walking too quickly, *tajjet tikle sollan,* is considered unattractive. The *alāššo,* the indigo-dyed veil, is the favorite piece of clothing in the Kel Alhafra woman's wardrobe: it leaves a delicate blue sheen on the skin. However, the light-blue "bazin",[119] *ubukār,* is also very popular. In general blue is the color favored for clothing, *nəsofāɣ tādalāt dāɣ ini,* although apart from the blue staining of the skin, the women could not explain this color preference.[120]

Along with elaborate hairstyles all of which have a specific form and corresponding name (*tayārye, itəl n-bəbba* etc.), for celebrations, the women decorate the soles of their feet and the palms of their hands with henna, *ɣimmunāt ifassān-nāsnāt d-itəfran-nāsnāt.* They wear rings, *tāḍhuten* (sing. *tāḍhut),* and earrings made of silver, *tizābaten* (sing. *tazbit),* necklaces with silver ornaments, *taššaw əhanāt timāɣwānen n-āzrəf,* silver bracelets, *iḍkar,* or bead chains, *temaɣwānt* (pl. *timāɣwānen),* made from carnelian, turquoise and other

---

119 "Bazin" is the term for a colored cotton material, produced in Africa or China, various qualities of which are sold on the markets throughout Mali.

120 Kriss writes that in Islam, the property of warding off evil is ascribed to the color blue. See Kriss and Kriss-Heinrich, *Volksglaube im Bereich des Islam,* vol. 2, 4.
For the Kel Alhafra, however, blue, *tādalāt,* stands for fertility, for green pastures (the Tamasheq use the same word for green and blue), for *akāsa* (the abundant season of the rains, milk and butter), as well as for the natural world, the profane life of the here and now in contrast to the sacred and the hereafter, which are represented by white, the color of death, *tamāllāt.*

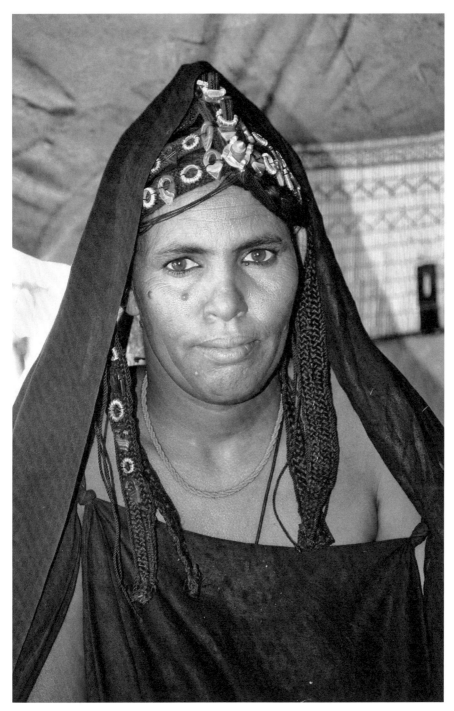

Figure 3.18. *Kel Alhafra woman with blue necklace,* kufya, *of plastic pearls, and a bridal piece of artificial hair into which small silver rings,* tikārkāruten *(sing.* takārkārt*), and* zākkāten *(sing.* zākkāt*), carnelian stones in the form of the cross of Agadez, have been woven (In Killa, November 2005).*

stones that they find in the sand at the sites inhabited by former cultures, *tezəmbaẓ*. However, because many families can no longer afford to purchase silver jewelry, women today often wear necklaces made of light-blue plastic pearls which they call *kufya*. Although Mariamma and Zainabu say that gold, *orāy*, is not a traditional precious metal among the Kel Alhafra, *orāy wār iha āladāt-t wa nanāy*, one increasingly sees gold jewelry being worn by Tamasheq women who live in the cities.

When it comes to the outstanding virtues that go to make up beauty of character, *tihussay n-tašni*, these are all closely related to goodness, *hārātān ihuskātān*, love, *tārha*, friendliness, *zārho*, happiness, *tābayort*, knowledge, *tāmusne*, wisdom, *tamella*, and truth, *tidət*. A woman of inner beauty is a presentable woman, *tamāḍt ta fārorāt*, one who stays within the encampment, *tāqimāt dāy aməzzāy*, who is cheerful and approachable, *ijraẓ-ənnāt iman-ənnet*, laughs a lot and is full of charm, *təlla tājomāst*, is welcoming to everyone, *tihe amājaru alwāqq fuk*, attentive and caring toward her children, *təjəmmiyāt i-aratān-ənnet*, and keeps her tent clean and tidy, *təšəšdəj d-təsədəw ehān*. *"iwar tāt zārho"*, "she is good" (in the sense of respectable, noble and highly esteemed), the Kel Alhafra say of a woman who takes good care of her husband, *təjəmmiyāt i-āhalis-ənnet*, and respects both the elderly, *təsimyār imyārān*, and her parents-in-law, *təsimyār iḍulan-ənnes*. What is not admired is a woman who talks too much: this characteristic can all too easily degenerate into *terk mājārād*, ill speech, and attract or enact the evil eye, *təšoṭṭ*. A woman of good character will speak with dignity and with calm, and only when her words have been carefully considered and her phrases well formulated.

For the Kel Alhafra, a respected person is one who can control everything that leaves his or her body including words, opinions and feelings, *iyulaf n-iman-ənnes*. Honorable behavior, *ātteqal* (pl. *ātteqalān)*, discretion, *ufur* (pl. *ufurān*),[121] dignity and prudence, *āššāk*, respect, *təmyār* (pl. *timyāren)*, and modesty, *tākrakəṭṭ* (pl. *tikrukaḍ),*[122] are as much hallmarks of a person's beauty as physical assets.

---

121 The verbal noun *ufur* is derived from *effer*, which literally means "to conceal, cover, keep secret and hidden from others". See also Foucauld, *Dictionnaire Touareg-Français*, vol. I, 334f. *hārātān iffarān* is the name given to things that, out of a sense of decency, one keeps to oneself.

122 *tākrakəṭṭ* (pl. *tikrukaḍ*) is derived from the verb *kərukəḍ*, meaning "to be bashful, to feel ashamed, or to behave in a reserved manner out of a sense of respect toward the other". The Kel Alhafra understand *tākrakəṭṭ* primarily as a sense of modesty and reserve in order not to draw the attention of a stranger to physical or spiritual nakedness. *"wār təssanād tākrakəṭṭ?"* they reprimand someone who has behaved in an unseemly or impolite way, "Aren't you ashamed of yourself?" For both sexes, *tākrakəṭṭ* is considered as a form of dig-

Topography of the organs

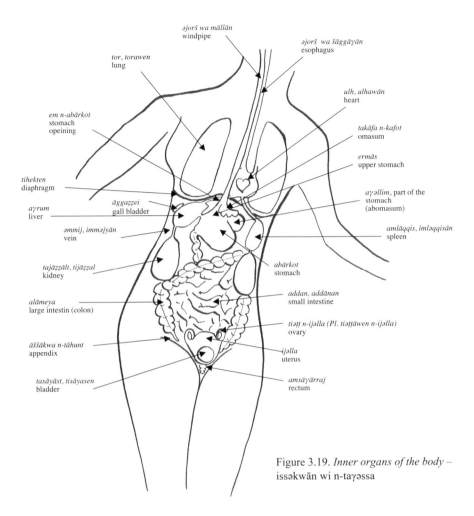

Figure 3.19. *Inner organs of the body –* issəkwān wi n-taγəssa

The Kel Alhafra will always name the heart, *ulh* (pl. *ulhawān*), as the most fundamental organ of the body, as it is the source of inborn warmth and the seat of the soul, *iman*. When asked, most Kel Alhafra locate the heart either in the center of the thorax below the breastbone (sternum), which in Tamasheq is

nified and respectful behavior, especially toward parents-in-law, older people and strangers. See here also: Casajus, *La tente dans la solitude*, 222; Robert F. Murphy, "Social Distance and the Veil", *American Anthropologist* 66 (1964): 1257–1274; Susan J. Rasmussen, "Female Sexuality, Social Reproduction, and the Politics of Medical Intervention in Niger: Kel Ewey Tuareg Perspectives", *Culture, Medicine and Psychiatry* 18 (1994): 433–462; Edmond Bernus, *Touaregs nigériens. Unité culturelle et diversité régionale d'un peule pasteur* (Paris: Harmattan, 1981) 156.

known as *tāsokālt n-iman,* "the spoon of the soul", or in the left thorax, where the pulse can be heard. The heart is framed on both sides by the lungs, *torawen* (sing. *tor*), considered the second most important organ. The diaphragm, *tihekten,* separates the thorax from the digestive tract, with the two organs lying below the diaphragm, the liver, *ayrum,* and the stomach, *abārkot,* also deemed highly important in the organ hierarchy. The stomach is either localized to the upper area of the abdomen or occupies its entire central region.

The Kel Alhafra extrapolate their knowledge from the inner organs of the ruminants they breed and slaughter, such as sheep, goats, cattle and camels, to human anatomy. In the Kel Alhafra view, therefore, the human possesses not a single- but a multi-chambered stomach. However, the human stomach is not divided into four parts (rumen, second stomach, omasum and abomasum) like that of goats, sheep and cows, but has only three sections, like that of the camel, the animal placed by God at the top of the animal hierarchy. Like the camel, the human has no second stomach (the two forestomachs take over its role), but just an omasum, *takāfa n-kafot,* an abomasum, *ayəllim* and a rumen, *abārkot.*

The liver, *ayrum,* is always positioned to the right of the stomach, with the gall bladder, *āggaẓẓei,* adhering to it. The spleen, *amlāqqis,* lies to the left of the stomach, although it is occasionally positioned somewhat vaguely in the right side of the body. The entire abdomen is filled with intestines, and here the Kel Alhafra distinguish between the large intestine (colon), *alāmeya,* the small intestine (intestinum tenue), *addānan,* and the rectum, *amsāyārraj.* The appendix is localized in the inguinal region on the right of the body; the Kel Alhafra name for it, *āššākwa n-tāhunt,* means literally, "bag of stones", indicating their recognition that stones may collect there, sometimes with fatal consequences. The intestines are flanked on the left and right sides of the body by the kidneys, *tijāẓẓāl,* while the bladder, *tasāyāst,* lies above the rectum. Situated above the bladder is the uterus, *ijəlla,* with its eyes, *tiəṭṭāwen n-ijəllan,* the ovaries.

No Kel Alhafra named the human brain as a central bodily organ, and in fact it was not even mentioned by the majority of my interviewees.[123] The pancreas is also not apparently known as a digestive organ, a finding also noted by El Mehdi Ag Hamahady in his 1988 study, "Nosographie tamashèque des gastro-enterites dans la région de Tombouctou", undertaken in the districts of Timbuktu, Diré, Goundam, Gourma-Rharous and Niafunké.[124]

---

123 Mohamed Ousmane, in his study in the Haoussa and Gourma region of Mali, also found that not all of his interviewees named the brain as an essential human organ: "The brain was not mentioned by everyone: only the Imouchars, the Bellahs and the Imrad referred to it." Ousmane, *La médecine traditionnelle,* 19.

124 "Some anatomical organs are little known: the sphincters and the pancreas." Ag Hamahady, *Nosographie tamachèque,* 17.

3.3.3. Body functions
The body's internal metabolism
In the universe of the Kel Alhafra, in their real lifeworld, their tents and their environment, there exists a closed divinely willed order that is mirrored within the human body. Ideally, the structures and functions of the entire organism are coordinated with one another, *taslāt fuk təla edāgg-ənnes dāy tayəssa*, and every part of the body is perfectly designed and regulated for its specific role.

As mentioned above, the heart, *ulh*, is considered the most significant bodily organ. It is the seat of both, the soul, *iman*, and the divine breath, *unfas,* and boosts every process of the body as a driving force, source of life energy and inborn warmth, *āṣṣahāt*. Together with the lungs, *torawen* (sing. *tor*), which flank the heart and are connected to it via veins, *imməjyān* (sing. *əmmij*), the heart is responsible for the circulation, *ibardāš n-ašni*, and respiration, by pumping air and blood through the veins, *itajj unfas d-ašni dāy imməjyān*. The heart, the Kel Alhafra say, is the motor of the body, *ulh sund moter n-tayəssa,* a source of power like the blacksmith's bellows that make the charcoal glow, *ulh sund tishāḍ n-enhāḍ ta təsrəy tizuẓam*, or like a pump that brings water from within the earth to the surface, *sund pômp itajj aman n-ider fāll ākal*. The heart is responsible for the life drive, *āṣṣahāt,* for nutrition, *asəmmənsu,* for growth, *tadāula,* and not least for sensory perceptions such as feelings of love and desire, *tārha,* which are inseparable from reproduction and reproductive events. All the veins of the body meet in the heart; a specific "vein", the windpipe, *əjorš wa māllān,* brings air to the heart which transmits it via another vein to the lungs, which then inflate. On breathing out, *asunfəs,* the used air is expelled back along the same route and out through the nostrils, *inābajān n-tinšar* (sing. *anābaj n-tinšar*). However, it is not only the lungs that are supplied with air by the heart, *aḍu wa n-unfas,* the entire body, from the toes to the skull, *har tinsawen tajj takārkort,* is filled with the life-giving breath, *unfas,* that is distributed in the blood and air through the system of veins. If the breath is circulating, the whole organism can function and all the organs can work, *issəkwan iššāyālān d-unfas*; if the breath stops, death is the consequence, *a-fāl imda unfas a-bās illa taməttānt*.

Another major organ is the liver, *ayrum,* which is like a fire, *sund efew,* and with the assistance of the breath coming from the heart, is responsible for the combustion of food (the used air produced by this process leaves the body like the smoke from a fire, *sund aho n-efew,* through the mouth or the nose, but this exhalation from the liver often has an unpleasant smell). During digestion, *asəmməšəl n-isudar day-tayəssa,* food passes along the gullet, *əjorš wa šāggāyān,* to the omasum, *takāfa n-kafot,* where it remains for a while until the mouth of the stomach, *em n-abārkot,* opens and it is transported on to the abomasum. A second digestive process takes place there, after which the material moves on to the rumen, *abārkot,* where small dilations on the stomach wall, *ixšəmyəšamān n-abārkot,* assist in food uptake. In the stomach and intestines, *addānan,* the food is separated into a liquid, *hārāt ābduj,* and solid waste, *hārāt aṣṣuhu.* Via veins, the liquid reaches the liver, where it is transformed into nourishment for the blood. The solid waste is passed out of the body as feces, *isbəkkitān* (sing. *asbəkki*). The digestive liquid that reaches the liver is filtered there into the components of the blood and into waste that is transported to the kidneys, *tijāẓẓāl,* (sing. *tajāẓẓālt*), and then to the bladder, *tasāyāst,* from which it leaves the body as urine, *āwas.* The liver is thus responsible both for the nourishment and cleansing of the blood, *asəmmənsu d-əšəšdəj n-ašni,* and well-nourished, clean blood is a sign of vitality, *āṣṣahāt,* and health, *āssexāt.* If food is metabolized poorly, the blood becomes weakened and impure, which debilitates the entire organism and can result in sickness.

The heart is also connected to the brain, *akəlkəl,* but for the Kel Alhafra, the latter is not involved in bodily functions but is rather the locus of memory, *tasāktot,* of thoughts, *inəzjam* (sing. *anəzjum*), and of reason, *tayətte.* The spine, *tazārrāt n-ārori,* and the spinal cord, *akəlkəl n-ārori,* are seen as extensions of the brain, from which the nerves, *iẓārwan* (sing. *aẓār*), spread out "like branches on a tree", *sund iləktān n-emāyt.* The brain is connected to the heart via veins, and if this connection is disrupted in any way, the affected individual is no longer capable of thinking, *wār ādoobed ansənəzjəmu*; the same holds if the brain itself is injured.

The Kel Alhafra perceive the human organism as a self-contained whole, a system created by God just like the universe, in which each individual element possesses an immanent sense in a context of mutual dependence, even though this sense is not always apparent to human beings. The Kel Alhafra could never tell me anything very exact about the function of the spleen, *amlāqqis,* or the gall bladder, *āggaẓẓei,* and ideas about how the brain works were, for the most part, vague.

Dealing with the body's secretions and excretions

The body as a self-contained organism, *tayəssa,* is powered by the divine breath, *unfas,* and needs food, *isudar,* to maintain its innate lifewarmth and energy, *āṣṣahāt.* This metabolic process creates wastes that leave the body either through the nose and mouth or via the anus and urinary tract. Air that has been used up in the body's circulation, *aḍu wa n-unfas,* is expelled either during exhalation, through the mouth and nose, *āsunfas,* or it is forced out during belching, *tujreken* (sing. *tujrek*), or in breaking wind, *tixādasen* (sing. *taxādast*). In general, used air is considered unclean, *wār šādij,* and the Kel Alhafra never exhale into a vessel from which one will drink or eat or on hot food to cool it. If a child burns itself while playing, the mother will never blow comfortingly on the painful spot but will offer the child a toy or something sweet as a distraction. Air that is expelled after transformative processes in the liver and stomach is not suppressed as it is in European and North American culture but is often released through loud belching. Likewise, although intestinal wind is viewed as unclean, breaking wind is not viewed as explicitly offensive. Spit, *ilāddan* or *imətman,* as a bodily secretion is also considered *wār šādij*, unclean, but tobacco consumers in particular expel a targeted stream of spit anywhere and often, including during conversations in or around the tent, although the spit is always quickly covered over by sand with a rapid movement of the hand. In this way, salivary mucus, *təšānɣešt* (pl. *tišənɣaš*), is left in the immediate area in which a family lives and mingled in the sand where children play. *inšeran*, nasal mucus, that accumulates in the nose during a cold or an allergy is, like spit, deposited either in the sand or smeared on tent posts in the individual's immediate environment.

Around every Kel Alhafra tent, there is a circle with a radius of three to six meters, *asəfraḍ*, that is regularly cleaned of animal waste, thorns and other litter with the help of a small broom. Men and women move somewhat beyond this circle in order to urinate, *itajjān āwas-nāsān s-ajāma n-asəfraḍ*, to the north or northwest; one should not urinate in the direction of Mecca. Defecation is also done in these cardinal directions, usually further from the tent. Feces, *asbəkki* (pl. *isbəkkitān*), are usually buried by women, but men and children seem to be less conscientious about this; although men often urinate and defecate a long way from the encampment, children's feces in the vicinity of the tent are a magnet for flies, *eẓẓ* (pl. *eẓẓān*), which then go on to settle on food. Children, as well as the sick and the old who are not very mobile, will relieve themselves wherever they happen to be; if they do so in the tent, the soiled sand is collected with a small wooden shovel, *āsaltəf*, and deposited in a container, usually a leather sack made especially for this purpose, *ejābeš*, which is then emptied outside the *asəfraḍ* in the northwest at the "refuse site", *ɣor edāgg wa n-erdān*

If blood, *ašni* (pl. *išnitān*), leaves the human body, either during a nosebleed, *ahunšar*, or through a wound, it is swabbed with a piece of cloth that is later burned in the direction of the *qiblāt* or buried outside of the male-connotated side, south of the tent. As a life-juice, blood is especially attractive to the *kel tenere,* and if care is not taken, it will fall into the wrong hands and cause significant harm. It is for this reason that menstruating women have to take special measures to protect themselves (discussed in more detail in section 3.4.2.1.)

Sweat, *tide* (pl. *tidawen*), is perceived both as a sign of strenuous physical activity but also as waste from an overheated body that is out of equilibrium and is attempting to cool itself with the body's water. Certain illnesses can be "evaporated" from the body by sweating, and to stimulate this process, the sick person will be wrapped in a warm blanket. Sweat from a sick person is carefully washed off and the polluted water is thrown away northwest of the tent. However in the heat of the Azawad, and especially during the burning hot months of *ewelān*, sweat is a constant companion and no special attention is paid to it as a body waste.

Other wastes due to bodily indisposition or illness, such as vomit, *ibsan,* or diarrhea, *tufit*, are dealt with in the same way as urine or feces. Wound pus, *arəssod̦*, is wiped off with a cloth that is then burnt or buried.

Everything that leaves the body as an excretion or secretion and returns to the environment is only touched with the left hand and is viewed by the Kel Alhafra as dirty and impure, *innokāl d-wār šādij*; this includes any human sperm, *amān n-āhalis* or *aššāhwāt,*[125] that is spilled and does not enter the female body for the purpose of conception.

There is one exception here: tears, *aməțț* (pl. *iməțțawān*) are not regarded as impure. They are aroused by the heart and are an expression of great joy, *tādawit*, or despair, *ərjum*, mourning, *tākmo n-iman*, or pain, *tezz̦ort*. Wherever possible, however, tears, as a sign of strong emotions whose public exposure is considered unseemly, are hidden from others, even by older children and adolescents as a form of self-control, *iɣulaf iman-ənnes*. Anyone who cries at the smallest provocation is scorned by the Kel Alhafra as *asəmməțțu* (pl. *isəmməțțiwān*), a "crybaby".

The Kel Alhafra have high standards for control of the body, and from an early age, children are taught to bring their bodily processes under control, *taɣlift*, and these requirements for personal self-control, *iɣulaf n-iman-ənnes,* increase with age and with one's position in the social hierarchy.

3.3.4. Borders of the body

The Kel Alhafra classify their lifeworld in the same way that they ascribe to the universe a divinely willed and immanent order, and as I have outlined above, not only is the tent a representation of this universal order, the body is also embedded within it and seeks throughout life to maintain a balance between the bipolar powers that characterize it.

This dialect of complementary phenomena in their lifeworld is also reflected in the Kel Alhafra view of the body's borders. Following Douglas, the north, which stands for the woman's side of the tent (the feminine, fertility, an inseparable bond with nature and intimacy), would be ascribed to the "informal realm", where bodily control can be relinquished and where, within a

---

125 *aššāhwāt* is a word borrowed from Arabic: *šahwa* (pl. *šahwāt*) means, among other things, "yearning", "desire", "longing", "passion", "lust".

proximate zone of personal trust, roles may be relinquished.[126] In contrast, the south stands for the "formal realm", the male half of the tent which is open to guests and strangers, for activities that are oriented toward the outside, for control of the self and the body, an area from which impurities like bodily wastes are excluded and emotions are hidden behind the veil. The south represents culture, *idommān*, in the sense of an elevation of the human above the natural condition through training and development of spiritual and moral potential, and *tamusne*, which can free the body from its fleshly state and transform it into a pure and ethereal form. This public forum is marked by personal and social distance, and is one in which roles are clearly assigned: borders separating bodies are precisely maintained, and individual bodily expressiveness is subordinated to socially accepted behavior and norms.

Proximity and distance in everyday life

Table 3.4. *Proximity and distance in everyday life*

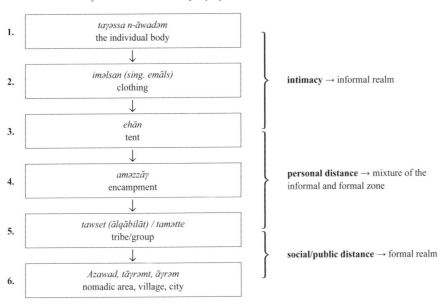

Of the four symbolic, concentric circles of space and distance that surround the individual body in the system elaborated by Hall – "intimate distance", "personal distance", "social distance" and "public distance" – only three re-

---

126 See Douglas for a description of the symbolic relationship in the opposition, "formal-informal". Mary Douglas, *Ritual, Tabu und Körpersymbolik* (Frankfurt am Main: Fischer, 2004) 107–108.

gions appear of actual significance for the Kel Alhafra.[127] The contours of the individual's body, *elām n-tayəssa*, set the first limit, but the skin never completely closes off the inner body from its surroundings; the body's openings allow constant exchange between inside and outside. To prevent interference in this sensitive mechanism of exchange and to ensure its natural flow, the body's orifices are protected in various ways. Using special diets, *išəkša*, amulets, *tikarḍiwen n-oyān*, stones, *timāywānen*, holy and magical formulae, *surātān d-tināfalalen*, or incense, *aḍutān*, a Kel Alhafra seeks to safeguard the exchange between inside and outside and to mitigate disturbances. Certain parts of the body are especially vulnerable, and a taboo[128] is placed on their being viewed by another person. This applies to the buttocks and lower abdomen, which are always covered, even in the intimate space of the tent. A woman's belly, in particular, the vessel of life and death that is considered to be a direct bridge between the body and the macrocosm, between becoming and passing away, and between this world and the hereafter, must be hidden from any ill-meaning glances and is always covered.

In the familiar world of the tent, the Kel Alhafra cover the taboo areas of the body, but in the immediate family circle, external appearance is now and then neglected, less attention is paid to neat dress, and the hair may be disheveled and uncombed. The tent represents a border that exceeds that of the body but whose woven matting, *tāsajit* (pl. *tisajiten*), encircles and shields the informal area of intimacy from the outside. No later than after the evening prayer, *amud wa n-təsoḍəsen*, guests and strangers leave the tents they are visiting and relinquish the private sphere to the occupants until sunrise, *ayyān ejādāš n-ehān har isunf tajj ajmoḍ n-tāfuk*. On the one hand, the tent is the shelter for the core family, for close family members and is a space for physical intimacy. But during the day, the southern half of the tent in particular is the reception area for visitors and guests. This opens the tent temporarily for relationships with others, and a transition is made from intimacy to interactions requiring a degree of dis-

---

127 Among middle-class Americans, Hall identified four symbolic circles that surround and position a human body. He distinguished between an "intimate distance" (0–45 cm), a "personal distance" (45–120 cm), a "social distance" (1.2–3.6 m) and a "public distance" (3–7.5m and over). For Hall, the latter is the area in which no social or personal interactions take place. See Edward T. Hall, *The Dance of Life: The Other Dimensions of Time* (Garden City NY: Anchor Press/Doubleday, 1983).

128 By taboo, *ārid* (pl. *āridān*), the Kel Alhafra understand, "Things that are not possible in our society" – *"hārātān waddey imukānān dāy tamətte ta nanāy"*. *ārid* is a condition conferred or induced in a being or a thing by a special spiritual power that always originates from the impure sphere of the *kel tenere*. Foucauld translates *ārid* as "souhait (ou prédiction, ou prévision, ou conjecture qui renferme un présage (quelconque, bon ou mauvais) (souhait, ou prédiction, prévision, conjecture) qui, par lui-même, est de bon ou mauvais augure)". Foucauld, *Dictionnaire Touareg-Français*, vol. IV, 1569.

tance. Although these encounters still take place within the protective space of the tent, they are regulated by certain social conventions. If a stranger drinks tea with the male head of the tent, his wife either leaves the tent and visits a neighbor, or she can demonstrate to the stranger her reserve, *tākrakəṭṭ,* by turning her back and covering her face with her veil when she speaks. Nevertheless, even here the borders are not static, and a visitor who begins by entering the "formal", southern half of the tent may be suddenly received into the intimate family circle and into close physical proximity.[129]

A Kel Alhafra child grows up in this informal and intimate space, which extends for a child to every tent in the encampment and to the living spaces of relatives. In adolescence, however, when his sensory and intellectual capacities are developed, a young Kel Alhfra male will leave and spend nights away from the maternal tent, *ifal ehān n-ma-s,* either alone or in the company of his peers. Only when a young man marries, *etār n-ehān* (literally, "to ask after a tent"), does he return to the protective intimacy of a woman's tent. A woman, in contrast, never sheds the symbolic skin of the tent. When a young woman leaves the maternal dwelling to marry, she is usually already the owner of a tent she has crafted with her own hands.

A Kel Alhafra encampment usually comprises a family collective of three to eleven tents that travel together. The space between the tents is such that one can recognize one's neighbors when they are standing outside them but cannot hear what they speak: *tādoobād ad tənhəyād anhārāj-ənnāk, mušām wār səjedād a-wa ijann.* The distance between two tents also depends, though, on the individual relationships between the tent inhabitants. All the inhabitants of an encampment cultivate personal contacts with each other, but here, outside the intimacy of the family tent, roles are clearly expressed, and social conventions prevail along with essential social controls. It is beyond the scope of this work to go into kinship relations, social hierarchies and a close analysis of social norms among the Kel Alhafra, but the personal space of the encampment is a zone of perpetual interchange between inside and outside, between intimacy and social monitoring, between familiarity and distanced respect. There is nothing static about this interchange, and it varies according to the situation, the atmosphere and the social standing of the actors. There is also brisk exchange between the various encampments with mutual visits of often entire or several days in a neighboring encampment. For such visits, a Kel Alhafra woman usually takes her youngest

---

129 Lambs, *ikrāwatān* (sing. *akrāwat*), and kids, *eɣāydān* (sing. *eɣāyd*), are sometimes allowed into the intimate areas of the tent, for example when they are sick, when they are being raised by hand or for other special treatment; otherwise, animals like sheep and goats spend the night outside, near the tent, but are not tolerated inside it.

children with her and spruces herself up, washes, and puts on her best veil to make a good impression on her kin. She will also usually take a small gift along, such as butter, meat, rice, tea, sugar or dates from her own stores.

When Kel Alhafra meet at festivities such as weddings, *izləyān* (sing. *āzli*), baptisms, *isəmawān* (sing. *isəm)*, or funerals, *tifəyyeden* (sing. *tafəyyet*), at religious festivals, *imaddān* (sing. *amud*), or at political meetings, *tamādāšt dāɣ tamətte fāll-folitik*, they will always recognize kin among the throng. In this setting, however, personal relationships retreat into the background. The experience of the dialog, *edāwānne*, in such a context, constructs the shared ground: the people that have come together move in the same environment, use the same objects, share the same basic principles and values, and coexist in one and the same world. They have formed alliances to face the immense challenges of the desert and have fought together for their rights and mutual survival. Here, individuality is surrendered to a group-based identity, because only within the group can each man or woman find protection, *taggazt*, security, *āṣṣater*, and care, *tamədda* (pl. *taməddawen)*[130] – no one can survive in the desert alone. A strong tribe, *tawset* or *ālqābilāt*, protects its members, *tawset ta təjənniyāt əddināt-ənnes,* and threatens with retaliation, *eɣa* (pl. *eɣatān)*, anyone who attacks one of its people. In return, the tribe expects loyalty from everyone, and each member must bow to its regulations and norms.[131]

In the vastness of Azawad, the Malian government, *ālhukuma wa n-Mali*, based far away in the capital of Bamako, has little to offer the Kel Alhafra: *"wār təlla ālhukuma diha",* they say, "here there is no government". In situations of hardship, it is not the state that rushes into the desert with aid but members of the tribal fraction that fulfill the state's role. It is only through this solidarity, this mutual support, that the tribal association can function: the individual is strengthened by group membership, and the fraction by its individual members; the collective overall is nurtured by symbols and rituals. Like the universe as a macrocosm and the body as a microcosm, the tribe as an entity is created by the cooperation of its individual parts, in which the individual is dependent on the whole and first gains an identity through the role he or she plays within the group structure. It is in this realm that the social controls are most strongly felt: the individual is fully absorbed by the group, and the "collective we-consciousness"[132] is placed above that of the single "ego", such that

---

130 *tamədda* (pl. *taməddawen)* is the verbal noun from *māddu*, "to unite against something" or "to be protected by someone".

131 On the relationship between individual and tribe, see also Ali Al Wardi, *Soziologie des Nomadentums* (Neuwied: Luchterhand, 1972).

132 As a collective we-identity Assmann understands: "the image that a group constructs of itself and with which its members identify. Collective identity is a question of the identifica-

each one understands his or her respective gender specifically as belong to the men, *meddān*, or the women, *tiḍeḍen*, and plays the appropriate role in conformity with the tribal organism.

If a Kel Alhafra male leaves the tent, *ehān*, encampment, *aməzzāy*, or the protection of the tribe, *tawset* (a rare occurrence for a woman unless she marries a man outside her own group), he puts on his best clothes, *itajj anākābbaənnes wa ojarān n-tihussāy*, carefully arranges his face veil, *itajj ayewədənnes*, attaches a dagger to his belt, *itajj abṣar dāy taməntaka-ənnes*, saddles his camel, *itajj tārik dāy amənis-ənnes*, and stashes his gun in a saddlebag, *itajj ālbarroḍ-ənnes dāy āššākwa n-amənis*. Only male Kel Alhafra travel alone and expose themselves to the dangers, *mišitān* (sing. *miši*), confronting them outside the protective spaces of the tent, encampment and tribe. This "public" zone, which extends from the vast desert of Azawad northwards to the Algerian border and to places like In Salah, and also southwards to Ber, Gao, Timbuktu, Gourma-Rharous or even Mopti, is out of bounds for independent discovery by a Kel Alhafra woman. A man however, well-equipped and armed, may dare to enter these strange environments, but even here he will always seek out personal relationships. A "public distance" in Hall's sense, in which no social interactions take place between individuals, is rarely relevant for the Kel Alhafra. Absolute depersonalization and alienation between people does not exist in their world. Even in places where he has neither kin nor acquaintances, a Kel Alhafra male will find co-religionists who offer him a familiar base and points of contact through shared symbols and through Mecca as a global focus. It is the forces of nature, *mišitān dāy ajāma*, the *kel tenere* who lie in wait for him in lonely spots, and God's tests and punishments, *iṭṭusān* (sing. *aṭṭas*) *n-māssināy*, that are the threats a male Kel Alhafra must face. The limited recourse he has for protecting himself and fending off these forces lies in his trust in God, *tafləst dāy māssināy*, which sets him on the righteous path, so that he will not be tempted or misled by corrupt powers, *wār nəsəfrəy*[133].

Disturbances of proximity and distance during illness
Among the Kel Alhafra, curative and care activities are the responsibility of women: *"wāddey əššāyāl n-āhalis"*, they say with a smile, "it not the concern of a man". It is the woman who medicates, treats, feeds, washes and in general

---

tions made by participant individuals. It does not exist "as such" but only to the extent to which particular individuals lay claim to it. Its strength or weakness depends on its vitality in the consciousness of the group members and on its ability to motivate their thinking and actions". Assmann, *Das kulturelle Gedächtnis*, 132.

133 *nəsəfrəy* means "to mutually lead one another astray", in which an *anāfrəy* performs an incorrect act that transgresses the prevailing moral edicts.

takes care of a patient. Sick people are never left to their own devices, a female member of the family will always remain with and take care of them. This is also the case in those rare situations when a sick person is receiving treatment in the health care center in Ber or at the hospital in Timbuktu. Male Kel Alhafra will visit, enquire about his health and provide some company, but it will always be a woman who concerns herself with the sufferer's physical well-being. The sick remain in the protective environment of the tent if they are not mobile, and the members of the tribe demonstrate their support through visits. If the illness is classified as *torhɘnna ta tinsɘlsit*, "a contagious disease", the Kel Alhafra take care that the sick person does not use the same bowl and the same spoon as other family members, a precaution known as *"aẓɘlāy n-ākoss"*, "separating the bowls". However, my question about exposure to infectious diseases received the somewhat resigned response, "the disease exceeds our means", and solidarity with the sufferer always takes precedence over the possibility of infection. However, if a Kel Alhafra knows that she or he has an infectious disease and deliberately passes the infection on to others, a liability is incurred, *āmarwas* (pl. *imarwasān*), for which one must account alone before God on the day of judgment, *ašāl wa n-tebādde*.

Sick children always remain in the care of their mother, and if she visits a neighboring encampment, she will take the sick child (if it can still be carried) with her, despite the fact that it may infect other children. A Kel Alhafra child is never isolated, even when sick: *"wār nādoobād"*, the women say, "we cannot do that", and *"aratān imiɣatārān s-ɘddināt a-san ijān ɘnniyāt"*, "children need the proximity of people so that they feel comfortable". However, if an obviously epidemic disease breaks out in an encampment, neighboring encampments suspend their visits as much as possible to avoid bringing the disease into their own tents. Even during such events, though, contact cannot be totally cut off. Daily tasks must be performed, and the animals watered at the wells. Activities that require reciprocal assistance must continue.

Attitudes to those with physical and mental disabilities

In the Kel Alhafra conception, disability is the result either of *ālhāqq*, God's justice, for reasons that are not always evident to humans, or is due to the meddling of the *kel tenere*, when certain social regulations have have been disregarded or abused.[134]

---

134 As a consequence of *tɘšoṭṭ*, the evil eye, or breaking a taboo, *ārid*, the *kel tenere* can cause disability to an unborn child, or exchange a newborn at birth for one of their own *ǧinn* class. To avoid the interference of the *kel tenere*, sexual intercourse should never take place in the open air, a pregnant woman ought not to spend any time alone in nature, nor should she ever undress fully, and the body should always be cleaned of impurities, *āmaḍas*.

When the Kel Alhafra speak of *bəddən (bəddənān)*, this designates physical damage of the parts of the body required for support or movement or of the individual organs, damage that limits the range of possible physical activities. Someone who is physically disabled, *anābdun* (pl. *inəbdan*), such as a blind person, *emādderyəl*, someone who is deaf, *amāẓẓaj*, or mute *amədəmdəm*, is neither categorized as "abnormal" nor ill-treated. The infirmity may be inherited, *itra dāy imārawān-ənnes*, due to prenatal damage as the result of a shock, *tarəmməq*, due to an unfulfilled wish, *tārha*. It can be from a sickness, *torhənna*, an accident, *ejāḍāl*, or a violent act, *tahhāyt*, but the head and the intellect retain their clarity, *eyāf d-tayətte-ənnes wār iyšaḍān*, and so the individual remains a full-fledged member of society.

The Kel Alhafra also consider that cognitive disability is caused by the *kel tenere*, who, in the case of *amdun* (pl. *imdunān*), have penetrated an unborn child and taken possession of it. By *amdun* the Kel Alhafra understand "someone possessed by a harmless *ǧinn*", who although not endowed with the same intellectual capacities as most humans is, nevertheless, never of a bad character, *wār tāšne-ənnes tallābasāt*.[135] In this connection, the Arabic term, *buhlul* (pl. *bahālīl*), sometimes crops up, which, with the meanings of "fool" and "clown", reflects the unserious and animated aspect of the *amdun* within Kel Alhafra society. An *amdun* is not evil, *wār əššaḍ*, but the Kel Alhafra will refer to him as *abudəl*, "of no use". This relieves him of the burden of making decisions or working and allows him a certain freedom to move relatively unmolested between encampments, asking for a bowl of milk at any tent.

The perfidious *ǧinn*, however, can ambush human beings in every daily situation and attempt to overpower them in a weak moment. Particularly susceptible are those who are constantly worrying and wallowing in their problems, *zənəzjəm dāy ālhumum*, those who think too much, *amzuzāw tayətte-ənnes*, who neglect themselves, *wār ikkul iman-ənnes*, or who withdraw from general social contacts, *ikkas iman-ənnes dāy tāwset*. Those who want things they cannot have, *irha ajāraw hārātān s-wār adoobed ajāraw-nāsān,* or who do not have their passions under control, *wār adoobed tijāwt n-ənniyāt ijann*, can also be targets. A slight cognitive change first becomes noticeable with *ālwāswāsāt*, vicious insinuations, with delusions and obsessions caused by Iblis, by a lack of willpower, *wār ila derhan ajjen*, or insufficient self-control and unseemly behavior, *wār ijəmmək a-wa-s-ənta*, which is frowned upon, but tolerated by others. The Kel Alhafra call such people, *āwadəm wa iyšaḍ n-tayətte* – "someone whose

---

135 In contrast to Christian conceptions, the spirit or demon, *ǧinn*, need not necessarily be of an evil character when, in the Kel Alhafra understanding of possession, it penetrates the human body and speaks or acts in place of the individual's suppressed or spellbound soul, *iman*.

reason is disturbed" – causing contrary behavior in the sense of *addey dāγ āladātān-nānāγ*, "not according to our rules and customs" (i.e. conduct outside the common understanding of *inimāhāl*, "appropriate, average and normal").[136]

The Kel Alhafra only begin to speak of insanity, *ālšin* (literally, spirit or demon) or *ušəḍ*, in reference to a mental illness when someone lives entirely in their own world, has entirely lost their reason, speaks to him- or herself, no longer participates in the social life of the group and is often malicious, *tašne-ənnes tallābasāt*, and may be violent. As someone who is psychically sick, an *amušāḍ* (pl. *imušāḍān*) is always associated with dark powers and leads a marginal existence outside society, in the care and company of only his or her closest kin. The Kel Alhafra told me, though, that *imušāḍān* of this sort *"ār ilan tiγārras"* – "do not live a long life", and soon return to their own world, *"ad ijəššān āddunya-nāsān šik"*.

For the Kel Alhafra, mental illness is a possession, *ālšin,* a debilitation of the spirit, *tayətte*, and the soul, *iman*, that results from spiritual erring, *anāfraγ n-tayətte*, moral guilt, *ābākkaḍ*, or as an apostasy from God, *ālžahil*, which exposes one to the influence of evil spirits, *ālwāswāsāt n-kel tenere*. Possession is, nevertheless, curable. It can be treated by a marabout who, as exorcist, can channel divine powers to drive the demon out of the possessed body. Those suffering from epilepsy, *ayəttus*, as well as the old who become demented, *ijmatān n-ənniyāt*, are also considered to be possessed by a *ǧinn,* and only the divine power of the holy verses of the Koran can help them.[137]

3.3.5. The body in space and time

Unlike the linear or chronological time of clocks and calendars whose regime is imposed on the human body in industrial society, the Kel Alhafra comprehension of time is first of all cyclic. Time is tied to nature, the seasons that are determined by the stars, the climate and the growth of plants, but also it is tied to the animals that, like the Kel Alhafra themselves, must adapt to these changes in order to survive.

For the Kel Alhafra, a human life begins on earth at birth and, likewise, *akāsa,* the rainy season, represents the beginning of a new pastoral cycle. The

---

136 Values and norms among the Kel Alhafra are often conveyed through stories, *infusen* (sing. *tanfust*), and proverbs, *oẓẓawān* (sing. *oẓẓ*), that paraphrase the rules for everyday communal life, educate listeners in the making of judgments and decisions, and provide guidance toward and along the path to "just dealings".

137 For the treatment of the mentally ill, *imušāḍān*, specific verses of the Koran, for example, are written in ink by the marabout, dissolved in water and given to the sick person to drink, or amulets, *tākarḍiwen*, containing appropriate surahs are worn against the body. Such treatments usually provoke, in the first instance, an intensification of the symptoms as the demon seeks to defend itself against the divine power before a recovery gradually sets in.

season of fertility, of lush meadows and release from dependence on the wells, *tajəllāwt n-unwan*, starts with the appearance of the *šāttehāḍ*,[138] "the sisters of the night" or Pleiades, which first appear in the early morning hours of June or July in the eastern night sky. The Pleiades bring clouds and rain, *tijārāken d-ijənnawān*, and when the first drops fall, the Kel Alhafra refer to these as *"iməsirādān n-šāttehāḍ"*,[139]- "the ablutions of the sisters of the night", a celestial cleansing at the end of a cycle before entering a new fertile phase. Once *akāsa* is established in August, and if enough rain has fallen so that the animals can take up a lot of moisture just by eating juicy plants and do not have to be watered every day, the constraining link to the wells can be unfastened: *azzāmān n-unwan imda*, the "time of the wells" is over and the nomads can start moving in search of the best pasturelands.

akāsa is followed by *ɣarat*,[140] introduced by the star *ɣuššāt* (Canopus) in the east. This announces the time of the fever, *azzāmān wa n-tenāde*, when in September, the last rains fall.[141] The earth is still damp and the malarial mosquitoes begin to spread. During October and November, a low season for the Kel Alhafra, which they call *ɣarat jərəs*, the temperatures gradually begin to cool, the rains cease, the earth dries out and the "time of the wells", *azzāmān wa n-unwan,* sets in again. Now the nomads begin to settle down in the richest pastures of northern Azawad, hoping to survive the approaching, meager months without too much hardship. In the cold season, *tajrəst,* that lasts from the middle of December into February, the temperatures can fall to 0 °C, and humans and animals suffering from the frosty conditions usually remain in one spot. *tajrəst* is followed by *afāsko,* the season of winds, of sand and dust storms from March to April, when the days get warmer, but the nights remain

---

138 *šāttehāḍ,* the seven stars of the Pleiades represent in the stories told by the Kel Alhafra seven sisters who wear a single, shared garment, *karše,* and are the wives of *Amānar* (Orion). The individual sisters (stars) are called: *Ārajāwāt, Assākāwāt, Allāɣāwāt, Mātarājā, Mātasāksāk, Mātalāɣla* and *Faḍimāta.*

139 According to Klute, the Kel Adaɣ call rain that falls during the dry season, *ewelān,* "*iməsserədn ən-šat-ahaḍ*", "corpse-washer of the sisters of the night", because the Pleiades have now disappeared, i.e. died. Like a corpse-washer, this rain prepares the "daughters of the night" for their grave. Georg Klute, *Die schwerste Arbeit der Welt. Alltag von Tuareg-Nomaden* (Munich: Trickster, 1992) 71.
       The Kel Alhafra said, however, that they would speak of *iməsirādān n-šattehāḍ* on two occasions: once in May, when the Pleiades disappear in the west and can leave behind clouds and rain, and a second time in June/July, when the "sisters of the night" return. They make no mention, however, of a "corpse-washer".

140 *ɣarat* is also used to described a human's tiredness and exhaustion during *ɣarat māllāt,* the "white autumn", the second half of the season, *ɣarat,* when the plants have already dried out and no more rain falls.

141 The appearance of *ɣuššāt* (Canopus) shortly after sundown in the west announces, according to the Kel Alhafra, the end of the rains.

comfortably cool. The various species of acacia blossom, but this is also the season of the bothersome flies, *eẓẓan*, that pester humans and animals alike.

The transition from *afāsko* to the hottest season, *ewelān*, takes place in May. Now the animals must be watered every day, the milk stores have run out, and the nomads start to suffer from the heat and a monotonous diet. The Kel Alhafra families move with their sheep and goats to the vicinity of a well where enough *afāẓo (Panicum turgidum)* grows, which they use to construct a pleasantly cool hut, *abugi*, to escape the insufferable heat of their tents. During *ewelān* the men often move north with the camels, sometimes to Algeria, in search of better grazing land, while the women, children and old people remain behind longing for the onset of a new rainy season, *ašāraju n-akāsa*, which will herald the rebirth of nature. However, it is only after enduring and surviving *tišwāyšwāy*, the difficult transitional season between *ewelān* and *akāsa* in June and July, the time of the parched earth and hunger that humans and animals can look forward to recovery and revival in a fresh pastoral cycle that begins with the new rains.

On the one hand, time, *ālwāqq* or *azzāmān*, is experienced as a periodic emergence, maturation, degeneration and disappearance, analogous to the seasons, the female fertility cycle, or the biological aging of a human being; on the other, rites accompany the transitions of birth, adolescence, adulthood, old age and death by ceremonially reproducing and maintaining the cycle of

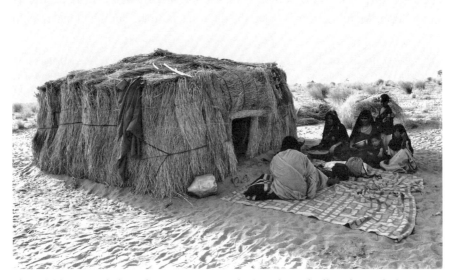

Figure 3.20. *Hut made from* afāẓo *(Panicum turgidum) used as a dwelling during the hot months of* ewelān *(In Agozmi, March 2005).*

the world order in the face of a general tendency toward decay. Rites, like the veins of the circulation, guarantee the circulation of a shared meaningfulness on which the structure of the Kel Alhafra lifeworld depends. This aspiration toward coherence is reflected in the ritual repetition of prayer,[142] which organizes the day, and in the celebration of religious festivals that follow a lunar calendar and endow the lifeworld with a ceremonial infrastructure.[143]

Although the conception of time by the Kel Alhafra is primarily oriented by cyclic and ritual repetition, it is also punctuated by special or exceptional events, by personal relationships and specific interactions that then persist in living memory. When asked a Kel Alhafra will rarely have any idea how old he or she is, but can sometimes mention an event that took place just before or after their birth. "I was born in the year that the automobile flew", – *"arwey dāy awātay wa təforrād torāft"*, an old woman told me, from which one can conclude that in the accounts of her kin, she was born around the time when the first airplane was sighted in the region, i.e. circa 1932. Time here is not a continuous linear flow but is arranged by memories that provide points of orientation in the past. The distant past is often ordered by catastrophes *musibātān* (sing. *musibāt*): the year of the great drought, *awātay wa n-mānna*, of the locusts, *awātay wa n-tišwālen*, of the measles epidemic, *awātay wa n- tassididet,* etc. In contrast, the more recent past is described with reference to events concerning kin, the encampment and the tribe: in the month Alhassan returned, *iyor wa dāy əqqālid Alhassan,* in the week that Ahill's donkeys disappeared, *usubu wa rāḍḍa išāḍān wi n-Ahill*, on the day that the Algerian lorry stopped at the well, *ašāl wa ittus torāft ta n-Alžer γor anu*, etc.

Rites anchor transitions in the everyday temporal cycle, while on synchronous and diachronous levels, one-off events and celebrations shape the coherence of the group.[144] However it was only after drought, war and occupying powers forced the Kel Alhafra into a confrontation with other societies and other ways of life that they began to develop a consciousness of their own identity and space held together by a shared symbolic system. Kel Alhafra who emigrated to Libya or attended schools in the refugee camps in Algeria and Mauritania encountered a significantly different concept of time there. They experienced, first of all, a distantiation from nature and, in

---

142 Each day is subdivided by five prayers: *amud wa n-tifāwt* – the morning prayer (between 5:00 and 7:00), *amud wa n-tezzār* – the midday prayer (between 12:00 and 14:00), *amud wa n-takāṣt* – the afternoon prayer (between 16:00 and 17:00), *amud wa n-almāẓ* – prayer at sunset (between 18:00 and 19:00), *amud wa n-təsoḍəsen* – the prayer before going to sleep (between 20:00 and 22:00).

143 On "ritual coherence" see Assman, *Das kulturelle Gedächtnis*, 89.

144 See Assman, *Das kulturelle Gedächtnis*, 89.

social structures governed by chronological time, a weakening of their bond
to the periodic coming and going of the seasons in Azawad. Simultaneously,
a space was created in which they could make comparisons and reflect: for
many, life in the desert, unlike that of those settled in villages and cities,
appeared as "wild" and as "untamed" as nature itself (and thus incorporated
into their own self-conception the very images that were being projected
onto them): *"dāy ajāma ijraw āwadəm iman-ənnes a wa irha itajj"* – "in the
desert everyone is free (can do what they want)". This encounter with the
significantly different, with the Other, the "cultivated", *kel ayrəm*, increased
the need for familiarity, for membership of their own group, and for their
own living space. Kel Alhafra who live as nomads nowadays in the Azawad,
are proud to belong to the *kel ajāma* (even if, in the cities, this term is often
used pejoratively in the sense of "untamed savage"), proud to belong to those
of the desert, to those of the vast, uninhabited and empty spaces. In contrast
to the *kel ayrəm*, to the villagers and townspeople, the *kel ajāma* know how
to orient and assert themselves in the endless spaces of an unpredictable nature and a hostile desert.

As the pastoral cycle is regulated by growth and decay, the human is
also subordinated to fate, *tāyrəst*,[145] that accompanies the individual from
birth to death. Like every other creation, the human is subject to divine rule,
temātert n-Māssināy, and divine authority, *alāmār*, exercised by a God of justice, *māssināy n-ālḥāqq*, whose eyes see everything, *tiəṭṭawen n-Māssinināy
ihannāyān hārātān fuk*, and who never commits wrong. As a source of moral
values, life in this world, *tāmudre fāll tesāyt n-ākall fuk*, is closely connected to the next world, *ālaxirāt*, and every Kel Alhafra acts in compliance with
ālžānnāt, paradise, and avoids everything associated with *ālžāhānnām*, hell,
because *"taməttānt ad ikka"*, "death will come".[146] For each human there is a
day preordained by God, *ašāl wa n-tāyrəst təmda*, on which he or she will die
and must answer for his or her deeds in this world. Death is inevitable, and for
the Kel Alhafra a continual companion that can strike at any age. Many chil-

---

145 The Kel Alhafra emphasize that although *tāyrəst* as human fate determines the longevity of
     every individual, it is never arbitrary because it is always under God's control.
     tāyrəst is equivalent to the Koranic concept *dahr*, the lifespan of each individual determined
     by God, which comes to an end at the moment of death, *taməttānt* (Arabic: *'ajal*). On the
     Koranic conception of *dahr* and *'ajal* see Toshihiko Izutsu, *God and Man in the Koran: Se-
     mantics of the Koranic Weltanschauung* (North Stratford: Ayer, 1998).
146 See surah 21:35: *"kullu nafsin ḏā'iqatu-l-mauti wa nablūkum bi-š-šarri wa-l-ḫayri fitnatan
     wa 'ilaynā turǧa'ūna."* – "Every soul shall taste of death; and We try you with evil and good
     for a testing, then unto Us you shall be returned." But see also surahs 4:78, 62:8, 67:2.

dren do not reach their fifth year, but the Kel Alhafra will never speak of "a high child mortality rate", but, rather, of *"tayrəst təmda ɣās"*, "the predetermined time of death has arrived/the life determined by God has drawn to a close, that is all".

Once the lifespan ordained by God is accomplished, the angel of death Izra'īl collects the soul, *iman*, from the human body and conducts it to heaven. There the hour of divine justice awaits it, *āssayāt wa n-āššāreya*, and it will learn if God has forgiven all its sins, *ibākkaḍān* (sing. *ābākkaḍ*), and is destined for paradise. Then it returns for a brief while to this world. If however the soul belongs to the damned, *ināmāšrayān* (sing. *anāmāšray*), it is immediately refused admittance through the lowest of the heavenly doors and is lead back to earth to join all the other wrongdoers, *fāll ākall yor edāgg wa n-ināmāšrayān*.

After a corpse has been buried, *ānjālos wa n-amāsəstān*, "the angel who asks questions" interrogates the dead in the grave: *"mi māssināy-ənnāk?"* – "who is your God?"; *"mi ānnābi-ənnāk?"* – "who is your Prophet?"; *"ma-mos āddin-ənnāk?"* – "what is your religion?"; *"əndek teje ta təha ālqiblāt?"* – "to what does the direction of your prayer point?". If the deceased answers correctly *(Āḷḷahu, Moxāmmād, ālislam, s-emāynāj)*, he will hear the promise of paradise, *mārušāten n-ālžānnāt*; incorrect answers, on the other hand, will be rewarded by torments, *ālyazzābān* (sing. *ālyazzāb*), in the grave.[147]

The souls wait until the judgment day and enter the eternal world of paradise, *dāy ālaxirāt n-ālžānnāt*, or roast in hell's fires, *dāy temse n-ālžāhānnām*. Not all sinners, *ināsbākkaḍān* (sing. *anāsbākkaḍ*), though are condemned forever to the torments of hell, because God is just, and after serving the sentence for their sins, he sometimes allows believers, *inəsləmān* (sing. *anəsləm*), the desired entry into paradise.[148]

In the Kel Alhafra conception, modeled on that of the Koran, the moment of death is not a definitive endpoint but a transition between the two worlds, between the here and now and the hereafter, *āddunya* and *ālaxirāt*, during which the soul enters the eternal world, while the dead body in the grave without soul, *iman*, without divine spirit, *unfas*, or living warmth, *tākusse*, becomes pure material and decays.

---

147 On the interrogation in the grave, see: Koran, surahs 8:50, 16:32, 41:30, 47:27.
148 On the notion of the waiting time until the Last Judgment, see: surahs 10:45, 20:103, 79:46.

3.4. Cultural expression of the female life cycle

Table 3.5. *Female life cycle*

Period during the life cycle		Duration	Changes
ebenu	Fetus	1–120 days (3 × 40 days)	Perception of pregnancy *ajmoḍ n-abārkot*
ara (pl. aratān)	Child	ca. 120–280 days (40 × 7)	Birth - *tiwit*
itiwāt (pl. itiwātān)	Newborn	1–40 days	End of confinement *təzjar n-amẓor*
āmankas (pl. imānkāsān)	Infant	7 days to 2 years	Weaning *isəmda n-āsənkas*
tamārkəst (pl. timārkāsen)	Small child	0–5 years	Walking *ilamādan tekle*
talyāḍt (pl. tilyāḍen)	Child, girl	5–12 years	Second dentition *ismaskān isenān wi n-axx*
tābārmawāḍt (pl. tibārmawāḍen)	Adolescent	12–20 years	Menstruation *iba n-amud*
tamawāḍt (pl. timawāḍen)	Young adult	18–30 years	End of growth *isəmda tadāwla*
tamaḍt (pl. tiḍeḍen)	Woman	30–50 years	Motherhood *tamāḍt ta n-anna*
tamɣārt (pl. timɣāren)	Old woman	≥50	Menopause – *tijbəs* Death – *taməddānt*

3.4.1. Childhood – *amārkəs*

In Kel Alhafra society, one is not born but becomes a woman. From birth, *ti-wit*, through baptism, *isəm*, breastfeeding, *āsənkas*, and the first years of life, children of both sexes are cared for in the same manner, except that on the day of her baptism, *ašāl wa n-isəm*, seven days after birth, during the ritual washing, *ālwālḷa*,[149] and shaving of her hair, *telāẓe*, a small part of the hair, *taššəkoḍt*, is left on the back part of the head.[150]

---

149 For a precise description of the ceremony of the first ritual washing and name giving for newborns, see Walentowitz's work on the Kel Eghlal and Ayttawari Seslem in Azawagh, Niger. Walentowitz, *Enfant de soi*, 412–413.
150 In contrast to the Kel Eghlal and Ayttawari Seslem in Azawagh, Niger, the Kel Alhafra do not refer here explicitly to a haircut, but in general to a "shaving" of the head hair. On the name-giving ritual, see Walentowitz, *Enfant de soi*, 172–173.

Until about two years of age, while they still have no self control over their excretory functions, children are usually left naked, *isafān*, and remain in the care of their mother, *anna*, an older sister, *tamāqqārt*, or a close female relative, *tāmarawt*, who carries the infant, *āmankas*, around with her. The child is only separated from an adult when it is put to sleep lying on its back on a piece of cloth, *fāll isəftāy*, or, more rarely, in a cradle, *dāy asəkənsəki*.[151]

In this period, the mother breastfeeds the child on demand assuming she does not become pregnant again during its first two years.[152] *"axx wa n-tālxamilt wa lābassan i-āmankas fāl a-s səjrəw-ənnes tufit ta n-lāho"*,[153]– "a pregnant woman's milk makes the baby sick and causes diarrhea", the women explain. In such cases, to wean the child early, the women spread pepper, *ižəkimba* (*Xylopia aethiopica*), on the breast, or distract it with something sweet, like sugar, *əssukar*, or a date, *tehāyne*. If a child is weaned before what is considered the ideal period of two years, during the changeover in diet, the women feed it pounded millet, *enāle taddāhān*, or rice, *tafāyāt*, with some chopped meat, *isan taddāhān*. Diarrhea, *tufit ta n-lāho*, in such cases is common and is treated with a herbal infusion made from water, *aman*, and *akāmen* (*Zornia glochidiata*). Once weaned, the infant, *āmankas*, becomes a small child, *amārkəs*, and learns to walk, *ad əlməd tekle*, taking a further step away from susceptibility to the *kel tenere* to which a child crawling on the ground is particularly exposed.

The Kel Alhafra pamper and spoil their children, who are allowed to move freely around the tent and encampment. In large families, one of the children will often be brought up by childless kin or by the grandparents.[154]

The older the children get, the more their gender-specific worlds begin to separate. While a young boy will soon join his older brothers watering animals at the well and tending the small livestock, a girl remains with her mother in the tent and is soon participating in the women's activities: prepar-

---

151 A Kel Alhafra child is never put to sleep lying on its stomach because body openings like the nostrils and mouth would be in direct contact with the earth and more easily accessible to penetration by the *kel tenere*. For this reason also, the head of a sleeping child in the dorsal position is always covered with a cloth, and indeed adults also never leave their heads uncovered in sleep.

152 Experts in the Koran among the Kel Alhafra explain that the ideal breastfeeding period of two years is derived from the following Koranic surah: *"wa-l-wālidātu yurḍi'na 'aulādahunna ḥaulaini kāmilaini li-man 'arāda 'an yutimma-r-raḍā'ata 'alā-l-maulūdi lahu ..."* – "Mothers shall suckle their children two years completely, for such as desire to fulfil the suckling." However, "... if the couple desire by mutual consent and consultation to wean, then it is no fault in them" (2:233).

153 *lāho* is the term the Kel Alhafra use to designate the milk of a pregnant mother.

154 In families with many children, a grandchild, *ahāya* (pl. *ihāyawān*), raised by its grandparents, is perceived by the Kel Alhafra as being especially coddled.

ing food, undertaking tasks in and around the tent, learning handicrafts, taking care of her younger siblings, and submitting to maternal authority in the female sphere of tent and encampment, *tārday i-anna-ənnes dāy ehān d-i-tiḍeḍen n-aməzzoy fuk*.

Kel Alhafra children are exempted from religious practices like prayer, *amud* (pl. *imāddān*), and fasting, *āẓum* (pl. *iẓāmmān*) After their circumcision, *illui*,[155] between the sixth and eighth year when they lose their milk teeth, young boys, *ilyāḍen* (sing. *alyāḍ*), in small groups start learning to read and write the Koranic surahs on wooden tablets, *isəllumān* (sing. *asəllum*), if there is a Koranic scholar, *ālfaqqi* (pl. *ālfāqqitān*), in the encampment who can teach them the recitation and copying of the texts. Girls, *tilyāḍen* (sing. *talyāḍt*), take part in these lessons more rarely – for them, preparation for religious exchange in the outside world is less important than preparing themselves for life as a woman and mother within the tent.

From about her seventh year, a girl begins to let her hair grow, and from age ten at the latest, it will no longer be cut. The Kel Alhafra refer to the hair cutting as *asəṭṭəwi*,[156] "the forgetting". While the shaving of the hair henceforth belongs to the past, *telāẓe ta ayy-tāt γās*, a girl now becomes increasingly conscious of her shame, *tākrakəṭṭ*, and inspired by her older friends, *timidawen* (sing. *tamidit*), sisters, *šātma* (sing. *wālātma*), or mother, *anna*, enters into the transition phase from childhood liberty to self-control, *iγulaf n-iman-ənnes*.

---

155 The ritual circumcision of Kel Alhafra boys is undertaken by men of the encampment, preferably they say, seven years, seven months and seven days after birth, *əssa iwətiyān, əssa orān d-əssa išilān*. Kel Alhafra girls are not circumcised.
As is well-known, the number seven, *əssa*, has long been associated with special powers and effects, and it also plays a role in their interaction with nature and the human biology of the Kel Alhafra: a pregnancy lasts 4×70 days from conception to birth; the baptism takes place on the seventh day after birth; at seven years, a boy is circumcised, and a girl lets her hair grow; at 2×7 years, a boy receives the face veil, *aγewəd*, and the girl the *alāššo*; at 3×7 years, an individual becomes a fully fledged member of the society, etc. Such subdivision of the life cycle is known from Greek antiquity and was later taken up by the Arabs, in particular 'Arib and Tabari.
For comparison with the hebdomadal division of the Greeks, see Franz Boll, "Die Lebensalter. Ein Beitrag zur antiken Ethologie und zur Geschichte der Zahlen", *Neue Jahrbücher für das klassische Altertum* 16.31 (1913): 89–145, 114–124. On Arabic representations, see: 'Arīb Ibn Sa'īd al-Kātib al-Qurṭubī, *Kitāb Ḫalq al-ǧanīn wa -tadbīr al-ḥabālā wa-l-maulūdīn. Le livre de la génération du foetus et le traitement des femmes enceintes et des nouveau-nés*, eds. Henri Jahier and Abdelkader Noureddine (Algiers: Publications de la faculté mixte de médecine et de pharmacie d'Alger, 1975/1956) 6:40, 3-11. Ṭabarī, Abū l-Ḥasan 'Ali Ibn Sahl Rabban, *Firdausu-l-Ḥikmat. Die propädeutischen Kapitel aus dem Paradies der Weisheit über die Medizin des 'Ali Ibn Sahl Rabban aṭ-Ṭabarī*, Translated and commented by Alfred Siggel 1953 (Mainz: Akademie der Wissenschaften und der Literatur, Abhandlungen der geistes- und sozialwissenschaftlichen Klasse 14, 1953) 357–463.
156 *asəṭṭəwi* is the verbal noun from *səṭṭəwu* (causative), "to cause to forget, to forget".

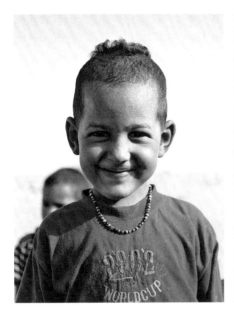

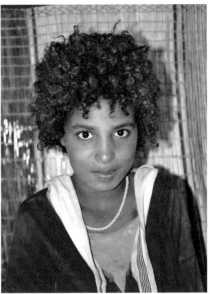

Figure 3.21. talyāḍt – *girl with* taššəkoḍt, *the part of the hair on the back of the head that is not shaved after the baptism (Buneyrub, October 2005).*

Figure 3.22. *From age 10 at the latest, a girl's hair is no longer cut. The Kel Alhafra refer to the last cutting of the hair as* asəṭṭəwi, *"the forgetting" (Buneyrub, October 2005).*

3.4.2. Puberty – *ābārmawāḍ*

Gradually, a young girl learns not only feelings of shame, *təjəš tākrakəṭṭ*, and learns coquetry. She begins to flirt with boys, *sant āddālān d-meddān*, to move differently and to cease behaving like a child, *ənniyāt aba-s tajj imərumorān wi n-ara*. She has her hair braided, *sassākna eγāf-ənnes*, and pays attention to her appearance, *təjənniyāt iman-ənnes*, so that she stands out to the world of boys and men, and can have an existence outside the maternal tent and the feminine sphere.

A *tabārmawāḍt* has left childhood behind but is as an adolescent not yet fully established in the new life of a woman. Her breasts develop, *asədwəl n-ifāffān*, hair grows in the armpits and pubic area, *kəlləf d-amẓādān wi n-tidāydāγt d-n-āšinšād*, and her character also begins to change, *tāšne tamāskal*: one moment she will be cheerful and affectionate, *ijraz-ənnes iman-ənnes d-iwar tāt zarho*; the next she is aggressive and negative, *ti lābassāt d-wār tāt iwar zarho*; she promises things she immediately forgets, *janna hārātān tiji*; daydreams, *tihurja*; and, her feelings swing between generous love and adoration, *tārha māqoorāt d-tārha n-āwadəm*, to hate and absolute disdain, *tokāḍ āwadəm d-itajj-as sund akli-ənnes*. She begins to challenge maternal authority in the tent, rebels and is disobedient, *wār tārdeγ i-anna-ənnes*, seeks her freedom, and develops a curiosity about the male adolescents around her, *təṭṭiwāsān i-imiwāḍān jer imāzzayān*. During this transition phase, when the adolescent is neither a child nor a woman, is outgrowing her mother's care and authority in the tent, but is not yet mistress of her own, she makes a step outside and begins to present herself to the male world as a demure, beautiful, desirable and mysterious woman, *tuffart*, awaiting discovery and, through the social integration of a marriage, *aẓli*, to be borne into a new phase of her life.

Menstruation and the meaning of *tāyimit* or *iba n-amud*

During adolescence, the woman's body becomes more fragile, *tafəkka təlāmḍe*, the female organs being more vulnerable than the male's, and in the Kel Al-hafra view, during menstruation, the bodily fluids enter a state of imbalance that places the entire organism in a state of "heat", *wa n-tākusse*.

Kel Alhafra girls usually experience menarche, *ajmoḍ n-tāyimit*, sometime between the ages of 9 and 13. Although this event used to be marked by the ritual handing over by the mother to her daughter of the latter's first veil, *ekāršāy* or *alāššo*, today many girls start wearing the indigo-dyed veil when their body first starts showing signs of their womanhood (i.e. some time before menstruation). After the first menses, *tənhāy tāyimit*, the *tabārmawāḍt* finally leaves childhood and from now on is more closely surveilled by the community to ensure that she does not become pregnant unintentionally, which would ruin her chances of marriage.[157]

Menstruation is usually referred to by the Kel Alhafra as *tāyimit*, meaning "to sit oneself down, to repose, to take time out". The woman wears an old "pagne",[158] *tasedibəlt*, or places scraps of cloth between her legs, and for the first two of the two to eight days of bleeding, she usually remains sitting in or near the tent, *təqqima dāy mey dādes n-ehān*.

---

157 Rasmussen also notes that among the Key Ewey in the Aïr region in Niger, there is no specific ritual accompanying menarche: "Yet menstruation is symbol-laden and recognized as a sign of change, and at puberty a woman undergoes a clear social as well as biological transition, although there is no ritual for first menses." Susan Rasmussen, "Lack of Prayer: Ritual Restrictions, Social Experience, and the Anthropology of Menstruation among the Tuareg", *American Ethnology* 18.4 (1991): 760. In contrast, Figueiredo-Biton observed that among the Kel Adagh in Mali, at menarche, girls "receive their first veil (ekarshay)", and at the same time, a new specific, hairstyle symbolically marks the transition from childhood to womanhood. See Cristina Figueiredo-Biton, "Initiation sentimentale et sexuelle chez les Touaregs du Mali", *L'autre* 4.2 (2003): 225–237.
   Among the Kel Alhafra, however, the two characteristic hairstyles for women, *tayārye* and *itəl n-bəbba* are, like the gift of the *ekāršāy*, braided for her daughter before the first menses by the mother when she feels the time is right.
158 "Pagne" is the term for a piece of cotton that is worn especially by women in West Africa like a wrap-around skirt around the hips and covering the rear of the body down to the knees.

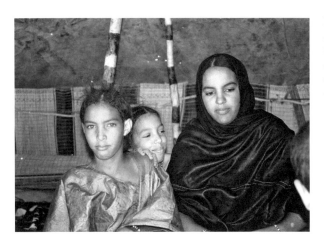

Figure 3.23. *A girl,* talyāḍt, *(left) and an adolescent,* tabārmawāḍt, *(right), can be distinguished by their clothing and their hairstyle. (Inkilla, November 2005)*

For the Kel Alhafra, menstruation serves the purpose of removing surplus blood that, because of her tendency to have a damp-cold constitution,[159] collects continuously in a woman's body and is removed in a kind of self-cleansing during her periods, so long as she is not pregnant. This cyclic cleansing process causes a regular disturbance of the thermic equilibrium which is not equivalent to a sickness as such but can be accompanied by belly pains, *tākmo n-tāsa,* nausea, *tākmo n-ulh,* headaches, *tākmo n-eɣāf,* and emotional discontentment, *ənniyāt wār ihuskāt,* because the body has become overheated, *aswəs n-taɣəssa.* (Only when a woman's cycle does not occur within what is considered a regular range of 25 to 29 days is a woman viewed as "sick".) To restore the balance between hot and cold, *tākusse d-təssəmḍe,* a menstruating woman takes care not to eat any foods designated as "hot", *issukas,* in order to avoid stoking further the body's fire. She will also not wash during the first three days of her menstruation, *wār təsirād,* because a body removing excess blood has "opened", *taɣəssa tamera,* and if she undresses, she will place herself at the mercy of harmful powers.

Unlike the Aïr Tuareg studied by Nicolaisen and Rasmussen, no special domestic restrictions are placed on Kel Alhafra women during menstruation, such as bans on touching food or food containers, on harvesting, or on drinking milk from dams.[160] They are however forbidden to partake in religious ritual practices such as prayer, *amud,* or fasting during Ramadan, *āẓum dāɣ ārrāmāḍan,* because a menstruating body is considered to be sullied, *ikordāt,*

---

159 In the Kel Alhafra conception, because of her moist-cold constitution, the woman is under the influence of the moon, which has an effect on the growth and fertility of moist things.

160 Nicholaisen writes: "... (menstruating women) may not drink the milk of animals that have just had young nor water from leather sacs." Nicolaisen, *Essais sur la religion,* 122. And Rasmussen has observed that: "... menstruating women are not supposed to harvest crops or to touch specific leather containers." In: Rasmussen, 1991, "Lack of prayer", 752.

by the menstrual blood, *āšni wa n-tāɣimit*.[161] Thus, the Kel Alhafra also describe menstruation as *iba n-amud* – "loss of prayer" – although unlike willful neglect of prayer there is no requirement to redeem or make up for the loss.[162]

To avoid forfeiting its ethereal purity, the religious world, which is placed above nature and is free of carnality, must not come into contact with a menstruating woman. She is therefore also forbidden to touch the holy book of the Koran or to wear amulets with Koranic surahs, *tikārḍiwen n-oɣān* (these are only worn by Kel Alhafra women after they have entered menopause).

Tied to her natural cycle, during menstruation, a woman retires into the feminine area of the tent and is also taboo for a man: the Koran forbids sexual intercourse with a menstruating woman.[163] If this precept is ignored and a woman becomes pregnant after an impure coitus, the resultant child can succumb to all sorts of ills, because the Kel Alhafra consider that healthy development of the embryo can only occur when there is a balance between *tākusse* and *təssəmḍe* in the entire body, which is not the case during menstruation.

Most girls marry before they reach menarche, *dat ajmoḍ n-tāɣimit*, and certain husbands do not wait until their wives begin menstruation to have sexual intercourse with them, *wār əqqalān meddān ajmoḍ n-tāɣimit n-tiḍeḍen-nāsān*.

Disturbances during menstruation

adku wa n-tāɣimit / tezzort n-ārori: "abdominal cramps while sitting / back pain"
DYSMENORRHEA

During menstruation many women suffer from pain in the lower abdomen, *tezzort n-adku*, or groins, *tezzort n-ārori*, which the Kel Alhafra women recognize as being gynecological in origin, *dāɣ əssəbab n-torhənnawen n-tiḍeḍen*.

As a remedy, slightly heated cow urine is mixed with butter, *āwas n-tās ikkusān d-udi*, a few days before menstration and introduced into the vagina. If the pains are bad, the woman takes a hip bath in luke-warm water containing leaves of the *ahəjjar* plant (*Acacia adansonii*).

---

161 In contrast to Figueiredo-Biton's description of the Kel Adagh, Kel Alhafra women do not view their condition during menstruation as "closer to the sacred", but quite explicitly as "unclean", *inokall* or *ikordāt*. Cristina Figueiredo-Biton, "Initiation sentimentale et sexuelle chez les Touaregs du Mali", *L'autre* 4.2 (2003): 227.

162 The term noted by Figueiredo-Biton as in use among the Kel Adagh to describe menstruation, "*təməzgidda*" – "mosque" – finds its equivalent among the Kel Alhafra, *tamāsjida*, but is rarely used. See Figueiredo-Biton, 2003, "Initiation sentimentale", 228.

163 Here, Koranic scholars among the Kel Alhafra refer to the following surah: "*wa yas'alūnaka 'an-l-maḥīḍi qul huwa 'aḍan fa-'tazilū-n-nisā'fi-l- maḥīḍi wa lā taqrabuhunna ḥattā yaṭhurna...*" – "They will question thee concerning the monthly course. Say: 'It is hurt'; so go apart from women during the monthly course, and do not approach them till they are clean" (2:222).

iba n-amud wār dāɣ ālwāqq-ənnes: "the loss of prayer that is not according to its time"

IRREGULARITY OF THE CYCLE

May Kel Alhafra women experience an irregular cycle, *iba n-amud wār dāɣ ālwāqq-ənnes*, i.e. periods that to not recur regularly every 25 to 29 days, the failure to menstruate, *iba n-tāyimit*, even in the absence of pregnancy, *mušān wār ila abārkot*, or spontaneous mid-cycle bleeding.

The women view these irregularities as being gynecological in origin, referring to them in general as *torhənnawen n-tideden*, "women's ailments", or *torhənnawen n-təssəmde*, "sicknesses of the cold" (see chapter 4.1.2.1.). But frequent sexual intercourse, *anəməns s-ijāt*, a poor and monotonous diet, *išəkša wār olaɣnān*, overheating or undercooling of the body, *taɣəssa wa n-təssəmde mey wa n-tākusse*, as well as bathing in cold water, *āsirād dāɣ aman issəmdān*, can also cause disturbances in the cycle.

As therapy for irregular cycles that produce bodily hypothermia, *taɣəssa wa n-təssəmde*, and thus a failure to menstruate, a young animal (preferably a goat that is not more than one year old and whose meat in considered "hot") is slaughtered, cut into four parts and cooked in a sandpit until the meat falls from the bones. A stock is made by mixing the meat with *əššāɣ* (wormwood, *Artemisia santonica*), *ālḥālba* (fenugreek seeds, seeds from *Trigonella foenum graecum*), *boɣlām* (cork from the cork oak, *Quercus suber*) and butter, and consumed for a period of three days. This is followed by a three-day diet of pounded and cooked millet, *əsink n-enāle*, mixed with fresh milk, *axx kafayān*, and butter *udi*, a combination to which a "hot" character is again ascribed. If necessary, the women repeat this latter "hot" therapy for up to nine days.

If an irregular cycle is consequent to a bodily overheating, which produces, according to the Kel Alhafra, heavier bleeding, the women prepare a drink with a "cold character", *wa n-təssəmde*, from camel milk, *axx wa n-toḷmen*, and *ālmuxāynes* (*Cleome bradycarpa*), and drink this between and after every meal for three to nine days.

3.4.3. From adolescence through young adulthood to womanhood –
tabārmawāḍt, tamawāḍt d-tamāḍt

It is not uncommon for Kel Alhafra girls to be pledged in marriage to a cousin immediately after birth, and they marry from age ten onward. For the Kel Alhafra, a *tabārmawāḍt* should be living with her husband when her menses begin, otherwise she risks becoming a *tamāḍt tā tijitāɣ*, "a woman to whom something has been added", a woman with an illegitimate child who will spend her live as a social outcast without any hope of marriage. "With us, marriage is not an affair of love" – *"wāddeɣ āwharān tārha d-tādooben"*, the Kel

Alhafra say: its primary purpose is the economic and conjugal union of a man and woman, an act that secures their existence rather than fulfills private happiness. In marriage, the role of the young Kel Alhafra woman is always the passive one ascribed by society to the female – the receptive one. She lets herself be married, *tāsdoobān*, and is given in marriage by her parents, *imārawān-ənnes tāsdoobān*. In contrast, the boys and men, as representatives of the active principle, marry, *ad əjən aẓəẓlyān*, and take a woman, *adoobānan*, validating their existence, setting up a household, settling down, and anchoring themselves in the world of the tent. The woman may be the tent owner, but she needs a male protector, *āmagaẓ* (pl. *imagaẓān*), be it a husband, *āhalis*, father, *əbba*, uncle, *āŋŋāt-ma*, brother, *aŋŋa*, or another male relative, *āmaraw wiyāḍān*, in whose custody her tent stands. And without whose protection and support, she cannot justify her existence in her own dwelling.

It is outside the scope of this study to describe the marriage ceremony, *āddāl n-aẓli*, but after marriage, the young wife is integrated into the family of her husband and is expected to work for her mother-in-law, *taḍāggālt*. *"tamāḍt tārdayāt iḍulān-ənnes tamāḍt ta n-afāran"* – "a wife who obeys her parents-in-law is a good wife", the Kel Alhafra say; she has surrendered her personality, *hak iman-ənnes,* her loyalty, *erkāwāl i-iḍulān-ənnes,* and her trust, *tafləst,* to her husband's kin.

The Kel Alhafra are usually monogamous, and only sedentary and wealthy men or marabouts take more than one wife, though this is a relatively recent phenomenon, *hārāt wa išray*. A Kel Alhafra woman cannot tolerate living alongside a second wife, *wār tārda tijraw*, and so if a man does have several wives, they always live apart from one another in their own households. Divorce, *iməzzəyān* (pl. *aməzzi*), is frequent but not frowned upon. If a divorced woman, *tamāḍt tamizəjət,* is in good health she can soon expect to find another claimant to her hand, and if she brings children from a prior marriage with her, they are likely to be adopted by her new kin and are identified as *ijolan* (sing. *ājola*).

According to the Kel Alhafra, as soon as a married girl begins to menstruate, her husband will seek to make her pregnant, and so she will usually conceive during the phase of *tabārmawāḍt* between 15 and 18 years of age, becoming in the process a *tamawāḍt*, a young adult. An unmarried woman enters the phase of *tamawāḍt* at around 20 years and no later than when she stops growing.

However, to count as a woman, *tamaḍt*, in society requires sexual experience, at least one marriage and to have attempted to become a mother. Single women are rare among the Kel Alhafra; if a young woman is healthy, her parents will arrange her first marriage, and if a healthy woman of childbearing age is divorced or widowed, her kin will see to it that she remarries as soon as possible.

Pregnancy – *təla abārkot*

If amennorhea, *iba n-tāyimit*, lasts for more than a month, the skin becomes pale or almost transparent, *elām amšiši*, the breasts enlarge, *ifesān ifāffān*, and the nipples darken, *ikkāwālnen tidmuma n-ifāffan*, the Kel Alhafra women speak of *tinəhāytān*,[164] pregnancy, which is often accompanied in the first two weeks by nausea, *tākmo n-ulh*, nervosity, *akfor*, and various longings, *tārhawen* (sing. *tārha*). *"təla ənniyāt"*,[165] – "she has an intention (is pregnant)", say the Kel Alhafra, *"təla abārkot"*,[166] – "she has a 'paunch'", *"təla tāsa"*, – "she has a belly", and "will receive/have something" – *"ad təkrəš hārāt"*.

During pregnancy, there is a change in the rhythm of eliminating excess blood, which is no longer held back until menstruation and then suddenly discharged in a relatively large amount, often with cramp-like pains, *tākmo n-ārori*. If conception has occurred, a little of the excess blood is transported each day directly to the embryo, *ebenu*, in a painless process marked by amenorrhea, *iba n-tāyimit*. Henceforth the pregnant woman, *tālxamilt*,[167] "the one who is burdened with a heavy load", finds herself in a constant state of hotness, *n-tākusse*, and until the birth should avoid consuming foods considered hot, *issukās*, in order to maintain her thermal equilibrium.[168]

As soon as a Kel Alhafra woman is sure that she is pregnant – usually sometime within the first four months – she will start to speak of *"ara dāy tāsa-nin"*, "the child in my belly", and views the growing fetus, *ebenu*, as a human with an individual soul, *iman*, who, however, will only receive the divine life-breath, *unfas*, at the moment of birth.

Throughout her pregnancy, a woman temporarily becomes a "creatrice", a woman with creative power, *tamādt təla assəxlək*, in whose body new life is growing. In this state, she receives special consideration from those around her because she has entered a vulnerable condition between life and death, be-

---

164 Literally, *"ti nəhāy tān"* – "those we see/one sees". The Kel Alhafra explanation for this term is that in the early stages of pregnancy, a woman often feels nauseous and leaves the tent in the early morning hours and is seen by her neighbors; later the large belly, *tāsa māqoorāt*, betrays her condition.

165 *ənniyāt* (pl. *ənnyātān*) means literally, "intention" or "attention": *ila ənniyāt ad ajj inhaynānāy* – "he has the intention of seeing us", *"ija ənniyāt"* – "he takes pains", "he watches out", " he is careful".

166 *abārkot* is also applied to the paunches of small livestock. Foucauld describes *abārkot* as "paunch, stomach of ruminants without its contents, the membranous container only". Foucauld, *Dictionnaire Touareg-Français*, vol. I, 95.

167 *tālxamilt* derives from the verb *əlxəm*, meaning "to bind fast", "to stick to one another", "to smother in, provide, wrap in a weight".

168 In other, similar humoral systems such as those in Latin America described by Febrega, pregnant women enter a "hotter" condition than normal. See: Horacio Fabrega, *Disease and Social Behavior: An Interdisciplinary Perspective* (Cambridge MA, MIT Press, 1974) 239.

tween becoming and passing away, a state that is particularly attractive to assaults by the malicious *kel tenere*.

Pregnancy and birth place a Kel Alhafra woman at high risk, *iha miši dāγ təršen hārāt*. There are no prenatal examinations, and many mothers and children do not survive the delivery (see section "Peri- and postnatal complications"). Because of the many dangers, *mišitān*, to which a *talxamilt* is exposed during pregnancy, the Kel Alhafra consider that she should never spend any time by herself in lonely spots, *wār təqqim iman-ənnes dāγ ajāma,* and should not come into contact with a male stranger, *wār tədəsād āhalis wār təzzeyād*. At the same time, her kin and others in the encampment take pains not to frighten her, *wār əssərmān-tāt,* to offend her, *wār əmməjrādān hārāt wa ikma-ās*, or to wake in her any desires for what is unattainable, because unfulfilled wishes and shocks can provoke a miscarriage, *eha*.

A pregnant Kel Alhafra woman continues to perform the usual daily tasks, but takes care not to carry anything too heavy and, as the birth approaches, not to bend down too often. As the delivery day – reckoned as seven times 40 days since the "last washing", *āsirād wa n-ājilal*,[169] (40 weeks = 280 days) – approaches, if her mother is still living, the daughter goes to the former's encampment to deliver the child in the maternal tent, while the father remains behind to look after the other children.

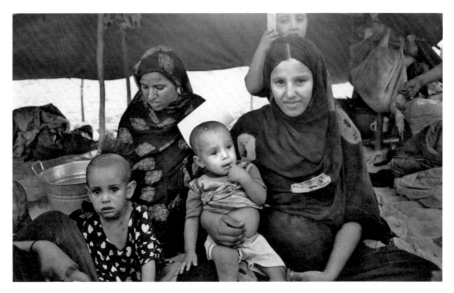

Figure 3.24. *Young Kel Alhafra woman with her first child (under two years old), who is already weaned, because the mother is pregnant again. The child died of meningitis,* eγāf wa lābasān, *shortly after this photograph was taken (Tin Timāγayān, 2005).*

---

169 *āsirād wa n-ājilal* is the ritual washing on the last day of menstruation.

Disturbances during pregnancy

iba n-ašni: "lack of blood"

ANEMIA

The Kel Alhafra women say that if a pregnant woman has pale skin, *elām-ənnes amšiši*, is often tired, *təlḍaš ālwāqq fuk*, weak, *tərəkkəm*, complains of headaches, *tākmo n-eɣāf*, and suffers from dizziness, *aɣālab,* she does not have enough blood, *wār tāt təha ašni inuflāy*. This means that the unborn child will also be undernourished. *iba n-ašni* can be very dangerous for the approaching birth, because the woman will not have enough energy to push the baby out and may die if she loses too much blood.

As a remedy, the pregnant woman is given more meat, *isan*, and other "well-nourishing" foods, *išəkša wi olaɣnen*, to eat.

tawārāɣwārāɣ: "those whose skin turns yellow"

In Tamasheq, *"wārāɣwārāɣ"* means "to spin and look in all directions", a bodily movement that causes dizziness, *aɣalab*, nausea, *tākmo n-ulh*, and a yellow skin discoloration, *elām ārāɣān*. Such symptoms occur especially during the sixth to ninth month of pregnancy, *ɣor talxāmilt dāɣ iyor wa n–sāḍis har iyor wa n- tāẓa*. Women who do not get enough exercise, who do not take a walk every morning, *wār ətīkelnāt hak tifāwt*, and who do not eat enough meat, *wār ākšenāt isan inuflāyān*, are most likely to present with this condition.

tākmo n-ulh/tājlifāt (pl. *tājlifāten*): "pain of the heart" or "a feeling of reluctance"

NAUSEA

During the first three months, a pregnant woman can suffer from nausea and vomiting, *tākmo n-ulh / tājlifāt d-ibsan*, especially in the morning just after she has risen, *s-tifāwt ḍarāt tənkār*. Severe vomiting may cause belly pains, *tākmo n-ermās*, and the *talxāmilt* can no longer eat, *wār tādoobād tetāte*, which may lead to undernourishment.

To prevent nausea, a pregnant woman avoids all foods classified as "hot", and before getting up tries to eat a little salted, cold millet leftovers, *əsink wa n-enāle sammeḍān d-tesəmt n-ašāl āndin*.

təlleɣāf or aɣālab (pl. *iɣālabān*): "the bouncing of the head" or "the dominated and besieged being"

VERTIGO

Like nausea, the Kel Alhafra women say, vertigo usually occurs during the first three months of pregnancy, *dāɣ kārad orān izjarān*, but can also result from *tawārāɣwārāɣ* or *iba n-ašni*, anemia.

aẓāndi

HEMORRHOIDS

During the late stages of pregnancy, the unborn child presses against the organs in the abdomen and can, according to the Kel Alhafra women, provoke hemorrhoids, *aẓāndi*. Constipation, *tāyārt n-tāsa*, literally, "the closing of the belly", is a frequent problem during pregnancy, and this also may also induce the development of hemorrhoids.

Therapy to relieve constipation comprises a laxative made from the leaves of the *tāhahist* (*Cadaba glandulosa*), *ahārjəjəm* (*Cassia italica*) and *balāssa* (*Commelina forskalei*) plants, together with *ākāmen* (*Zornia glochidiata*) seeds. Although hemorrhoids are usually surgically removed or cauterized, neither treatment is applied during pregnancy.

The Kel Alhafra report that pregnant women also suffer from thromboses, *ālfay,* and *tāhafnent.* For more about these, see the descriptions in chapter 4.1.1.

On the causes and handling of miscarriages, see following sections about early abortion, miscarriage and stillbirth, and about causes of miscarriages.

Birth and confinement – *tiwit d-amẓor*

When the labor pains begin, *əššāyāl wa n-təršən hārāt*, a couple of older women "with experience", *tiḍeḍen ti təknāt tamusne*, arrive to help the mother-to-be, *tenāmāẓẓort* (literally, "the suffering one"), give birth. Because there are no professional midwives or birth assistants in Kel Alhafra society, each woman learns from her own experience, *tamusne n-iman-ənnes*, how to give support during childbirth and applies her knowledge as appropriate.

To stimulate labor, the pregnant woman is first given liquefied butter, *udi ijzaynān*, to drink. Between the contractions, the "birth assistants" encourage her to move, *amrumar*, to take a walk, *tekle*, inside the tent. When the bearing-down pains begin, the woman finally lies down in the southern, "male" half of the tent, *teje ta n-ajuss*, on her right, strong side, and the southern part of the tent is screened off by a woven mat from the north, the direction of the *kel te-nere*. A neighbor holds the woman's head, while the mother or a close relative who has been selected as the main assistant, *tanākbālt*,[170] because of her "special experience", *tamusne tahuskāt*, sits at her feet and watches over the ex-

---

170 *tanākbalt* (pl. *tinākbalen*) means literally "someone who supports/welcomes" and derives from the verb, *əkbəl*, "to support", "to encourage", "to welcome". A *tamāḍt ta təkabbālāt* is a woman who assists during childbirth. She is sometimes also referred to as *tamyārt ta təyattāsāt tābutut*, "the old woman who cuts the umbilical cord" (see also next footnote).

pulsion of the baby, while the other women offer words of encouragement and murmur appropriate protective verses from the Koran.

A Kel Alhafra woman gives birth wrapped in her everyday *ekāršāy* lying on a spread-out cloth, *fāll isǝftāy*. Care is taken that she does not become disrobed, *wār tǝsaf,* during the birth process, so that she does not fall victim to the *kel tenere* during this critical phase. While she forces the baby out, the mother's legs are sometimes bound together to prevent excessive tearing of the perineum and vagina; any wounds, *ibiwǝsān* (sing. *ābiwǝs*), that do arise are not sewn after the birth but are left to heal of their own accord. As soon as the child has fully left the birth canal, the divine breath, *unfas*, enters the baby, as signified by the first intake of breath and the first cry. The *tanākbālt* then immediately cuts the umbilical cord to about 30 cm with a razor blade, *lam*, or a special, small knife, *tabṣārt;* the utensils are neither specially prepared nor sterilized in boiling water.[171] The "birth assistants" will wait for up to three hours for the appearance of the afterbirth, before they manually assist in its extrusion by massaging the mother's belly or gently pulling on the umbilical cord. Once the placenta, *timeḍen*, has been released, it is immediately removed from the tent and buried by the *tenākbālt* to the east, *s-emāynāj*, in the direction that is connotated as "holy", so that it can be reabsorbed into the cycles of nature untroubled and unmolested by the *kel tenere*.

The blood and mucus, *ašni d-tǝšānyǝšt*, are washed from the baby with lukewarm water, *amān alāmẓāyyān,* with special attention paid to nostrils, ears, mouth and eyes. It is then dried, wrapped in a cloth and given to the mother. One of the "assistants" discreetly announces the birth to the members of the encampment without mentioning whether it is a girl or a boy: *"tǝkrǝš hārāt"* – "she has obtained something", the Kel Alhafra say, *"tǝjraw anāftāγ"* – "she has received a guest". Only on its baptismal day, *isǝm*, will the encampment officially welcome this "guest" as a new member of the society. For the time being, as its first ritual of arrival in the religious community, the newborn, *itiwit*, is given some water blessed by a marabout to drink, *amān ǝlwǝlitān*, containing a mashed date, *tehāyne taddāhat*, that has been chewed by a man accorded specific religious powers, *ǝfaẓ tāt ǝlwǝli*: the Kel Alhafra call this act *"ewit n-ānya"* – "the rubbing of the palate".[172] Finally,

---

171 Because of this special act during which the umbilical cord is cut, the Kel Alhafra sometimes refer to a *tanākbālt* as *"tamγārt ta tǝγattāsāt tābutut"* – "the old woman, who cuts through the umbilical cord".

172 The custom of *ewit n-ānya* is apparently a widespread ritual of welcome in Islamic soicieties; in this context, Koranic scholars among the Kel Alhafra quote hadiths from *al-Buḫārī* and *Muslim*. See Ṣaḥīḥ al-Buḫārī: 5467, 5476, 3909. Muslim: 2144.

the *tanākbālt* who has cut the umbilical cord and assisted the child in starting its life whispers the call to prayer in the baby's right ear, *tajtāntān ewit n-āyora dāy timāẓẓuj n-ara.*

The baby is not breast-fed for the first 24 hours, *wār isənkās dāy sānatāt timārwen d-əkkoẓ āssayātān ḍarāt itiwit.* If it cries too much, the women give it a little drink of sugared water, *aman d-əssukar*, prepared with slightly pounded leaves of the *tāhahist* plant (*Cadaba glandulosa*), a mashed date, *tehāyne taddāhāt*, or *tafəngora*, pulverized fruit of the baobab tree (*Adansonia digitata*).

For the Kel Alhafra, mother's milk, *axxfəf*, as the potential nourishment for the unborn child, is produced in a protracted brewing process in the body. During pregnancy, the menstrual blood is divided into three portions: one nourishes the fetus, *isudar n-ebenu*, a second is converted into milk, *iməskāla s-axx*, while the last is discharged as lochia, *ufəy n-āšni wa n-āmẓor.* In the production of colostrum, *edāyās*, this process of brewing and transformation is still incomplete, *aswəs wār imda*, hence its impure, yellowish coloration and occasional contamination with mucus, *təšānyəšt*, and blood, *ašni*. Foremilk is thus considered unsuitable as food for the baby.

Lying-in, *amẓor*, lasts for 40 days, *əkkoẓāt timārwen išilān.* It is a time for the mother to return to her pre-pregnancy condition, to regain her thermal equilibrium and to recuperate, *təsonfāḍ n-tamaḍt ta təkrəš hārāt.* During this period, she and the child are in a particularly fragile state and are rigorously supervised and cared for by the encampment women. The mother should eat her breakfast at the same time every day, *tinimāhal a s-takkāl tajumjemtənnes hak ašāl ālwāqq sund wadey*, may not wash while there are vaginal discharges, *wār təsirəd dāy āmẓor*, and must ensure that she is always within the protective environment of the tent by sunset, *tinimāhal a s-təḍu tāfuk təla yorənnes.* Food for the young mother is usually prepared by the *tanākbālt*, the

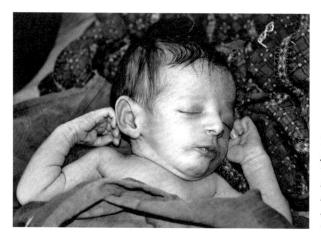

Figure 3.25. *Five-day old girl before her baptism, when she will receive the ritual washing,* ālwāḷḷa, *head shave,* telāẓe, *and her name,* isəm *(Indiārrān, October 2005).*

woman who cut the umbilical cord, and the woman in childbed always eats her meals – comprising foods considered especially nutritious, such as milk, *axx*, meat, *isan*, and butter, *udi* – apart from others. During confinement it is important that she gains weight, *tinimāhal ad timɣar dāɣ āmẓor*, so that she produces enough milk for her child. She breastfeeds the newborn on demand and if she does not have enough milk, the child is given goat or camel milk, *axx n-taɣat meɣ axx n-toḷḷemt*; if it refuses these, it is offered sugared water, *aman d-əssukar,* with *tāhahist* (*Cadaba glandulosa*) instead.

The infant is not washed until the seventh day after birth, the day of its naming, *ašāl wa n-isəm*. Fine sand or powdered *tāhahist* are sprinkled on the navel wound so that it dries out and heals. During the baptism, *isəm*, the child receives a ritual bath, *ālwāḷḷa*, its head is shaved, *telāẓe*, and the eyes are outlined in antimony, *taẓolt*, to protect it from the evil eye, *təšoṭṭ*.

During her confinement, the mother also takes the precaution of painting the rims of her eyes with antimony and wears neither perfume nor jewelry, so that she does not attract the evil spirits to which she is all too susceptible during this vulnerable phase. Like a menstruating woman, she does not wash or participate in prayer, because her body has been rendered unclean, *inokāl*, by the birth and the outflow of lochia, *ašni wa n-amẓor*. By 40 days at the latest, when the flow of lochia has ceased, and the body has recovered from its "hot" to its normal condition, the woman leaves her lying-in bed, *təzjar amẓor*, washes herself, *təsirəd tafəkka-ənnes fuk*, has her hair braided, *sassākna eɣāf-ənnes*, puts on the new clothes her husband has given her to celebrate the birth, *tājimās iməlsan išrāynān wi ikfa āhalis-ənnes*, and returns with the child to her own tent and her husband's encampment, *taqqāl aməzzāɣ wa n-āhalis-ənnes*. However, young mothers often do not stay the full 40 days in their own mother's encampment, especially when they already have children, and return to their family as soon as the vaginal discharges cease, which can be within one month of the birth. If she has a good husband, *āhalis wa ofān*, he will wait for three months after the birth before he seeks sexual intercourse with her again, but, the women say with a smile, men often cannot wait that long, *"meddān wār ādooben oɣāl"*.

Peri- and postnatal complications

iba n-timennāḍ n-təršen hārāt: "the failure of the pains in the attempt to possess something"

WEAK CONTRACTIONS

If the contractions, *əššāɣāl wa n-təršen hārāt*, are too short, too weak, too infrequent or fail to appear altogether, the Kel Alhafra women speak of *iba n-timennāḍ n-təršen hārāt* – "the failure of the colic that accompanies the pains to possess something", which can lead to a delay in the opening or expulsion phase. If the birthing process seems to have come to a standstill, two women take hold of the pregnant woman and force her to move and to run, *tinimāhal a-s-tətajj imərumorān*, give her water blessed by a marabout, *aman əlwəlitān*, or liquified, hot butter, *udi ijzaynān d-ikkusān*, to drink, and massage her belly so that the intestines empty, in the attempt to hasten the birthing process. According to the Kel Alhafra women, *timennāḍ n-təršen hārāt* is especially common among primiparas, and young women sometimes experience contractions for 24 hours or longer. Women who have already had one child usually have less trouble during subsequent births.

iba n-timennāḍ n-timeḍen: "failure of the contractions that expel the placenta"
RETENTIO PLACENTAE

If the placenta, *timeḍen*, is not expelled within the expected time period (one to three hours after birth according the the Kel Alhafra women) and either does not or only partially detaches from the uterus, this can lead to heavy bleeding, *allāɣ n-ašni*. As in the case of weak contractions, *iba n-timennaḍn-təršen hārāt*, the mother is given a drink of hot liquid butter, and her belly is massaged to encourage a strong contraction that will detach and expel the afterbirth. If these attempts fail, after the cervix has relaxed, *ḍarāt asənnārkəb n-em n-tazəzjart n-ijəlla*, the birth assistant pulls gently on the umbilical cord, *temeḍt*, and if this still does not help, she finally places her hand into the body and pulls the placenta out of the womb (though this is a procedure only a "very experienced assistant", *tanākbālt ta təkna tāmusne hullān*, can perform).

ejāḍāl n-ehān: "fall or collapse of the uterus"
INVERSIO UTERI

According to the Kel Alhafra women, the uterus turns inside out, *ejāḍāl n-ehān*, when a birth has not gone well, *kunta əššāɣāl wa n-təršen hārāt āṣṣohen*, the mother is weakened by a succession of too many births, *as tamāḍt ta rəkkəmāt n-āssāmārkəs*, when a child is pulled forcibly out of the birth canal, *kunta ukās n-ara d-āṣṣahāt*, or when, to expel an undetached placenta, too much pressure is applied to the uncontracted uterus and the umbilical cord. The birth assistant immediately reverses the uterus, raises the mother's legs, binds them together and leaves the *tenāmāẓẓort* lying on her back until the uterus has restabilized.

ara wār dāɣ edāgg-ənnes: "a child that is not in its place"
POSITIONAL AND PRESENTATION ABNORMALITIES

If, feeling the belly, the "birth assistants" recognize a breech presentation (i.e. with the baby's pelvis, which feels larger than the head, at the level of the superior strait of the maternal pelvis), two women take hold of the pregnant woman under the arms, shake her, rub butter into her buttocks and smack her in the small of the back and around the buttocks to encourage the child to turn. If it is lying horizontally, only a very experienced *tanākbālt* will place her right hand into the birth canal and attempt to turn the child.

If the child is blocked in the pelvis, *ara irmamān*, the women say that they can do nothing and do not interfere, *wār taḍis*. Either the pregnant woman dies or she survives, and the outcome lies in the hands of God alone, *ihan dāy ifāssan n-māssināy*.

ibiwəsān (sing. *ābiwəs) / tāɣārawiten* (sing. *tāɣārawit*): "lesions"/"those reduced to silence"

Vaginal and perineal tears

During the late stages of birth, or when a child is pulled with a degree of violence out of the birth canal, tissues around the vulva and in the perineal area often tear, especially in young mothers. These wounds, *ibiwəsān* (sing. *ābiwəs*),[173] are not sewn, are very painful, and if urine, *āwas*, or lochia blood, *āšni wa n-āmẓor*, enters the gaping tears, they may develop an infection, *ātunjar*.

To treat the blood-encrusted wound site that is often contaminated with meconium and feces, it is smeared with hot cow's butter, *udi n-tas ikkusān*. When an infection is severe, the woman sits in a tub of lukewarm water containing *ālmuxāines* (*Cleome bradycarpa*) and *ākāmen* (*Zornia glochidiata*). If the vulva is internally damaged, the women prepare suppositories of butter, *udi, ālmuxāines, ākāmen* and *ālɣānfar* (cloves), which are introduced into the vagina. A few women told me that sometimes the tears do not mend, resulting in incontinence, unpleasant odors and great inconvenience to the affected women. Such fistulas are known in Tamasheq as *tāɣārawiten* (sing. *tāɣārawit*),[174] "those reduced to silence", of which no mention is made in public and which are borne with enormous feelings of shame.

allaɣ n-ašni / ufəy n- ašni: "the difficult stopping of bleeding / the flowing out of the blood"

Peri- and postnatal hemorrhage

The emergence of the head is often followed by heavy bleeding, *ufəy n-ašni*, but this may also occur when the uterus is weakened or the placenta prematurely detaches or does not detach at all. The women call such an event *allāɣ n-ašni*, "the difficult stopping of bleeding", and consider it highly dangerous, *iha miši māqoorāt*, because the hemorrhaging woman is losing her life juices.

---

173 *ābiwəs* (pl. *ibiwəsān*) is the verbal noun from *əsəbiwəs* – to hurt oneself.
174 *tāɣārawiten* (sing. *tāɣārawit*) stems from *ɣārāwwāt*, meaning "reduced to silence".

To halt the bleeding, the woman takes a hip bath in lukewarm water to which have been added cow dung, *timāry* (sing. *temāryit*), and leaves of the *təsuya* plant (*Picris asplenioides*). Sometimes cow dung is mixed with *təsuya* and placed directly on the belly.

itunjārān (sing. *atunjār*): "the flaring up again/the relapse"
INFECTIONS

The term *itunjārān* (sing. *atunjār*) is used by the Kel Alhafra to describe various infections. Breast infections, *atunjār n-ifāffān*,[175] can develop during breastfeeding. As a remedy, the women prepare of paste of pepper and water, *ižəkimba d-aman*, which they massage into the breast, or a compress of *ahəjjar* (seed capsules from *Acacia nilotica*) mixed with goat or camel dung, *eyərrajān*, which is placed on the infected site to withdraw "heat" from it.

When the women speak of *atunjār n-ābiwəs n-təršen hārāt* or *ihədədutān* (sing. *ahədədu*) (swelling, abscess)[176] they are referring to an infection of the birth wound(s), which is often accompanied by fever, *tenāde*. Therapy here comprises hip baths as for the treatment of *ibiwəsān*, or, alternatively, the mother sits over a sandpit of smoldering camel dung, *eyərrajān* (sing. *ayərraj*), so that the smoke can enter her body. However, these remedies are not always sufficient and often the mother must simply wait, *əqqəl yās*, until the infection heals of its own accord.

tāhafnent
By *tāhafnent* the Kel Alhafra understand a condition of weakness, *arəkkəm*, or loss of force, *iba n-āṣṣahāt*, occasionally accompanied by fever, *tenāde*, which has been provoked by the waste from poorly digested foods that poison the body internally. (I will return to this clinical picture in more detail in chapter 4.1.1.).

If a birthing mother has *tāhafnent*, she is often too weak for labor, *əššāyāl wa n-təršen hārāt*, suffers from a rapid pulse and nausea, *tākmo n-ulh*, vomits, *ibsan*, has difficulty breathing, *wār tādoobed sənfəs*, and gradually loses her forces, *tarəkkəm*. The assisting women encourage her, feed her a laxative, *isəssənkar*, of butter, *udi*, minced meat, *isan taddāhān,* and *tājārt* leaves (*Maerua crassifolia*), *ifrākitān n-tājārt*. However, the Kel Alhafra women say that, here again, it lies in God's hands whether the mother and child survive.

---

175 *atunjār* is the verbal noun from *ənjər*, meaning, "to fall sick again", "to flare up", "to suffer a relapse".

176 *ahədədu* (pl. *ihədədutān*) is derived from the verb *hədədəy*, meaning literally, "to swell", "to be swollen".

ālfaγ: "the exploding/detonating"

THROMBOSES

Shortly before the birth, but also during the period of confinement, a woman can suffer from nausea, *tākmo n-ulh*, vomiting, *ibsan*, and pains in her thighs, lower legs or soles of her feet, *təkm-e taγma-ənnes, elāγ-ənnes d-itəfrān-ənnes*. The Kel Alhafra call this disorder *ālfaγ*,[177] which translates literally as "the exploding/detonating", and regard it as an escalation of *tāhafnent*. Women who are overweight or who have too little exercise are particularly suscepti- ble to *ālfaγ*, whose symptoms include yellow eyes, *tiəṭṭawen ti tāraγnen*, yel- low gums, *tihayniwen ti tāraγnen*, a yellow skin, *elām āraγān*, and swollen feet, *iḍāran isəkəfān*. The woman drinks an herbal infusion of the leaves of the *ājar* tree (*Maerua crassifolia*), eats lightly mashed whole millet, *tājārāft jārāft n-enāle*, and forces herself to take more exercise.

aḍu: "air"

For the Kel Alfhafra, *aḍu* refers to air that circulates in the organism, *dāγ tayəssa*, in the stomach, *dāγ tāsa*, and thorax, *dāγ tarāja*, and can impede bodily functions.

If a *tenāmāẓẓort*, a woman in labor, suffers from *aḍu*, it can block the labor pains, and if the contractions fail to appear, then the child's life is in danger. Such a woman is given a cathartic made from butter, *udi*, *ālmuxaynes* (*Cleome bradycarpa*), *ahārjəjəm* (*Cassia italica*), *ālišwaḍ* (fine leaves of the *tebāremt* plant, *Cymbopogon schoenanthus*) and cow urine, *āwas n-tas,* while at the same time the assistants massage her lower abdomen to stimulate contractions.

Early abortion, miscarriage and stillbirth – *āšušəf, eha d-oγšad n-tiwit*

If the fetus, *ebenu*, is expelled during the first four months (3×40 days) of a pregnancy, the Kel Alhafra speak of *āšušəf* (pl. *išušəfān*), an early abortion, in which the embryo is described as *āššāf*, "the one that swims in a fluid". Loss of the fetus during this stage of pregnancy is frequent according to the Kel Al- hafra and receives no special attention or mention by the women concerned: the bleeding is treated as a heavy menstrual bleeding, and the accompanying pain may indeed by misrecognized as dysmennorhea or as a menstruation with pain that is noticeably more severe than usual.

Only when the child's body is further developed, between the fourth and seventh month (after the last "day of washing", *āsirād wa n-ājilal*, the end of the last menstruation), and the embryo is recognized as a child, *ara*, with a di-

---

177 *ālfaγ* is the verbal noun derived from *əlfəγ*, meaning "to burst", "to explode", and "to detonate".

vine soul, *iman*, do the Kel Alhafra women speak of *eha* (pl. *ehatān*), a miscarriage. At this stage of the pregnancy, the fetus has not matured sufficiently, *wār inŋŋān inuflāyān* (literally, "they are not sufficiently cooked"), for the child to have enough force to participate actively in the birth. Hence loss at this stage is not viewed as a normal birth event but is perceived as a miscarriage, *eha*, and the woman wraps the fetus in a cloth and buries it east of the tent outside the *asəfrāḍ*, the cleaned circle around the tent.

Children that are born dead after the seventh month of pregancy are *aratān immutnān*, "dead children" of *"oyšad n-tiwit"*, "a disturbed birth". Because such children are fully developed and basically capable of life, they have the right to a proper burial and are washed, wrapped in a cloth and buried in the direction of the *qiblāt*. However only a newborn that dies during or shortly after birth having already received the divine breath, *unfas*, and has breathed independently for a while, is treated as a discrete personality and is accorded the full mourning rites with sacrifices and prayers.[178]

Causes of miscarriages

tarəmməq:[179] "anxiety, shock, agitation"

The Kel Alhafra women say that most miscarriages are caused by an event that provokes strong emotions in the pregnant woman. These strong emotions heat up an organism already in a hot state due to the pregnancy, leading to blockages or, through "overcooking", *aswəs n-tayəssa*, to spontaneous evacuation. "The belly empties itself", *sātf n-tāsa*, and the fetus is lost in the bleeding.[180]

Mariamma told me how, during her last pregnancy, she was searching for wood not far from the encampment: "Suddenly, quite nearby, a gun went off; the noise startled me so much that I began to bleed at that very moment", – *"sallāy i-amāslu n-ālbārroḍ i-ohazān, isārmāy-ahi hullan a-fāl ālwāqq ti-dāy*

---

178 On the beliefs and practices around premature births among the Tuareg in Azawagh (Niger), see Saskia Walentowitz, "L'enfant qui n'a pas atteint son lieu. Représentations et soins autour des prématurés chez les Touaregs de l'Azawagh (Niger)", *L'autre, cliniques, cultures et sociétés* 5.2 (2004): 227–242.

179 *tarəmməq* is the verbal noun from *ərməy*, meaning literally, "to be excited, concerned, shocked".

180 The concept of *tarəmməq* is apparently also perceived as a basic cause of miscarriage among the Tuareg in Azawagh (Niger): "An emotional shock (*teremméq*, litt. 'fright') on receiving bad news, like that of the death of someone close, constitutes another cause of death *in utero* and premature birth. It is thus necessary to protect the future mother from situations that might engender strong emotions, especially during the first four months of gestation, because during that time the uterus can open suddenly and the child, which is in the phase of passing from a liquid to a solid state, risks 'falling out'." Walentowitz, "'L'enfant qui n'a pas atteint son lieu,'" 230.

ufəy n-ašni isənta".[181] Others tell of arguments with their husband or a neighbor, hearing bad news, or similar shock-like events that provoked miscarriages.

tārha or derhan: "strong desire, passion"

Like *tarəmməq*, vehement desire, *tārha*,[182] or strong wishes, *derhan*, during pregnancy can provoke a miscarriage.

The Kel Alhafra women say that a pregnant woman who experiences strong desires that are not fulfilled becomes stiff focusing on her wishes. As a result, her heart becomes cramped, precipitating a state of shock in her body, the outcome of which is, once again, evacuation of the fetus. If bleeding has already started in a woman who has succumbed to *tārha*, this will, however, stop immediately if she gets what she is longing for. For this reason, a pregnant woman should never be refused anything, and everyone in the community takes great care not to arouse unrealizable longings in her.

ejāḍāl: "fall"

If a *tālxamilt*, a pregnant woman, falls from a donkey, *ejāḍāl n-ešāḍ*, or from a camel, *ejāḍāl n-amənis*, or trips and falls over somewhere, such a fall, *ejāḍāl*, according to the Kel Alhafra can cause an "emptying of the belly", *sātf n-tāsa*, a miscarriage.

issukās: "hot foods"

If the body of a *tālxamilt*, which is already in a hot state due to the pregnancy, receives additional heat through food, it can overheat, *aswəs n-tayəssa*, and attempts to return to its thermal equilibrium by expelling blood. However, during this compensatory bleeding, the fetus is also flushed out.

The Kel Alhafra women report that eating habits have changed significantly in recent years. Before the droughts and political troubles, they nourished themselves almost exclusively on milk, *axx,* butter, *udi,* and meat, *isan.* Since the decimation of their herds, however, this diet is no longer available to them and they must consume too many new and "hot" foods, *imənsiwān wi n-əšrāynān d-ikkusnān*, such as oil, *sund dilwil*, millet, *enāle*, rice, *tafāɣāt,*

---

181 Interview with Mariamma Wālāt Muḥammad, Inkilla, November 2006.

182 In Tamasheq, *tārha* also means "love", the term always being understood as embracing the notions of desire and striving for union with the desired one, a state that can quickly lead to a morbid fixation, which as a pathological condition is referred to using the same term, *tārha*. In her work on traditional medicine among the Tamasheq in the Timbuktu region, Le Jean describes *"tārha"* as a "malady of the heart", also known as *"al waswasat"*. The Tamasheq disapprove of excessive emotions that can turn into such fixations, viewing them as the work of the antagonistic Iblis. *al-waswasa*, the diabolic suggestions lead to passions that like a *ǧinn* can take hold of a person and make him or her mad. See Le Jean, *Médecine traditionelle*, 84.

pasta, *mākkāruni*, and tea, *ātay*. Such a diet is in their view very detrimental, *a iha aḍārora*, to the body's inner thermal equilibrium.

terk mājārāḍ d- tǝšoṭṭ: "bad speech and the evil eye"
If someone shows anger towards a *tālxamilt* or speaks badly of her, "her soul aches", *tākmo n-iman-ǝnnes*, she is emotionally wounded, a situation that, as in *tarǝmmǝq* and *tārha*, can provoke strong emotions, during which the heart cramps up, and blockages or a state of shock develop in the body which can lead to a miscarriage. Jealousy, *tiṣmiten*, of a pregnant woman in particular has the effect that *tǝšoṭṭ*, the evil eye, activates the *kel tenere* whose pernicious powers can rob the prospective mother of her child.

Greater contact with the outside world
The Kel Alhafra women say that they used to live much more isolated lives in the desert. Today lorries from Algeria come to the wells to sell goods, *ašāli malanāt i-torfen anu imarān šanšen-in d-ǝddināt-i hārātān-nāsān*, the young people go to the cities, *imiwāḍān ǝjǝlān ajāma ǝkkān iyǝrmen*, and the men seek work elsewhere, *meddan immayān ǝššāyāl dāy iyǝrmen*. Since their contact with the outside world has increased, diseases have become more common and include those they have never experienced before, *torhǝnnawen wār ti nezzāy*, and there have also been more miscarriages.

During the drought of 2005 when a plague of locusts crossed over the land consuming everything in their path, airplanes sprayed the area with a white powder, *torfen n-išǝnnawān osānāt-dd dāy awātay wa ti tǝlla tašwālt, ǝjjanāt ta hārāt n-ejel wa māllān fāll ihǝkšān*. The camels ate anything that the locusts had left behind, including the residues of the powder, *ikšan tan imǝnas*, and the goats and sheep also grazed among the dead insects. "Afterwards, not only did the animals have more abortions, our women also suffered from more miscarriages" – *"dāy awātay-dāy ḍarāt awen ihan ehatān ājootnān dāy irǝzzejān hakǝd yor tiḍeḍen-nāsān"*.

Therapies for bleeding during pregnancy
If bleeding occurs during pregnancy, the women attempt to arrest it by drinking several times a day a decoction of henna powder, *ejel wa n-hālla*, dissolved in water. Henna (*Lawsonia inermis*) is considered "cooling", *wa n-tǝssǝmḍe*, and should help the body to compensate for the excessive heat.

Fertility, contraception and sterility – *āsāmārkǝs, iba n-asǝmru d-ajǝjru*
If a woman bears a child every year without interruption, she is known among the Kel Alhafra as *tamāḍt asǝmmārkās*, "a woman who is very fertile". *"tǝla tišer"*, "she is fertile", the women whisper behind their hands, but never

out loud, in order not to provoke the *kel tenere*. The evil eye, *təšoṭṭ*, lurks in *asəmmārkās*, in the state of permanent pregnancy, the women say. Nobody wants to be pregnant and bearing children all the time: "this weakens not only the woman, but also her children" – *"išəlḍaš tamāḍt d-aratān-ənnes daɣ"*.

Many women do not get pregnant while they are breastfeeding, *wār təla abārkot kunta tamāḍt tāsənkas*, but for a *tamāḍt asəmmārkās*, this rule does not apply, and she can do nothing about her perpetual fecundity. The Kel Alhafra have heard of *timāɣwānen*, pills that can prevent conception, but they themselves know of no chemical or biological contraceptives, nor of any plants or plant extracts that can be used to prevent pregnancy.[183] "If we knew of something, no woman would bear an illegitimate child", they observe with a smile, *"a-fāl nəsan-t wār təlla tamāḍt tijitāɣ wāla"*. To prevent a pregnancy, it is, rather, the husband who must be abstinent, though he rarely can be, or he must practice coitus interruptus or a sexual practice known as *jer tāɣmiwen*, "between the thighs", or *jer tibəlloḍen*, "between the buttocks", in which a man does not penetrate the woman but reaches orgasm between her thighs or buttocks.[184]

A *tamāḍt təjujārāt*, a woman who cannot become pregnant, is not considered by the Kel Alhafra as sick and is not excluded by the society. Sterility, *ajəjru*, can, according to the Kel Alhafra, affect both men and women, but such a problem is never discussed openly. A man's sterility becomes obvious when he has many wives but none of them become pregnant until they have left him. Male sterility is considered untreatable, *wār ihen isəfrān*; female sterility, on the other hand is viewed as a temporary condition that can be rectified.

The women state that they know neither the causes nor treatments for *ajəjru*, *wār nəsan əssəbab wāla isəfrān*; sometimes a woman simply turns into a stone, *sund tāhunt*, when her husbands approaches, and in this "petrified state" she cannot become pregnant.

3.4.4. Old age and death – *amɣār d-taməttānt*

After menstruation stops around 50 years of age, a woman leaves the reproductive phase of her life and becomes a *tamɣārt*, an "authority", "a respected

---

183 Hureiki writes, however, that the Tamasheq can provoke abortions for example by using the sap, leaves or charred wood of the *torša* bush (*Calotropis procera*), or with the sap of the bitter colocynth (*Colocynthis vulgaris*). See Jacques Hureiki, *Tuareg, Heilkunst und spiri- tuelles Gleichgewicht* (Schwülper/Hülperode: Cargo Verlag, 2004) 163. The Kel Alhafra women, however, say that they would know if a plant was capable of such effects, *kunta təlla tisāɣta tāssohet sund wadeɣ, nəsan-t*; the plants mentioned by Hureiki can provoke vomiting, *ibsan*, but not complete "emptying of the belly", *sāṭf n-tāsa*.

184 See here also the descriptions by Edmond Bernus, *Touaregs Nigériens. Unité culturelle et diversité régionale d'un people Pasteur* (Paris: L'Harmattan, 1993) 158 ; Henri Lhote, *Com- ment campent les Touaregs* (Paris: Susse, 1947) 505, on the Tuaregs in Niger.

woman", who possesses "stature", "importance" or "prestige", *təla təmɣāre d-təmmənya*.

"tamɣārt tijbəs", the Kel Alhafra say, "the old woman is wearing a belt", she is "dried out". Released from the cyclic bondage to nature, "her belly is tied up" – *"tāsa-ənnes tijbəs"*. She will no longer menstruate or get pregnant again, so can devote herself without restrictions to prayer and celebrating the religious rituals and can wear amulets containing Koranic verses, *tikarḍiwen n-oɣnawān*, because her body is no longer in an "impure" condition. *"iba s-təha tiḍeḍen"* – "she no longer possesses that which classifies her as a woman", the Kel Alhafra say, and a *tamɣārt* thus takes on an almost gender-neutral position in society, her voice is heard, she can say what she wants and what she thinks, *tādoobād ad tānn a wa tārha dāɣ d-a wa ta s-təjānn*, can receive strangers, *tādoobāad ad asəlkāḍ i-inaftayān*, support her neighbors, *tādoobād ad tilal n-inhārājān-ənnes*, make decisions, *tādoobād ad təja a wa tārha wāla tasəstān n-āwadəm*, rebuke her sons, who usually live in the same encampment, *tādoobād ad tānn i-aratān-ənnes a wa ajjen*, and boss around her daughters-in-law, *tādoobād tāhkāmāt tiḍulen-ənnes*.[185]

The older a Kel Alhafra woman becomes, the more she involves herself in religious activities, and as her life approaches its end, she increasingly engrosses herself in her dialog with God through prayer. According to the Kel Alhafra, God has determined the day on which each individual's life will necessarily end, *tāɣrəst təmda*: *"tamudre ti jəzələt taməttānt ijma tāt āššāk"* – "life is short, of death there is no doubt". Old people appear not to fear death: they often suffer from various ailments that their difficult existence in the desert only accentuates, and they see in death a relief from earthly hardships. *"taməttānt ta rāqisān, tamudre ta təẓẓəwāt"* – "death is easy, life is hard", an old lady told me; she was not afraid of her end in this world and placed her trust in God and his mercy, *"wār əqsudāɣ taməttānt, əfləsāɣ dāɣ Māssināɣ d-ānnoɣmāt-ənnes"*.

If someone in the encampment is dying, kin visit to provide assistance and support during the last hours and to take leave of the dying person. *"ānš-ahi"*, "forgive me (what I have done to you)", they murmur to each other, so that the dying person is at peace with those closest to her before the soul leaves the body. If a child dies, its soul will go directly to paradise. In the case of an adult, the good and bad deeds in this life, *timašālen d-terk timašālen*, will be

---

185 Rasmussen describes the transition from the reproductive to the post-menopause phase of a woman's life among the Kel Ewey in Niger in the following article: Susan Rasmussen, "From Childbearers to Culture-Bearers: Transition to Postchildbearing among Tuareg Women", *Medical Anthropology* 19.1 (2000): 91–116.

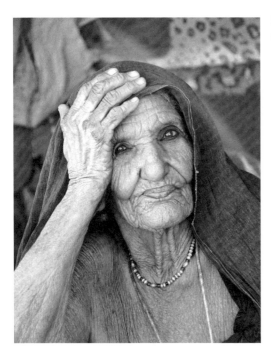

Figure 3.26. tamɣārt *in an encampment at Tin Timāɣayān (October 2005).*

weighed against each other on judgment day, *āssayāt wa n-ālxisab*. (On the fate of adult souls in the next world, see section 3.3.5.).

When a woman dies, her body is washed by female kin. When a man dies, his last washing is performed by male members of the encampment. The sand on which this washing has taken place, *āsəssarād*, is shoveled up and deposited north of the encampment. If a close relative has died, Kel Alhafra will often travel enormous distances to offer their condolences to the bereaved, *āšəwwəškən*.

After the washing, the corpse is wrapped in a cloth and, whenever possible, carried on the day of death itself by the men to the cemetery, *tifəska*, if there is one close by. Otherwise the men dig a grave, *aẓekka* (pl. *iẓəkwan*), east, *s-emāynāj*, of the encampment. The body is placed on its right side in the grave, with the head in the south and the face turned toward Mecca. It is then covered with clean sand, and a large stone is placed at the position of the head and feet (for women, the Kel Alhafra place two stones at the foot of the grave). The grave site is finally covered with thorny twigs to deter wild animals, *tiwāɣsen* (sing. *tawāqqāst*), from interfering with the corpse. Graves are not individually identified, and after the burial they are neglected. The deceased are honored, instead, in such religious festivities as *ālmoulud*, during which after a communal prayer, a memorial procession takes place to a nearby cemetery.

Women do not accompany the funeral cortege to the cemetery and remain behind together in the tent to quietly mourn and lament. When the men return, an animal belonging to the dead person is sacrified, *tākaffart*,[186] cooked, and eaten by the guests in a commemorative meal, *ākarrad*.[187] For seven days after the death, the surviving kin drink *aman n-ahəjjar* (water containing *Acacia nilotica* seed capsules) every day in memory of the deceased. Traditionally, a goat or sheep should also be sacrificed and consumed on the seventh and 40th day after the death, but the Kel Alhafra say that this custom is usually disregarded today because they no longer own enough animals.

If someone dies of a serious disease, their clothes and belongings are burned after death. Places where people died, *idggāān wi n-nānmetān*, are avoided because they are sites that attract the *kel tenere*: *"edāgg dāɣ ətfā n-iman iqsud-t iman"* – "there, where a soul has been spilled out, other souls are afraid", the Kel Alhafra say. The names of the dead are no longer spoken aloud after they have passed away, and photographs are burnt: to name something is to bring it to life, and a dead soul must be allowed to continue its eternal existence in the next world unmolested by the living.

3.5. Health in everyday life

3.5.1. Hygiene – *ašəšədaj*

Body hygiene

The Kel Alhafra rise in the still comfortably cool early hours before dawn to milk their herds, make butter and prepare millet for breakfast. Everyone washes their face and hands before the first prayer, *dat amud wa n-tifāwt hak āwadəm əsirād idəm d-ifassān-ənnes*. Afterwards, the women or older girls shovel the *təsātfi,* the sand in which small children have urinated during the night, out of the tent and hang the soiled bedding to air and dry in the sun. The face and hands of children are also washed in the morning, but never their entire bodies, to avoid their catching cold in the sometimes freezing first hours of the day.

In general, the Kel Alhafra pay more attention to their outer appearance than to thorough bodily hygiene, and the people themselves confirm that they wash less often today than they used to: *wār nāsirād sund əmukān wa n-ihənnin*. They often find themselves far from a well, and water that has been laboriously brought to the encampment is valuable. However, even when the hair has not been washed, it is carefully braided, finger- and toenails are regularly cut short with a razorblade, and before a visit to a neighboring encampment, the thread-

---

186 *tākaffart* (pl. *tikaffaren*) refers to the sacrifice in commemoration of the dead person, from whose herds a goat or a sheep should be slaughtered on the first, seventh and 40th day after his or her death.

187 *ākarrad* (pl. *ikarradān),* the ritual commemorative meal for the dead means literally, "the binding together", "the bound being".

bare, everyday *ekāršāy* is exchanged for clean clothing. For the Kel Alhafra, a respectable outer appearance is tantamount to a healthy physical and spiritual condition, and only the ill and those with psychic problems neglect how they look, *āmarhinān wār ikkulān iman-nāsān yās.*[188]

Until an infant is about two years old it is constantly with the mother who cleans the child whenever it gets dirty, although urine-soaked garments are not necessarily seen as grounds for a wash. From two years on, when the mother is often caring for a new baby, "the child begins to flee the water", the Kel Alhafra say, *"ad sənt s-efel n-aman"*: it is no longer the focus of maternal attention or control and evades whenever possible the disagreeable procedure of being washed.

During the hot months of *ewelān* or *akāsa*, both adults and children sometimes pour water over one another's heads, but the purpose here is more to cool the sweating, overheated body and help it return to thermal equilibrium than to clean it. Adult women usually wash themselves thoroughly on the last day of menstruation, but otherwise just hands and face are cleaned before and after eating. Hands, face and feet receive a ritual cleansing before prayer, and a religiously prescribed ritual washing should also be performed after sexual intercourse.

Water is not only immensely valuable and the soul of life, *aman iman*. Natural water is also recognized by the Kel Alhafra as *aman n-tināriwen*, "water of the demons", which can elicit sickness. Because a naked body, according to the Kel Alhafra, magically attracts the *kel tenere*, and the exposure of body openings presents an evil *ğinn* with the opportunity to penetrate the body, great caution is taken with regard to cleaning the body. Furthermore, during the cold months, *s-tajrəst*, when the temperatures sink to 0 °C and people are particularly susceptible to cold-related diseases, they do their utmost to avoid additionally cooling the body with water.

The hair, from a western perspective, is also rarely washed. The Kel Alhfra women explain that frequent washing damages it, and that is why they protect their hair from the sun and dry air by greasing it with butter, *udi*. They also delouse it on occasion and braid it into elaborate and long-lasting styles. When they wash their hair, the women add to the water the plant *taləggid* (*Cyperus jeminicus*), which is purported to make the hair smooth and glossy.

---

188 The healer Fadi Walett Faqqi corroborates the statements made by the Kel Alhafra: "The state of one's hair, fingernails and teeth is considered an indicator of an individual's physical and mental health: unkempt hair, long and dirty fingernails, teeth yellow with tartar are the signs of someone who is seriously unbalanced." Walett Faqqi, *Isefran*, 12.

Teeth, *isenān* (sing. *esen*), are cleaned by adults with twigs from the *tešāq* and *ājār* trees (*Salvadora persica* and *Maerua crassifolia*), an antiseptic effect also being attributed to the "toothbrushes", *tisāqsānen* (sing. *tasāqsint*), fashioned from the *tešāq*. Women often clean their teeth additionally with charcoal so that they stay white and shiny.

When the Kel Alhafra move into the outside world, visit a neighboring encampment, travel to the market in Ber or even further, to Timbuktu, they put on their best clothes. The women wear their jewelry, wrap themselves in a cloud of perfume they have bought from the Algerian traders who stop occasionally with their trucks at the wells, and a neighbor braids their hair. On an everyday basis, however, they wear the same *ekāršey* day and night until it is falling apart. It may be washed every now and then, but given the value of water, only if there is enough of it around, and there is a well not too far away.

Hygiene in the tent and encampment

In the morning, the tent is tidied up and the bedding rolled up and stored above the floor on the *tijəttawen n-ilālān*, the wooden stakes in the northern and southern tent halves on which baggage and other items are hung so that scorpions, *tiẓərḍam* (sing. *tāẓarḍəmt*), spiders, *sorasān* (sing. *sorās*), small, black insects called *tigədugəden* (sing. *tāgədugət*), and snakes, *taššalen* (sing. *taššālt*), cannot hide in them. Then, a young girl or the tent owner herself cleans the tent floor with a small brush, *asəfrāḍ*, sometimes sieving the sand with a special sieve, *temey ta n-āsaltāf*, to free it of detritus, *erdān*. An area with a radius of about 3 to 6 meters around the tent, *asəfrāḍ*, is kept as clean as possible for prayer and to avoid sitting in places polluted by animals. Waste is always deposited in a northerly direction outside this *asəfrāḍ*, where hands are also washed, the mouth rinsed and dirty water is thrown away.

On Friday evenings and at dusk on nights with a new moon, the Kel Alhafra burn in their tents resin of the *adāras* tree *(Commiphora africana),* which they call *umm ālxer*, "the mother of well-being or happiness". The aromatic fumes, *aḍu*, are said to cleanse the tent of malign influences, protect it against assaults by the *kel tenere*, while at the same time exercising a healing effect on the soul.[189]

---

189 In his study on the Kel Dinnik and Kel Attaram in Niger, Bernus describes how the resin of the *adāras* tree is used especially in perfumes or as incense to pleasantly scent the air inside the tent: "The gum of the Adaras (metelkher) has a very special use: it is burnt, mixed with perfumes, inside the tent, releasing a fragrant smoke during gatherings." Edmond Bernus, "Cueillette et exploitation des ressources spontanées du Sahel Nigérien par les Kel Tamasheq", *Cahiers ORSTOM* 4 (1967): 43.

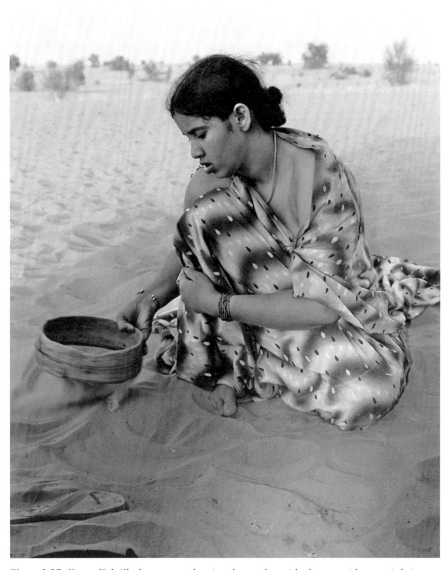

Figure 3.27. *Young Kel Alhafra woman cleaning the sand outside the tent with a special sieve,* temey ta n-āsaltəf *(In Astilan, February 2005).*

The Kel Alhafra live in close proximity with their animals, and although in general these are denied entry into the tent (unless they are sick or very weak), impertinent goats or sheep inevitably slip in unobserved every now and then to poke among the kitchen utensils and stores, leaving behind the traces of their invasion. Children often play in sand that has been soiled by animals and urinate and defecate in and around the tent. Most of the time, this waste is not removed immediately with the small shovel, *āsaltəf*, and attracts swarms of flies that can spread microorganisms (on the management of human excreta, see section 3.3.3.).

Vermin such as lice and fleas, which go under the general designation *tilken* (sing. *tillek*), are daily companions, and in the broiling midday hours when everyone seeks out the cool shadows of a tree or tent, children and women often delouse one another. Because of the almost permanent shortage of water, bedding and clothes infested by lice and fleas are not washed but are occasionally hung out by the women to air in the sun. With the Kel Alhafra living at such close quarters in the tents and encampment, vermin can spread rapidly, and entire families will often be affected by scabies, *ašyoḍ*, or by mycetogenetic dermatoses such as *ākorkor*.

In the pastoral cycle, the Kel Alhafra strike camp every 1 to 2 months in search of new grazing grounds and in this way regularly escape the encampments that have over time become soiled by both humans and animals. However, when they settle in villages or towns, they take the hygiene customs of the desert with them: they often do not construct latrines; they let the children urinate and defecate anywhere, and deposit, as before, their waste outside the *asəfrāḍ*. This behavior leads to overflowing mountains of refuse in the residential areas on the outskirts of Ber and Timbuktu, ideal breeding grounds for causes of fecal-oral infectious diseases.

Food storage and preparation

The Kel Alhafra keep food stores such as bags of rice and millet either on the baggage pole in the male side of the tent, *fāll tijəttawen n-ilālān ti n-āhalis*, or outside on a wooden tripod, *ijəttān n-āllon*, between the north of the tent and the kitchen area. Mice, *ikārran* (sing. *ākor)*, or the somewhat larger jerboa, *iḍawān* (sing. *eḍāw*), often get into the grain sacks, so many families own a cat, *muss* (pl. *mussāten)*, to deter these bold but unwanted rodents.

Vessels containing fluids are always covered with a lid, *eləffi*, and butter, *udi*, is also stored by the women in a closed bottle, *dāɣ buntāl*, or canister, *dāɣ bidon*. In general, the Kel Alhafra try to ensure that no foods or drinking water are left exposed for the *kel tenere* to settle in and enter the human body when consumed. The Kel Alhafra mention, however, that their traditional

wooden vessels like the large bowl for eating, *taẓāwat*, or the smaller containers, *ikassān* (sing. *ākoss*), in which food is stored are gradually being replaced
by *ikassān n-taẓoli d-n-mānna*,[190] metal and plastic containers, which drain the
foodstuffs of *ālbarāka*, their divine creative, procreative and healing powers.

The meat from slaughtered animals, *isan*, is dried outside the tents, at-
tracting countless flies, *ešan* (sing. *eš*), in the process. However, the women
carefully remove any maggots, *tiwǝkkawen* (sing. *tawǝkke*), before the meat
is cooked. Flour and grain sacks are often infested by worms, *tiwǝkkawen*, or
small, brown beetles, *tukmaten* (sing. *tukmat*), but again these are sieved or
picked out before the food is prepared.

Depending on the distance, the men fetch water from the wells either
daily or every other day, bringing it back to the encampment in goatskin
bags, *iddidān* (sing. *iddid*), or the inner tubes of truck tires, *šambǝrertān*
(sing. *šambǝrer*), and hang the containers on special posts for this purpose,
tijǝttawen n-iddidān. Evaporation keeps the water in the goatskin bags pleasantly cool, but the water in the black rubber tubes heats up and acquires an unpleasant taste, *aman dāγ šambǝrertān ihan terk temḍe*. Older Kel Alhafra especially are of the opinion that water stored in the truck tubes loses God's
blessing, *ālbarāka*, and makes people and animals sick. However *šambǝrertān*
are cheaper: the *iddidān* not only require the slaughter of a valuable animal,
they demand time and effort to make and must be regularly rubbed with butter for conditioning.[191] Thus young families in particular are slowly replacing
them with *šambǝrertān*.

There is large variation in the quality of the well waters in Azawad. Overall, the Kel Alhafra consider the water of their wells to be "palatable", *aman
wi n-unwan-nānāγ āẓẓidnen*, even though small, red worms are clearly visible in the water at Tin Timāγayān, and the water at Buneyrub tastes slightly
salty. Water is considered bad only when it is very salty or obviously polluted and tastes foul, *terk temḍe*, or smells strange, *aḍu n-aman irka*, as happens when a dead animal has fallen down the shaft into the well. More prob-
lematic is water from the river, *aman n-ejreu*, or from pools and puddles, *aman
n-iγārγārān d-iγātāllābān*, left behind after the rains, which animals drink and
people use to wash themselves. "The water of the south near the river is not
good" – *"aman wi n-ajuss s-tarrāyt n-ejreu wār olayān"*, the Kel Alhafra say,
and there are diseases lurking in it, *tǝhen torhǝnnawen dāγ aman wi-dāγ*. Some

---

190 The Kel Alhafra term for plastic is *mānna*, which means literally, "aridity", and derives from
     the fact that during droughts trees die off, there is no longer enough wood to make the cus-
     tomary eating and storage vessels, and these are replaced by plastic utensils.
191 The Kel Alhafra routinely grease their goatskin bags, *iddidān*, with *balāγa*, shea butter, to
     keep the leather supple and to prevent it from drying out and cracking.

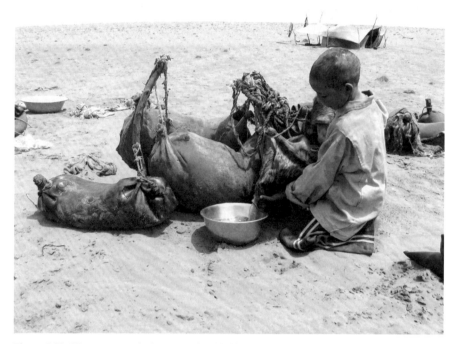

Figure 3.28. *Water sacs made from goatskin,* iddidān, *and rubber tubing,* šambərertān, *hanging on* tijəttawen n-iddidān, *special posts situated south of the tent (Buneyrub, June 2005).*

Kel Alhafra are convinced that the annually increasing prevalence of the fever, *tenāde,* at the end of the rainy season is attributable to the poor water quality; nonetheless, the suspected water is never boiled. Milk, *axx,* is likewise never heated over a flame and is processed raw, or immediately drunk as fresh milk, *axx kāfayān.* The Kel Alhafra are not aware that there are diseases such as tuberculosis and brucellosis that can be transmitted by the consumption of raw milk.

It is usually the men who slaughter the animals – although women do so in their absence – in the northeast, at some distance from the encampment. A fire is usually lit at the slaughter site, *edāgg wa n-ayārras,* and offal such as the liver, *ayrum,* kidneys, *tijāẓẓālen,* spleen, *amlāqqis,* heart, *ulh,* and lungs, *torawen,* are immediately roasted and eaten. The remaining meat is either cooked or dried, the intestines are rinsed and the stomach emptied and cleaned; apart from the hooves, *tinsāwen* (sing. *tinsāw),* horns, *iskawān* (sing. *isək),* the lymph nodes, *tifəyen* (sing. *tefāyt),* and the skin, *elām,* everything else from the animals finds its way into the Kel Alhafra kitchens.

Before they start cooking or handling foods, the Kel Alhafra always wash their hands. During the preparation of a meal, the women never clean a child or touch skins that have been tanned. Cooking is always done outside the tent and the women clean dirty dishes and utensils before they are used again. They also wash cereals such as millet and rice with water before the grains are ground in a mortar or before they are cooked whole. The Kel Alhafra rarely eat raw food (with the exception of *ašədder*, the millet drink for which the millet is pounded but not cooked), because in their opinion, raw and undercooked foods stick to the stomach wall and induce ulcers. There are neither vegetables nor fruits in Azawad and if the men go to market at the most they return with dried onions, *tayfart*, or more rarely tins of tomato purée, *tikbaten n-tāmati*, both of which can be stored and usually end up in a meat sauce. There are no vegetables in the traditional Kel Alhafra diet, but women who spent time in the refugee camps in Mauritania or Algeria, and learnt how to grow and prepare vegetables there, deeply regret that fresh products are neither grown nor available in Azawad. "If only we had tomatoes, cabbage, beans, epplants, carrots and potatoes, and could plant something" – *"əndār ənnəhāl yor-nānāy tāmati, šu, tadāllāyt, oberšin, karot, konbəter d-əndār nādoobed ad nādomm ilkāḍān"*, was the complaint of one young woman, "the settled people in Ber or along the river are much better off, they own gardens and can plant what they want" – *"əddināt wi iməzzāyān tāyrəmt n-Ber mey tarrāyt n-ejreu, əllant idāggān n-ādomm n-hārātān fuk wi irhanān"*. The older generation, though, do not want to know anything about these "vegetables", and would be quite content if the animals just provided enough milk for everybody once more, *"əjrazān-nānāy fālas irəzzejān ihen axx āttasān əddināt fuk"*.

3.5.2. Food customs in everyday life
Basic foodstuffs
axx:[192]milk

"aman iman, axx isudar" is perhaps the most well-known Tamasheq saying, *oẓẓ* (pl. *oẓẓawān*), "water is the soul (of life), but milk is nourishment (for the body)".[193] *"axx wa māllān wār t-illa wa ofān"*, the Kel Alhafra add, "there is nothing better than white milk", because milk refreshes the heart, the seat of the soul, *axx isəssmāḍ ulh wa edāgg n-iman*, provides the organism with en-

---

192 *axx* is used in Tamasheq to describe any substance with milky properties: *axxfəf* is mother's milk, *axx n-torša* and *axx n-təlaxx* describe the milky juices in the stems and leaves of the plants *Calotropis procera* and *Euphorbia scordiafolia*, respectively.

193 In Tamasheq, *isudar* means "food", "nourishment", but also "support" and "revival". The word *isudar* contains the verb *əddər*, meaning "to live", "to be alive", reflecting the vital, nourishing character of *isudar*, without which the human organism cannot work; instead of *isudar*, the Kel Alhafra sometimes also use the word, *taməddur* – "indispensable nourishment for the body's functioning".

ergy and builds up one's health, *axx ihe āṣṣahāt d-ihuskān i-assexāt*. Milk is the preferred foodstuff among the Kel Alhafra, and a well-nourished *tamyārt* at Tin Timāɣayān told me that she lived exclusively from milk and meat: "if there had been no more milk, I would have died long ago", *"a-fāl iba-s illa axx, tamdure-nin təmda"*, she said with a smile; she had never eaten anything else and if one day she were forced to, she thought it would signal her end. Today, however, many Kel Alhafra families can no longer speak as this old woman did – their herds are too small for milk to provide the basic, let alone the exclusive, non-meat foodstuff for months at a time.

The cycle of milk production by camels, cows, goats and sheep is a fragile one, dependent on the early onset of the rains, the amount of precipitation, the condition, distance and accessibility of the pastures, and the health of the animals. Even small variations in the system can have devastating consequences, as the late onset of the rains in 2005 and the locust plagues have shown. Just as disastrous and disruptive to milk production, though, are epidemics among the animals, or caterpillar, *tazləft* (pl. *tizəlfen*) (*Lymantria dispar*),[194] infestations in the pastures, after which, according to the Kel Alhafra, the ruminants suffer abortions.

The female animals give the most milk shortly after they have given birth; milk production then falls off gradually, usually stopping altogether when they are re-inseminated. Sheep and cows bear their young *s-akāsa*, in June and July, while goat kids are born *s-tajrəst*, between November and January (though some goats also have kids *s-akāsa*). If goat milk runs out in the hot months of the dry season, *s-ewelān*, humans and animals suffer from a "milk shortage", *iba n-axx*, until the return of the rains in June/July, *s-akāsa*, and the sheep start providing their milk, *axx n-tihātten*, again. Camels however not only have no fixed period of parturition, their duration of milk production is also the longest, up to 18 months.

Many Kel Alhafra do not own female camels though some men tend herds belonging to wealthy owners living in the towns. During the dry season, however, such herds are usually grazing in the far north of Mali or in southern Algeria and often have to travel enormous distances in the search for suffi-

---

194 The caterpillars of the gypsy moth (*Lymantria dispar*) can cause anything from extensive damage of leaves to total loss of the vegetation mass. If they have stripped the trees clean, food preferences become irrelevant and the caterpillars consume anything that is green, forming disordered, crawling columns along the ground in their search for food. Contact with caterpillar hairs can cause mucosal irritation or elicit local dermatitis. The caterpillars often bite through the stem of the leaf on which they are sitting, so that they fall together with the leaf to the ground. There, they are eaten by grazing animals. The Kel Alhafra consider the gypsy moth poisonous and capable of provoking abortions in the ruminants.

cient graze and browse. The men usually accompany the animals alone while the women and the children remain behind in the Azawad encampments near wells. Despite the long lactation period of the camel, the high mobility of the herds means that many families are deprived of the pleasures of their milk.

Tabel 3.6. *Annual lactation periods*

Animal Species	Month											
	Jan	Feb	Mar	Apr	May	Jun	Jul	Aug	Sep	Oct	Nov	Dec
Sheep								▒	▒	▒	▒	▒
Goats	▒	▒	▒	▒								
Camels	▒	▒	▒	▒	▒	▒	▒	▒	▒	▒	▒	▒
Cows	▒	▒						▒	▒	▒	▒	▒

If they are in good health and there is ample pasturage, sheep and goats can give birth twice a year (their gestation period is about five months).

The animals are always milked in the early morning when they have stopped ruminating, and at dusk when they lie down for the night near the tents to chew cud. It is usually the young boys and girls of the encampment who milk the sheep and goats, while men are responsible for milking the camels and the cows, collecting the milk in the *akābar*, the wooden container for milk. Women only do this work in the men's absence. After milking, the *akābar* is always handed over to the tent owner who pours the milk into a wooden bowl. She alone then decides on the distribution of fresh milk, *axx kāfayān*, and how much will be kept back and further processed into sour milk, *axx islayān,* butter, *udi,* and cheese, *tikāmmāren* (sing. *takāmmārt*).

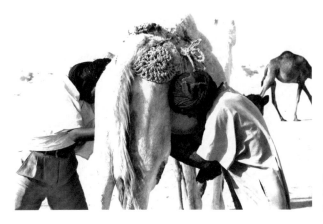

Figure 3.29. *Camels are always milked by two men (In Agozmi, March 2005).*

axx n-toḷmen: camel milk (lactation duration of mares: up to 18 months)
"axx n- toḷmen wa ofān", the Kel Alhafra say, "milk from the camel mare is the best". It is considered the most healthy and the best-tasting milk and to have a "cooling" character, *wa n-təssəmḍe*; it also keeps for a long time. However, the Kel Alhafra usually drink camel milk fresh as *axx kāfayān*, and men especially, with their somewhat "hot" and active temperament as inhabitants of the southern tent half, are happy to down liters of this cooling nourishment to thermally equilibrate their bodies. The Kel Alhafra do not pasteurize camel milk, and because it does not coagulate, they do not use it to make milk or cheese.[195]

axx n-iwan: cow milk (lactation duration of cows: 7–8 months)
Few Kel Alhafra families possess cows: "keeping cows is not really part of our tradition" – *"irəzzejan n-iwan wār dāy ālyadātān-nānāy"*, they say, because "cows have to be watered too often, and with our well system this is very difficult" – *"irəzzejan n-iwan wār dāy ālyadātān-nānāy"*. In addition, good pastures for cows tend to be found in the south, near the river. Cow milk is considered very fatty, and so it is usually made into butter, *udi*, or drunk fresh. Fresh, it is ascribed a "hot" character and is therefore particularly recommended for women suffering from gynecological illnesses classified as "cold". However, if the milk becomes stale, its character turns from "hot" to "cold" and it provokes *tāhafnent*.[196]

axx n-ulli: goat milk (lactation duration of goats: up to 5 months)
Goat milk is considered "hot", *wa n-tākusse*, and is highly appreciated by the Kel Alhafra because the mothers bear their young in the cold *tajrəst* months of November to January. Goat milk is also often used to prepare medication for "cold illnesses", *torhənnawen n-təssəmḍe*, but because of its "hot" character, when drunk on a daily basis it should always be diluted with some water.

axx n-tihātten: sheep milk (lactation duration of sheep: up to 5 months)
Milk from sheep is the least enjoyed of the milks because it "assumes the taste of the pastures", *axx n-tihātten ihe temḍe n-akāsa*, and sometimes tastes of a

---

195   In his article "Laits touaregs. Usages et symboles", Bernus writes that in Niger, "The Tuareg explain that characteristic [that camel milk does not coagulate] as due to the fact that the camel does not possess the fatty envelope (afadaghan) that surrounds the abomasum: 'the camel has sold it to the spines of the trees so that these do not tear its muzzle or tongue when it is eating the small leaves of the thorny trees'." Edmond Bernus, "Laits touaregs. Usages et symboles", in *Ressources vivrières et choix alimentaires dans le bassin du lac Tchad, eds.* Christine Raimond, Eric Garine, Olivier Langlois (Paris: Editions et Prodig Editions, 2005) 399–412.
196   See chapter 4.1.1. for a description of *tāhafnent*.

bitter herb; nevertheless, as the first milk after the poor months of the dry season, *ewelān*, its production by the sheep is awaited with longing. Drunk fresh,
the Kel Alhafra ascribe to it a "hot" character, *wa n-tākusse*, but if it is left
for a while, it cools down and becomes "cold", *n-təssəmḍe*. If the Kel Alhafra
have enough sheep milk, they prepare from it a dry and non-perishable cheese,
tikāmmāren.

āllon: cereals

For the Kel Alhafra, cereals represent a substitute food eaten only when they
do not have enough milk. If the rains come on time in June, the sheep begin
to give birth a month later (and goats can also have offspring twice a year, i.e.
also during the rainy season) and produce milk that, in a normal seasonal cycle, provides the main food source for the Kel Alhafra during *akāsa* (June to
August). Only when a family owns too few animals, or when a catastrophe
of some kind has stemmed or even halted milk production, do they see themselves obliged to switch to eating cereals. When milk is plentiful, cereals are
rarely consumed, and some people avoid them altogether; only from September, as the flow of milk ebbs do the Kel Alhafra supplement their milk consumption with cereals.[197] In the cold months, *s-tajrəst*, as the production of
goat milk declines, it is gradually replaced by cereals, and from the middle of
April until the beginning of the rainy season, *akāsa*, in June/July, cereals such
as millet, *enāle*, rice, *tafāyāt*, and flour, *ejel wa n-ālkāma*, become the main dietary component.

However, in 2005, when I was living with the nomads, a poor rainy season was followed by a plague of locusts, and as early as February, millet and
dishes made from flour were the main source of nourishment. From April until
June, nearly every encampment was without milk, and the people were weakened and haggard. Again, by February a year later in 2006, many families were
once more eating only millet. The Kel Alhafra told me that now, for six months
of the year they must depend on cereals as their staple food source, and the
millet, *enāle,* or flat bread, *tajəlla*, can only occasionally be supplemented with
a little meat or milk.

enāle: millet (100 kg: CFA 15,000–25,000)

Millet is the cereal most familiar to the Kel Alhafra – they have been buying it
for generations from traders from the south at the local Saturday market in Ber

---

197 During the transition from milk to cereal consumption, the Kel Alhafra recommend that one
stops drinking fresh milk, *axx kāfayān*, and switches to sour milk, *axx əssəlayān*, so that the
body is better prepared for the intake of the plant foods.

or the larger market in Timbuktu. "But in the last few years, the millet prices have kept rising", *"əqqimātnen n-enāle iẓẓəwātān n-iwətiyān wi išraynān"*, the Kel Alhafra complain. For many families, it is becoming almost too costly to purchase, and the men travel by camel or donkey into "the Dogon country" to acquire it more cheaply at source, but this deprives the encampments of valuable manpower for extended periods of time.[198]

tafāγāt: rice (100 kg: CFA 25,000–30,000)
"Rice has only recently appeared on our menus" – *"tafāγāt wār tāhojād dāγ imənsiwān-nānāγ"*, an old Kel Alhafra woman told me, "earlier, rice was the cereal of the wealthy" – *"tafāγāt ihənnin allon n-imenokālān"*. The rice the Kel Alhafra eat today is imported from countries as distant as Thailand and follows millet on their cereal preference list. However, because it is always more expensive than millet or flour, it is usually only served on special occasions, for guests or at festivities. Nevertheless, many old Kel Alhafra refuse to eat rice, disdaining it as "the diet of the people in the south" – *"amənsi n-əddināt wi n-ajuss"* and preferring instead the familiar millet, *"nāsof enāle fāw"*.

ejel wa n-ālkāma (farin): flour (100 kg: CFA 12,500-20,000)
The Kel Alhafra use flour, *ejel wa n-ālkāma* ("cereal powder") or *farin*, to bake a hard flat bread, *tajəlla* (pl. *tijəllāwen)*, in a sandpit. After it has been cooked, it is broken up into a bowl and served, like millet or rice, with oil, *dil-wil*, butter, *udi*, or a sauce, *aḍrəẓ*, poured over it. *tajəlla*, however, is served only to provide some variation in the diet or when millet is scarce. Flour is sold by Algerian traders, often directly to the Kel Alhafra from the trucks that stop at the wells (usually at Inokender). It is the cheapest of the cereals, and during food shortages, as in the first half of 2005 for example, for many families flour becomes the main dietary component over several months, because millet becomes rapidly unaffordable (in 2005, one 100 kg. sack cost CFA 30,000).[199]

---

198 The price of millet shows not only seasonal swings, it also varies depending on where it is cultivated. In the major arable zones in the south, it is generally cheaper than in the north, and so the Kel Alhafra travel in donkey or camel caravans as far as the Dogon country to exchange animal products and salt for the millet, or more rarely, to buy it with cash. During drought years, even this millet can become unaffordable, but is, or should be, offset by food aid and imports.
199 Interviews in In Astilan with Mariamma Wālāt Muḥammad, Tā'ana Wālāt Hameyya, Tin Albarāka Wālāt Hameyya, Ninde Wālāt Attta, February 2005 and February 2006.

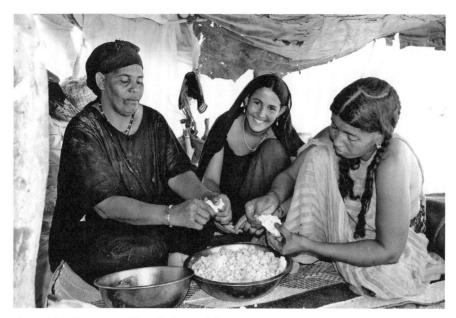

Figure 3.30. *Women crumbling flat bred,* tajəlla *(In Agozmi, March 2005).*

isan: meat

Meat is not a part of the daily Kel Alhafra diet. Families often do not eat any meat for several weeks until a special opportunity arises: guests arrive, there is something to be celebrated, a sick animal has to be slaughtered or a successful hunter brings his catch back to the encampment. Many families possess few animals of their own, and they are not allowed to eat the meat of the herds they tend for sedentary owners living in the towns. "There is too little meat today", the Kel Alhafra say, *"wār illa isan ajotnān",* and "we no longer have enough of it for a stock of dried meat" – *"wār nādobād əsāyār isan".* They believe, however, that meat should be eaten at least once a month, otherwise one falls sick and will suffer from *tākmo n-ulh* (nausea/heart trouble) and *tāhafnent.*[200] Going for more than 40 days without eating meat also brings bad luck.

Of the domesticated animals, meat from the pig, *əlxənžār,* dog, *edi,* cat, *muss,* and donkey, *ešāḍ,* is considered unclean and is proscribed. The Kel Alhafra enjoy eating meat from sheep and, most of all, that from camel mares, *isan n-tihātten mey isan n-toḷmen wi ofān,* to which they ascribe a "cold" character, *wi n-təssəmḍe.* Meat from the cow, *isan n-tas,* and the goat, *isan n-taɣāt,* however, is considered "hot". Not only is this less appreciated, when such

---

200 For descriptions of *tākmo n-ulh* and *tāhafnent* see chapter 4.1.1.

meat comes from animals more than one year old, it is believed to be responsible for the transmission of diseases that are classified as "hot".

The Kel Alhafra rarely eat fish, *imānan* (sing. *emān*), even when they are living temporarily near a river, or water pools during the rainy season. "Fish smell" – *"imānan ərkanān"*, the Kel Alhafra say, and, furthermore, they swim in natural water, *dāy aman n-tināriwen* (i.e in the element of the small demons), raising further doubts about their quality as a food.

Opinions about fowl are divided. Some Kel Alhafra view hens, *tikāzaten* (sing. *tekāzit*), as unclean because they pick up their food in the dirt of others. However, some nomad families moving in the southern Azawad keep a few small hens and a cock, *ikāzan* (sing. *ekāz*), which occasionally end up in the cooking pot.

It is mainly children and herdsmen who hunt birds, *ijḍaḍ* (sing. *ejāḍeḍ*), with slingshots. Buzzards, *ijuyas* (sing. *ājayəs*), quails, *tibārruten* (sing. *tābārrut*), guinea fowl, *tāylalen* (sing. *tāylalt*), spotted sand grouse, *takāḍuten* (sing. *takāḍut*), crows, *tekriten* (sing. *tekrit*), ravens, *eẓuyaj* (sing. *āẓayəj*), and ducks, *tikunšāmen* (sing. *tākunšāment*), are all considered suitable for roasting over a fire and eating. While herding small livestock, the young boys and herdsmen also catch lizards, *agezzamān* (sing. *agezzam*), jerboas, *iḍāwan* (sing. *eḍāw*), squirrels, *ikolān* (sing. *ākolān*), wild cats, *aydiwen* (sing. *ayda*), fennecs, *ikorsəyān* (sing. *ākorsi*), jackals, *ibāggan* (sing. *ebāgg*), hares, *timārwālen* (sing. *temārwālt*),[201] and in rivers of southern Azawad, turtles, *ikāyon* (sing. *akāyon*).

Meat from wild desert animals, *isan wi n-tiwāysen n-tenere*, such as the small dama gazelle, *ašənkaḍ* (pl. *išənkaḍ*), a somewhat larger gazelle species, *tenhert* (pl. *tinheren*), the dorcas gazelle, *edām* (pl. *idāman*), vultures, *išeyer* (sing. *ešeyer*), and anteaters, *idhəj* (sing. *adhej*), is considered particularly tasty and much appreciated because it has a largely "cold" character. However, such animals are now very rare in the Azawad, and they are rarely caught today.

tesəmt: salt

The Kel Alhafra flavor their food with rock salt from the mines at Taudenni that still gets transported to Timbuktu in camel caravans and gets sold at the local markets. They rarely use other seasonings when preparing their food. The iodine content of this salt is, however, quite low (0.02 ± 0.04 mg/kg). The human requirement for iodine lies at around 100–200 mg per day, and although

---

201 Many adult Kel Alhafra do not eat meat from hares, because they considered it to have a bad taste, *terk temḍe*, and also because hares, like women, menstruate, which in the Kel Alhafra view renders the meat unclean.

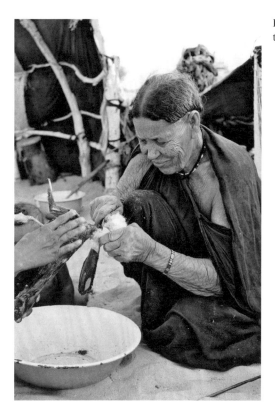

Figure 3.31. *Skinning a hare,*
temārwālt *(In Astilan, February 2005).*

foods such as milk, eggs and fish are good sources of iodine, they may be consumed little or not at all by the Kel Alhafra. Iodine deficiency increases the
risk of miscarriages and stillbirths and can cause defects during the development of the fetus.[202]

Meals – *imənsiwān*

The Kel Alhafra eat one main meal a day, either at midday or in the evening,
depending on when the family members are in the encampment. However,
they say that a person should eat something nutritious at least twice a day, *ilzam ad təkšəd sānatāt tāniwen dāɣ ašāl hārāt tāṣṣohāt.* They split up by sex
and age to eat: the young women eat together as do the children, the adult men
and the old people. Only when the nuclear family is alone together do they eat
from the same bowl, using beautifully carved wooden spoons or their right
hand. Before eating, hands are washed and the basmala is recited. The Kel Al-

---

202 See Claudine Prudhon, *La malnutrition en situation de crise. Manuel de prise en charge thé-
      rapeutique et de planification d'un programme nutritionnel* (Paris: Action contre la Faim,
      Karthala, 1995) 29.

hafra remain fairly silent during a meal and it is considered impolite to look at others while they are chewing food, *wār təsəjrād āwadəm wa itatt*. Each person should only take food from a shared eating bowl from that part that is nearest to them, and the distribution of meat or a sauce is solely the decision of the host or the head of the household. The Kel Alhafra attach importance to eating moderately, especially when one is not among one's own family, and in general they do not eat to full satiety, because "you must stop eating before your belly begins to press on you" – *"ilzam kāy ad təsəmdəd tetāte wār šādd əndi fāll tāsa-ənnāk"*. Having eaten enough, the spoon is placed to one side, the person rises, thanks God with a blessing and moves away to wash her or his hands. One should only drink after a meal, *ilzam-kāy ad təswəd ḍarāt tetāte*, the Kel Alhafra say, otherwise the stomach fills with water, *təḍnāyād tāsa-ənnāk s-aman*, and one will soon be hungry again, *təjlakād šik*. They also advise resting for a while after the midday meal before resuming activities, *id təkšəd amənsi sonfād dadāy əndi səntəd əššāyāl*, but not after breakfast or the evening meal: "after breakfast and the evening meal you must not sit or lie down but you must do something before you can take a rest again" – *"ilzam-kāy ad təknəd hārātān ḍarāt tājumjemt d-amənsi, wār tāqqimād d-wār təsonfād"*.

tajumjemt: breakfast

The Kel Alhafra rise shortly before dawn during the hot months of *ewelān*. The men milk the animals while the women begin pounding millet in order to cook *əliwa* (pl. *iliwatān*), a kind of millet or rice porridge. To prepare *əliwa*, the millet grains are hulled, *əsuṣṣābāt,*[203] and broken up in a mortar before being cooked to softness in some milk-water, *aman d-axx*, then seasoned with salt *tesəmt,* or sugar, *əssukar*. During the hot season, many women also prepare *ašədder* (pl. *išəddar*), a nourishing millet drink made from incompletely ground millet, *asəṣṣabu taddāhān ambānnān,* pounded cheese, *takāmmārt taddāhāt*, mashed dates, *tihāyniwen taddāhnen*, together with *tafəngora*, pulverized fruit of the baobab tree (*Adansonia digitata*) and red pepper, *ižəkimba* (*Xylopia aethiopiaca*). Some water is added to this mixture, and the mass is kneaded and formed into small balls, *tikrurəyen təndārrātnen*, that, when dried, can be stored for a long time. To make the drink, the *ašədder* balls, *tikrurəyen n-ašədder*, are dissolved in water, and a little milk, *axx*, or soured milk, *axx əssəlayān*, may be added. The drink is very effective in quenching the thirst and for assuaging hunger during the day. The Kel Alhafra appreciate

---

203 *əsuṣṣābāt* describes the action of pounding the millet to separate the grain from the bran (*asəṣṣəbu* is the verbal noun from *əsuṣṣābāt*).

ašədder particularly when they are traveling, *s-išilān wi n-āsikəl*, when food is short, *iba n-imənsiwān*, or when there is a lack of wood, *iba n-isāyerān*, because *ašədder* can be prepared without cooking and is quickly filling.

It is predominantly in the cold season, *s-tajrəst*, that the women also prepare *əsink n-enāle*, by pounding the millet grains into a powder, *ejel*, which they then cook in water, stirring continuously until it forms a thick porridge. This is then cooled and served salted in a wide bowl, *dāy tazāwāt*, with milk, *axx*, or butter, *udi*.

s-akāsa, during the milk-rich rainy season, many families also drink a bowl of fresh milk, *axx kāfayān*, or soured milk, *axx əssəlayān*, for breakfast, without any additional cereals. A morning cannot really begin, however, without the first glass of tea, *ālkisan n-ātay*, which every man drinks before he sets off for the wells with the empty water sacs, *iddidān mey šambərertān a wār iha hārāt*, and the donkeys, *išāḍān*.

amэkli: the midday meal

When the men return at midday, *s-tārhut*, from watering the animals at the well, *asəsu n-irəzzejān yor anu*, and with their asses heavily laden with filled water sacs, for fortification and refreshment, they often first drink some sour milk, *axx əssəlayān*, or *ašədder*.[204] When there is ample milk available, the midday meal is skipped. Otherwise the women may prepare *əsink n-tābālāttāst*, a millet dish made from whole, dehusked grains cooked to softness, *asəṣṣəbu saŋŋān*, served with either liquid butter, *udi imazlayān*, or a meat sauce, *aḍrəz n-isan*. Other popular midday dishes include rice with butter, *tafāyāt d-udi*, or *aman n-isan*, rice served with a meat sauce (in which the sauce, *aḍrəz*, is made from meat, *isan*, butter, *udi*, or oil, *dilwil*, with perhaps some dried onion, *tayfārt*, water, *aman*, and salt, *tesəmt*).

If millet is expensive and in short supply, the Kel Alhafra prepare a dough from white flour, *ejel wa n-ālkāma (farin)*, salt, *tesəmt*, and water, *aman*, which they bake in a sandpit under a layer of sand overlain with glowing charcoal. The flatbread, *tajəlla* (pl. *tijəlwen*), has quite a heavy texture and is considered somewhat difficult to digest, *tāẓẓāyt*. When cool, the Kel Alhafra break the bread into small pieces and pour butter, *udi*, oil, *dilwil*, or a meat sauce, *aḍrəz n-isan*, over it. As mentioned above, though, meat dishes are usually only served on special occasions, and the most common sauces are liquid but-

---

204 When their thirst, *fad*, is intense, the Kel Alhafra never drink water, which they consider only increases one's thirst. Someone who is very thirsty is first offered concentrated, undiluted sour milk enriched with *akāmān* (*Zornia glochidiata*) and red pepper, *ižəkimba* (*Xylopia aethiopica*), and only afterwards should he or she drink water, otherwise the symptoms of thirst such as dizziness, *təlleyāf*, or headaches, *tākmo n-eyāf*, are merely aggravated.

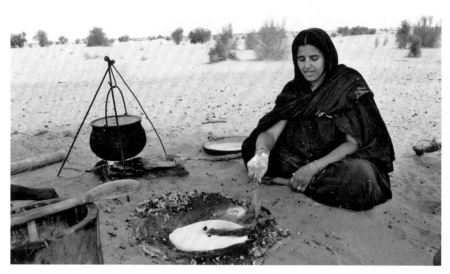

Figure 3.32. tajəlla, *a flat bread made from white flour,* ejel wa n-ālkāma, *water, aman, and salt,* tesəmt, *baked in a sandpit under glowing charcoal (In Astilan, February 2005).*

ter, *udi imaẓlayān,* oil, *dilwil,* sour milk, *axx əssəlayān,* or milk, *axx.* The midday meal is always rounded off with sweet tea, *ātay āẓẓidān,* and then during the often burning hot midday hours, the entire family takes a nap in the shadow of the tent.

amənsi: the evening meal

In the evening, when all the encampment inhabitants have returned from their daily tasks or a visit to a neighboring encampment, the Kel Alhafra usually eat *əsink n-enāle,* a millet porridge served with fresh milk, *axx kāfayān;* if they have not eaten anything substantial at midday, this will be accompanied by *əsink n-tābālāttāst,* millet with butter, or *tafāyāt d-udi,* rice with butter. Many Kel Alhafra are of the opinion that one meal a day is sufficient: "if you've eaten at midday, an evening meal is no longer necessary" – *"kunta təkšəd s-tārhut, wār imiyatār-ak ad təkšəd s-ehāḍ harwa".* The evening meal often ends with a glass of sweet tea, although many women do not drink tea at night, attributing a stimulating effect to the green tea from China: "if we drink tea at night, we do not sleep" – *"kunta nəswəd ātay s-ehāḍ wār nāṭṭās",* a young woman at Tin Timāɣayān claimed.

Nutrition of infants and children

Small children are usually breastfed until they are two years old, *tamāḍt təsənkās alyāḍ-ənnes har əssin iwətiyān,* assuming the mother does not become pregnant again, *kunta wār tənniyāt abārkot* (see chapter 4.4.1.). The mother's milk, *axxfəf*, however, is usually supplemented with animal milk, *axx n-irəzzejān*, especially the goat milk classified as "hot", *axx n-tayāt wa n-tākusse*, and the camel milk classified as "cold", *axx n-toḷmen wa n-təssəmḍe*, to restore the child's thermal balance as and when necessary. The women often enrich this milk with sugar, *əssukar*, or pulverized baobab fruit, *tafəngora*.

After the first six months, the women begin to feed the children *iləwa*, a millet or rice porridge, to which they often add *takrəttit*, small balls of fresh butter, or some liquid butter, *udi imaẓlayān*; in between, they always offer the child fresh milk, *axx kāfayān*, or sour milk, *axx əssəlayān*. From six months, *sādis orān*, a small child will also try out cooked meat pounded in a mortar, *isan saŋŋān d-taddāhān*, and from one year on, at midday the mother will offer the infant a porridge of cooked millet, *enāle n-imāndārrān*, or rice, *tafāyāt*, with crumbled cheese, *tikāmmāren taddāhān*, butter and milk, *udi d-axx*. Until it is two years old, however, small children only eat solid food at midday, in the evening they are fed milk, *axx*. Once weaned at around two years, *kunta ara əmmukās ḍarāt əssin iwətiyān*, the child is given the same food as the adults, *"ara wa ihan əssin iwətiyān tādobed tetāte sund ere iššāmān"*.

3.5.3. Cultural classification of foods

The dichotomy hot/cold – *tākusse d-təssəmḍe*

As already discussed in earlier chapters, the Kel Alhafra perceive the universe as an interaction of oppositional forces that together create a dynamic whole whose balance depends on a harmony among the individual parts. The human organism is a participant image of the universal macrocosm, a microcosm that, throughout life, strives to maintain the inner harmony as a thermal equilibrium,

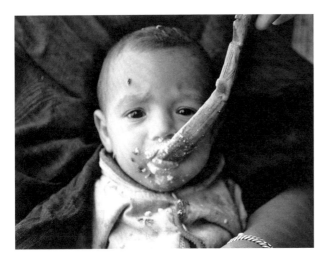

Figure 3.33. *A child under two years old being fed millet porridge,* enāle n-imāndārrān *(In Astilan, February 2005).*

constantly compensating for "cold" and "hot" influences. These influences comprise not only external surroundings – sicknesses and foods can also have an impact on the body's thermal balance. Since following their digestion, foods penetrate directly into the body, they can provoke a thermal disequilibrium triggering diseases. If a Kel Alhafra consumes too many foods with a "hot" temperament, the body overheats and contains excess energy, which gets expressed in illnesses of a "hot" character. If however, too much food of a "cold" character is consumed, the internal burner gets too low, and food, especially fat-rich foods, cannot be processed and transformed; they leave the body undigested, the organism is weakened and illnesses of a "cold" character ensue.

The Kel Alhafra classify foods into "hot/cold" categories, and thus a diet with "hot" or "cold" foods can compensate for thermal disequilibrium in the human body. Someone suffering from excessive heat and energy in the body eats predominantly foods classified as "cold", *isəssmaḍ*; if the body is "undercooled", "hot" foodstuffs, *issukās*, provide the counterbalance.

In general, the Kel Alhafra categorize fat-rich and not easily digestible foods as "hot", *isudar wi ədhənen d-āẓẓaynen wi n-tākusse*, while fat-poor and light foods are "cold", *isudar fāsusnen d-wār āẓẓaynen wi n-təssəmḍe*. Carnivorous wild animals, *tiwāysen ti tattānen isan*, are considered "hot", while herbivores, *tiwāysen ti tattānen taẓole mey tešše*, are innately of a cold nature, *ti n-təssəmḍe*. Everything that comes out of the river, from the south, is connotated hot, *hārātān fuk n-ejreu d-n-ajuss wi n-tākusse*, while everything from the north is cooling and cold, *hārātān fuk n-afālla wi n-təssəmde*. Raw cereals and seeds have a "cold" nature, *allonān wi n-təssəmḍe ar asγāl* (with the exception of Fonio), but move to the hot category when they are cooked and served with butter, *udi*, oil, *dilwil,* and spices, *beideitān*.[205] Fruit and vegetables, *ilkāḍān*,[206] are always classified as cold, *wi n-təssəmḍe*, because they contain a lot of water. Tea leaves, *āla n-ātay*, are likewise classified as cold, *wa n-təssəmḍe*, until they are brewed and served with sugar. Sugar, *əssukar*, always has a hot character, *wa n-tākusse*, as do oil, *dilwil,* spices, *beideitān*, and coffee, *ālqāhwa*.

Nevertheless, this classification system is not without exceptions to its rules, and when asked why Fonio, unlike all other wild plants, is classified as hot, the Kel Alhafra could offer me no explanations.

---

205 The Kel Alhafra have no term equivalent to spice (nor do they use what we call spices in their traditional cooking); they either use the Songhai word, *beideitān*, or paraphrase spices as *"hārātān wi tajj n-aḍrəẓ"* – "things which one puts in sauces".

206 The term *alkāḍ* (pl. *ilkāḍān*), was originally only used by the Kel Alhafra to describe wild fruits, but now that they trade and exchange on the markets in the larger villages and towns, today the term also covers cultivated fruits and vegetables. Only very recently have settled Kel Alhafra started to make a distinction between fruits, *ilkāḍān*, and vegetables, *legəmtān*.

Table 3.7. *Classification of foodstuffs*

issukās foods classified as hot	*isəssmaḍ* foods classified as cold
***axx* – milk**	***axx* – milk**
axx n-taɣāt – goat milk *axx n-tas kāfayān* – fresh cow milk *axx n-tihātten kafayān* – fresh sheep milk *axx əssəlayān* – bitter, full-fat sour milk **Milk products** *udi imaẓlayān* – heated butter *enetəš* – gently shaken milk that is not yet skimmed *enedu* – skimmed sour milk *afrar* - cream	*axx n-toḷmen* – camel milk *axx sāmmeḍān* – standing cooled milk *axx n-tas wi sammeḍān* – cooled cow milk *axx n-tihātten wi sammeḍān* – cooled sheep milk *axx əssəlayān* – sour milk, skimmed and diluted with water **Milk products** *udi* – fresh butter *takrəttit* – butter made from sour milk *tikāmmāren* – cheese
***isan* – meat**	***isan* – meat**
***isan n-irəzzejan* – meat from the herds** *isan n-taɣāt* –meat from the goat *isan n-teɣse* – meat from the kid *isan n-akrāwāt* –meat from the lamb *isan n-ebākār* – meat from the ram *isan n-tas* –meat from the cow *isan n-amənis* – meat from male camels ***tiwāɣsen fuk ti tattānen isan* – carnivorous wild animals** *isan n-ebāgg* – meat from the jackal *isan n-adhej* – meat from the anteater *isan n-aɣda* – meat from the wild cat *isan n-ahdal* – meat from the leopard ***isan n-ejreu* – meat from the river** *isan n-imān* – fish *isan n-ājamba* – meat from the hippopotamus ***iǰḍaḍ wa tattānen isan* - carnivorous birds** *isan n-tākunšāment* – meat from the duck *isan n-ājayəs* – meat from the buzzard *isan n-tekrit* – meeat from the crow *isan n-āẓayəj* – meat from the raven *isan n-ešeɣer* – meat from the vulture *isan n-tekāzit/ekāz* – meat from the hen/cock	***isan n-irəzzejan* – meat from the herds** *isan n-tihātten* – meat from the sheep *isan n-toḷmen* – meat from the camel mares ***tiwāɣsen fuk ti tattānen tāẓole meɣ tešše* – herbivorous wild animals** *isan n-temārwālt* – meat from the hare *isan n-ageẓẓam* – meat from the lizard *isan n-eḍāw* – meat from the jerboa *isan n-ākolān* – meat from the squirrel *isan n-tenhert* – meat from the dama gazelle *isan n-ašənkaḍ* – meat from the small gazelle *isan n-edām* – meat from the dorcas gazelle *isan n-amdāɣ* – meat from the giraffe *isan n-anəhil* – meat from the emu ***iǰḍaḍ wi tattānen tāẓole meɣ tešše* – herbivorous birds** *isan n-tabārrut* – meat from the wild pigeon *isan n-tāɣlalt* – meat from the guinea fowl *isan n-takāḍut* – meat from the spotted sandgrouse *tafārkit* – dried meat
***allon* – seeds/cereals**	***allon* – seeds/cereals**
təllumt – millet porridge *asɣāl* – Fonio (*Panicum laetum*) *horiamān* – *bərjut* seeds (*Echnochloa stagnina* seeds)	*enāle* – millet (*Pennisetum gamiensis*) *tafāɣāt* – rice *maṣar ṣāba* – maize *ṣāba* – sorghum *kuskus* – couscous *ālkāma* – wheat *farin (ejel n-ālkāma)* – wheat flour *mākkāruni/spagetti* – pasta ***allon n-tenere* – wild cereals and seeds** *waẓẓāj* – Cram Cram seeds (*Cenchrus biflorus*) *tašit* –*Eragrostis pilosa* seeds *tejābārt* – *Echinochloa colona* seeds *afāẓo* – *Panicum turgidum* seeds *tamāssālt* – *Limeum indicum* seeds *ajəruf* – *Tribulus terrester* seeds *abədebəd* – *Boerhavia coccinea* seeds *emeitāɣtāɣ* – *Agama colonorum* seeds

issukās foods classified as hot	*isəssmaḏ* foods classified as cold
	ilkāḏān – fruits/vegetables *šu* – cabbage *tāmati* – tomatoes *konkombər* – cucumbers *oberšin* – eggplants *laži* – okra *konbəter* – potatoes *tadāllāyt* – beans *tadāllāyt n-ikufar* – lentils *sālati* – lettuce *lāftānda* – pumpkins *ālbātana* – melon *betrav* – beetroot *karot* – carrots *māsāko* – sweet potatoes *tehāyne* – dates **ilkāḏān n-tenere – wild fruits** *iborāyen (sing. āborāɣ)* – wild dates from *tāborāyt* (*Balanites aegyptiaca*) *ibakatān (sing. abāka)* – Zizyphus saharae fruits *telajāṣt* – wild melon (*Citrullus lanatus*) *teɣrāggāyen* – fruits from the *ana* plant (*Leptadenia pyrotechnica*) *tarākāt* – Grewia tenax fruits *idumumān* – fruits from the *tādumut* tree (*Diospyros mespiliformis*) *ifārkitān n-infin* – Grewia villosa leaves *ifārkitān n-tanust* – Acacia senegalensis leaves *titanyen* – nuts from the wild date, *tāborāyt* (*Balanites aegyptiaca*) *tafəngora* – pulverised fruit from the baobab tree (*Adansonia digitata*)
Fat	
tadhunt – animal fat *esem* – animal fat melted on a fire that has re-emulsified *essem n-imānān* – fish fat *dilwil* – plant oil *essem n-irəzzejan* – animal fats	
Seasonings	
ižəkimba – red pepper (*Xylopia aethiopica*) *tayfārt* – onions (dried) *ālbəṣṣəl* – onions *tesəmt* – salt	
Stimulants/beverages/others	**Stimulants/beverages/others**
ātay – tea (green tea from China) *libton* – English black tea (tea bags from Nigeria) *asmād (pl. asmādān)* – alcoholic drinks *əssukar* – sugar *torawāt* – honey *matəji* – peanuts (roasted) *ālqāhwa ikkus* – hot coffee	*āla n-ātay* – tea leaves (green tea from China) *anāɣnāɣ* – fresh mint *ālqāhwa āssāmmeḏ* – cold coffee *matəji* – peanuts (unroasted)

Incompatibilities among foods

Certain food combinations are, according to the Kel Alhafra, predestined to elicit diseases of a "cold" or "hot" character, *torhənnawen n-tākusse d-təssəmḍe*, and every care is taken to avoid them during the preparation of meals. The worst combination is meat and fresh milk, *isan d-axx kāfayān*, which form an indi-gestible lump in the stomach that can block the entire digestive process. Also to be avoided are fish together with fresh milk, *wār tārḍed imānān d-axx kāfayān*, drinking tea with fresh milk, *wār təswed ātay s-artāyāt d-axx kāfayān*, sipping tea while nibbling on cheese from cow milk, *wār təswed ātay d-təkšed tikāmmāren ti n-axx n-tas*, seasoning undiluted milk, *wār təjjed hārātān wi n-aḍrəẓ dāy axx kāfayān*, or accompanying a strongly spiced meal with milk, *wār təkšed amənsi ihan iẓəkimba d-hārātān wi n-aḍrəẓ wiyādnen s-artāyāt d-axx*. In addition, cer-tain cereals should never be mixed together, *wār s-artāyāt allon*, because this provokes *aḍu*, or other digestive problems, *ātāxma*. Millet porridge should never be served with meat, *wār təkšed əsink n-enāle d-isan*, because meat must be ac-companied by whole millet, *tābālāttāst,* rice*, tafāyāt,* or bread, *tajəlla*. Sour milk should never be drunk immediately after the consumption of fresh milk, *wār təswed axx əssəlaynān ḍarāt as səswəd axx kāfayān*, and, as a general rule, a food classified as very hot should not be followed by foods of a "cold" character, *wār təkšed amənsi wa n-təssəmḍe ḍarāt as təkšəd amənsi wa n-tākusse*.

On a daily basis, however, the Kel Alhafra are always, though uninten-tionally, miscombining foods and paying the price in the form of health prob-lems. If Faḍimāta returns from a visit to a neighbouring encampment with di-arrhea, *tufit*, and vomiting, *ibsan*, the women will spend a long time discussing what she has eaten that day and which foods have provoked her indisposition through their incompatibility, before giving her advice on what cure she must use to restore her thermal equilibrium.

Food as medicine – medicine as food *(imənsiwan wi iha asāfar)*
Milk products
axx kāfayān (also known as *axx ikussān:* "hot milk"): fresh milk
With the exception of camel milk, the Kel Alhafra classify fresh milk as "hot" and use it as a therapy for "cold" diseases, *torhənnawen n-təssəmḍe*, such as *əjjəburu*, the common cold, *āmaẓla*, sinusitis, or *tijdil āwas*, bladder infection. *axx kāfayān* is also considered to be helpful for *dāmbāraku*, night sight (hem-eralopia), and, in general, to stimulate the appetite.

axx sāmmeḍān: no longer fresh, cooled milk
If milk is left standing for a while after milking and cools down it transforms from a foodstuff with a "hot" character to one with a "cold" temperament and is

used as medicine for illnesses classified as "hot", *torhənnawen n-tākusse*, especially digestive problems such as diarrhea with of a "hot" origin, *tufit n-issukās*.

axx əssəlayān: sour milk
Undiluted, sour milk always has a "hot" character but the Kel Alhafra attribute to it a neutralizing effect against poison, *āssām*, within the body. *axx əssəlayān* is administered to those with food poisoning, *āssām n-išəkša*, after someone has drunk polluted water, *aman ikordnān*, following plant poisoning, *āssām n-tāẓoli*, and for wound infections, *itunjārān*.

enetəš: lightly shaken milk that is not yet skimmed
enetəš is used as a medication agains "cold" diseases, *asāfar n-torhənnawen ti n-təssəmḍe*.

enedu: skimmed sour milk
enedu is used as a therapy for diseases classified as "cold", *torhənnawen n-təssəmḍe*.

axx n-tešāḍt: ass milk
Although the Kel Alhafra do not consider ass milk palatable, it is considered to be an effective remedy with a "hot" character, *asāfar n-tākusse*, against the highly infectious whooping cough (pertussis), *sāqqārnen*, which the Kel Alhafra say is a disease that afflicts not only children, but adults too.

axx n-taɣāt: goat milk
Goat milk always has a "hot" character, *wa n-tākusse*, and is used in various traditional medications against colds, *isefran n-təssəmḍe*; it is accorded a particularly soothing effect against coughs, *tāsut*.

axx n-toḷmen: camel milk
Camel milk not only refreshes the heart, *isəssmāḍ ulh*, with its "cooling" quality it quickly quenches a heavy thirst, *fad*, is considered to be a food that in general strengthens the constitution, *isudar n-āṣṣahāt*, helps against heartburn, *tākmo n-ermās* (which in the understanding of the Kel Alhafra can develop into gastritis), and is used as medication, *asāfar*, against the condition of *tāhafnent*.

udi: butter
udi is the general Tamasheq term for all kinds of butter. It is used both internally and externally against colds, *torhənnawen n-təssəmḍe*, ear inflammations,

tākmo n-timāẓẓujen, but also against various forms of allergy, *tādihātnen fuk*, and asthma, *təssah*.

The Kel Alhafra attribute to goat butter, *udi n-tayāt*, in particular, an efficient action against pimples, *isibān* (sing. *əsib*), and rashes. *udi n-tas*; butter from cow milk, in contrast, is employed to heal wound infections, *itunjarān* (sing. *ātunjar*), and lesions, *ibiwəsān* (sing. *ābiwəs*) in general, and facilitates the formation of scabs. Butter is also considered to be an effective medication for digestive problems such as belly pains, *tākmo n-tāsa*, or *aḍu*.

takrətti: small balls of butter produced when butter is shaken
The small, fresh clumps of butter that form when the butter sack, *ākāləkkol*, is agitated are for the Kel Alhafra a popular medicine with a "cold" character, used as a palliative against "hot" diseases, *torhənnawen n-tākusse*. These butter balls are also smeared on external wounds, *ibiwəsān* (sing. *ābiwəs*), to assist their healing.

udi imaẓlayān: cooked butter
For the Kel Alhafra, cooked butter has a strongly "hot" effect, *udi wa n-tākusse*, and is used against all sorts of "disease of the cold", *torhənnawen n-təssəmḍe*. *udi imaẓlayān* can also counter dehydration in diarrheal diseases of a "cold" origin, *tufit n-təssəmḍe*.

tikāmmāren (**sing. *takāmmārt*): cheese**
A "cooling" effect, *wa n-təssəmḍe*, is ascribed to the flat, yellow-white, hard pieces of cheese. *tikāmmāren* should help against the gripes, *tanānnāyāt*, and diarrhea, *tufit* (diluted with water against diarrhea classified as "hot;" supplemented by butter against diarrhea classified as "cold"), and quenches the "thirst" of an infant that is being weaned.

Meat

isan n-ebākār: meat of a young ram
The meat of a young ram, *ebākār*, is considered by the Kel Alhafra to have an especially "hot" character, *wa n-tākusse*, and is eaten over several days as a therapy against "cold" diseases, *torhənnawen n-təssəmḍe*.

isan n-teyse: meat from a kid
Kid meat is also classified as *issukās*, a "hot" food, and is cooked and eaten as a therapy for whooping cough, *sāqqārnen*.

isan n-akrāwāt: lamb meat
With a "hot", *wa n-tākusse*, character, lamb meat is especially used against bronchitis, *iḍmārān*, and other respiratory diseases classified as "cold".

isan n-timārwālen: hare meat
Like meat from a kid, the Kel Alhafra ascribe to hare meat a healing effect against whooping cough, *sāqqārnen.*

isan n-tihatten: sheep meat
Grilled sheep meat, *isan iknasnen wi n-tihātten*, is classified as "cold", *wa n-təssəmḍe*, and is used to heal the condition called *aḍkor*, a "hot" disease that precipitates internal blockages, especially of the digestive organs.

isan n-taɣāt: goat meat
For diarrheal diseases, *tufit*, intestinal infections, *itunjārān n-addānān*, and dysentery, *tanānnāɣāt*, "hot" goat meat is eaten for several days as a therapy.

aɣrum d-isan wār anəsses: liver and undercooked meat
(literally: "meat from which the water has not yet been removed")
Women in childbed, *tināmāẓẓoren* (sing. *tenāmāẓẓort*), are especially recommended to eat liver, *aɣrum*, and undercooked meat, *isan wār anəsses*, to replenish their blood content. In general, the Kel Alhafra ascribe to liver and undercooked meat a beneficial effect against anemia, *iba n-ašni*, and edema.

torāwen: lungs
According to the Kel Alhafra, consumption of animal lungs should help against asthma, *təssah*, and tuberculosis, *tāsut talābasāt.*

abārkot d-āddanan: stomach and intestines
Cooked stomach and gut walls are used by the Kel Alhafra to counteract digestive problems.

tāfārkit: dried meat
Dried meat is classified by the Kel Alhafra as "cold", *wa n-təssəmḍe*, and is used against "hot" diseases, *torhənnawen n-tākusse*, as well as in the diet of someone suffering from thromboses, *ālfāɣ. tāfārkit* is also used to stimulate the appetite.

tādhunt: animal fat
Animal fat is rubbed onto the irritant parts of the skin of those suffering from scabies, *ašyoḍ*, and dermatoses.

Plant products
tafāɣāt: rice
Rice is considered to be an effective remedy against all types of diarrhea, *asāfar n-tufit.*

enāle: millet
A millet dish will restore the thermal balance if there is too much "cold" in the body, it quickly stills hunger and it stimulates the appetite.

təllumt: millet bran
Millet bran relieves bodily congestions, and so is eaten as prophylaxis against *ālfāy*, thromboses. It also counters constipation, *oyān n-tāsa*, and in general stimulates the appetite. *"təllumt ar ulh"*, the Kel Alhafra say, "millet bran opens the heart", which means that eating millet bran makes one constantly hungry, and thus a diet with *təllumt* is eaten by women who wish to gain weight.

ātay: tea
"ātay asāfar n-alāḍḍeš" – "tea is a medicine against tiredness", the Kel Alhafra claim. It innervates the organism, including the digestive processes, and drives tiredness out of the body and spirit, *dāy tayəssa d-ənniyāt day*.

iborāyen (sing. *āborāy*)*:* wild dates
The fruit of the *tāborāyt* tree (*Balanites aegyptiaca*) is used as a general laxative, should help against constipation, *oyān n-tāsa*, and clean the digestive tract, *isirādān ātāxma*.

tarākaḍt: Grewia tenax fruit
The Kel Alhafra ascribe a thirst-quenching effect to the fruit of this mallow species.

Other

axxfəf: mother's milk
Mother's milk is viewed as an effective remedy for ear inflammations, *asāfar n-timāẓẓujen*, eye inflammations, *asāfar n-ahənnəj*, and against *tāməlle n-tiəṭṭ*, a white spot that spreads over the pupil and iris and can lead to blindness.

3.5.4. Malnutrition – *iba n-imənsiwān/ləbək*
The Kel Alhafra speak of *iba n-imənsiwān*, a "lack of meals", when there is no milk and therefore neither butter nor cheese in the encampment, *kunta wār t-illa axx d-wār t-illa udi d-wār ti-əllenāt tikāmmāren dāy aməẓẓoy*, when no animal can be slaughtered, *kunta enāye n-irəzzejān wār əmukān*, when cereal prices rocket, *kunta ālqimātān n-allon isiwāḍān*, and the grains become unaffordable, when, above all, food is in such short supply it must be rationed and people try to still their persistent hunger pains by filling their stomachs with *ašədder* or a watery *iləwa*. No one can eat to satiety, *əddināt wār s-ādoben*

tetāte har iywānān, they are constantly hungry, *ijlakān*, they become emaciated, *əlbakān*, weak, *irəkkəmān*, tired, *iḷḍašān*, and sick, *irhiinān*, and those without sufficient resistance, *āṣṣahāt*, die, *əmmutnān*. In the dry season especially, when food is scarcest, many families suffer from *iba n-imənsiwān*, and the Kel Alhafra say, *"tamudre s-ewelān tāṣṣohāt dāy tāfukk d-fad d-jələk"* – "life during *ewelān* is exhausting, accompanied by a burning hot sun, and continual thirst and hunger".

However, undernourishment is not only a seasonal phenomenon that leads to hunger, *jələk*, and dramatic weight loss, *ləbək*. The Kel Alhafra also describe other causes of *iba n-imənsiwān*.

ālxaufān n-ləbək – risks for malnutrition
mānna: drought

Under *mānna* (pl. *mānnatān*) the Kel Alhafra understand not only a regional and climatically conditioned drought due to a shortage of rain, but also a "general lack of everything that produces life", *"iba n-hārātān fuk dāy tāmudre"*. Swarms of locusts that strip trees, bushes and pastures clean, pests like the gypsy moth caterpillar, *tazləft* (pl. *tizəlfen*), that, especially during the dry season, *s-ewelān*, destroy the acacias that are so necessary for the animals' survival, catastrophes, *muṣibāt*, that devastate the rice and millet harvests in the south, *oyšad n-adomm wa n-enāle d-tafāyāt wi n-ajuss*, as well as rampant diseases among animals and humans, *təhen torhənnawen yor irəzzejan d-āddināt* – all of these are *āssəbabān n-ləbək ihee n-in mānna*, causes for a wasting away due to the lack of everything that produces life.

talāqqāwt: poverty

For the Kel Alhafra, *talāqqāwt* always designates poverty in the sense of food dependency. *"ilāqqāw"*, "he is poor", means that someone does not own enough animals to feed his family from the produce of his herds alone and most seek alternative ways of generating income to ensure their survival.

The Kel Alhafra calculate that the minimum number of animals required to support a family of average size (10 to 12 persons) is as follows:

Table 3.8. *Minimum assets required to feed an average family*

50 goats or sheep that provide milk
5 cows or 2 camel mares that provide milk
2 riding camels (for travel and transport)
5 male asses (for travel, transport and work at the wells)
3 female asses (for transport and well work; they are not used for travel)

A family lacking these assets is considered as *ejādāš lāqqāw*, a poor kingroup, and its male members are obliged to work for someone else. In exchange for food or for a very modest fee, the Kel Alhafra men of Azawad can assist in watering animals at the well each day, *asəsu n-irəzzejan*, tend animals belonging to someone else, *tamāḍent n-irəzzejan*, sell an animal on the market on behalf of its owner, *asikəl s-iwetān*, take over the daily tasks of a person who is absent, *assijāẓ i-āhalis asokālen*, run errands, *imašālan*, or tame camels and oxen, *assinān n-imənas d-iwdesān*. "No one will get rich from this kind of work" – *"ma taqālād ad ehāre dāy əššāyāl wadāy"*, the Kel Alhafra say, and usually the family just gets by, surviving as best it can on the means at hand. The oldest male member of one family, however, cited this saying: *"edām d-ākal-ənnet attaf-t amyar-ənnet"* – "the antilope takes care to remain on its land", and even when survival becomes very difficult, the older Kel Alhafra, at least, prefer a life in poverty to the uncertainties of living far from their familiar surroundings and ways.

ikənasān (sing. *akənnas*): conflicts

Conflicts are numerous in Azawad. They have many causes: disagreements about a well – who can water his animals first, where should a new well be dug – about access to the pastures, about stolen animals, about unacceptable political decisions, but also about rapes, raids and personal differences. The term *akənnas* encompasses *kanis*, rage, a fury that drives people to fight one another, *məkənnəs,* and to inflict suffering. *akənnas* is the opposite of *ālyafəyāt*, peace, and sometimes compels entire encampments to move or to flee from a conflict zone.

In the beginning of 2005, armed conflict developed in the western district of Oudéika between Kunta[207] and other Arab tribes, because the former did not accept the "democratic" election of a representative who was not one of their number. The Kunta took up arms and forced many Arab families to flee to the west. This led to a temporary nomadic overpopulation on the already sparse pastures around the wells of In Agozmi. Within a short time, the animals had consumed all the vegetation, further conflicts developed over the scarce natural resources and the Kel Alhafra began to suffer from hunger and food shortages. *"akənnas wār itəmmāḍrāy"*, the Kel Alhafra say, "a conflict is never small".

---

207 The Kunta are an Arabic-speaking group who live in the Azawad, Gourma, Adagh and Niger and identify themselves as descendants of Šayḫ al-Kabīr (died 1811). The Kunta are supporters of the Qādirīya Order and have always been politically active. See Charles Grémont, André Marty, Rhissa ag Mossa and Younoussa H. Touré, *Les liens sociaux au Nord-Mali. Entre fleuve et dunes* (Paris: IRAM/Karthala, 2004).

azəjor n-ākāll: emigration and transmigration

As mentioned above in the discussion about *talāqqāwt*, poverty, many Kel Alhafra families do not own enough animals to guarantee a livelihood. Although older people prefer to live in poverty rather than start a new life elsewhere, young men in particular prefer to seek their fortunes in the cities or abroad. Many go to Algeria or Libya to look for work, often leaving their families behind for months in the desert. The women and children stay in the encampment with relatives whose support they depend on to get by. "Some men don't even return" – *"illan meddān wi āba-s oyāl-dd ābādān"*, one woman complained, "they see a better life abroad and don't want to come back to us in the desert" – *"ihanāyān dāy ikāllān tamudre ta rāqqisāt āba-s oyāl n-ajāma;"* "but among us, the man is the shadow of the family" – *"māšan yor-nāy āhalis tele n-ejādāš"*, "and when he is away, then we can see where we stand" – *"a-fāl āba-s illa diha, nədob hanāyān əndek əmukān aməẓẓoy"*.[208]

atābatāt fall-iyen amənsi: unbalanced nutrition

If the Kel Alhafra have no milk and little meat during the dry season of *ewelān* (or even months earlier for many families), their diet will consist solely of millet, *enāle*, or flour, *farin*, with which they cook *tabālāttāst* or bake *tajəlla*, and serve with a little sunflower oil bought from the trucks of Algerian traders. On such a monotonous diet, which can last for weeks or months, the body, according to the Kel Alhafra, experiences "withdrawal symptoms", attributable to the renunciation of familiar foods such as milk, *axx,* meat, *isan,* and butter, *udi.* The Kel Alhafra call these "withdrawal symptoms" *amāyrəs*, meaning literally, "the crossing (of a difficult situation, of a difficult region)". *"ma təməyrāsād?"* – "what are you lacking?" they ask during periods of food transition. *"əməyrāsāy i-axx"* – "I lack milk", is often the reply. If the milk shortage in the encampment lasts for weeks, *amāyrəs* manifests itself: the skin slowly becomes darker, *elām ikkāwwāl*, the eyes become heavy, *təṭṭāwen aẓaynen*, and people suffer from headaches, *tākmo n-eyāf*, vomiting, *ibsan,* and fever, *tenāde*. This absence of the customary foods, *amāyrəs*,[209] which is accompanied by an overall debility, represents for the Kel Alhafra not only a threshold to malnutrition, *iba n-imənsiwān*, but also for diseases.

---

208 Interview at Tin Timāyayān with Həntu Wālāt Mustāfa, October 2005.

209 *amāyrəs* denotes a food transition, the giving up of food habits, but is also used for the symptoms that appear upon foregoing stimulants such as tobacco, tea or alcohol.

iba n-tāmusne: lack of knowledge

Ignorance, *ālžāhalāt*, often leads to poverty, the Kel Alhafra say, "we used to know much more about the processes of nature, about animals, about wild and medicinal plants" – *"ihənnin nəssan a wa itajjān dāy ajāma, nəzzay irəzzejān d-nəssan ihəkšān wi ihan isəfran"*, "but today we are gradually losing this knowledge" – *"ašāli-i-dāy nəttiwātān-in musnāt sund wadey"*. "Today everyone wants new things" – *"āmār-a-dāy əddināt fuk irhan hārātān wi išraynān"*, new impressions come from outside; people are becoming increasingly dependent on modern products and suffer from new diseases, *torhənnawen təšraynen*. Not only are these diseases unfamiliar, no one knows what to do about them, and many traditional remedies are suddenly no longer effective.

At the beginning of 2005, when the Kel Alhafra had nothing to live on except flour, *farin*, or millet, *enāle*, the children began to suffer from chronic diarrhea due to malnutrition, *iba n-imənsiwān*, in the face of which their mothers were helpless, lamenting that they were at a loss: "We don't know what we should do; we simply see our children slowing perishing before our eyes" – *"wār nəssan a wa əjjā, nəhannāy imutnān aratān-nanāy yās"*.[210]

Malnutrition of children

"Earlier children ate no cereals before they were 10 years old and lived only from milk, butter and meat" – *"ihənnin aratān wār tatten allon har mārāw iwətiyān, wār tatten ar isan, udi d-wār sassen ar axx"*, I was told by Ayšəni, a Kel Alhafra woman of about 75 years, "but today there is not enough milk" – *"ašāli-i-dāy wār t-illa axx ajen"*, "and the children like the adults are forced to eat just millet or flour, sometimes for months at a time" – *"aratān d-əddināt fuk əkšen enāle mey farin ilwāqqitān dāy awātay fuk"*.[211]

While I was doing research in the area around In Agozmi during March 2005, there were many families that had been living exclusively on a diet of cereals since January. They had no idea how they were going to survive the coming months until the rains began, when the sheep would start giving birth, and milk would become available once again. In many encampments, the women complained that their children were suffering from *sāqqārnen*, whooping cough, and were wasting away from the chronic diarrhea it caused.

In one encampment, at two hours walking distance from the encampment in which I was a guest, the children were in particularly poor health, and in one family, a four-year-old girl and an 11-month-old infant were dying.

---

210 Interviews at In Agozmi with Tiyāyya Wālāt Muttalāmīn, Tayyāha Wālāt Muttalāmīn, February/March 2005.
211 Interview at Buneyrub with Ayšəni Wālāt Alḥassan, October 2005.

Their mother told me that both had contracted *sāqqārnen*, whooping cough, a month previously, and the coughing, *tāsut*, vomiting, *ibsan,* fever, *tenāde,* and chronic diarrhea, *tufit,* had weakened them so much they would neither eat nor drink, *wār irhan imənsiwān d-wār irhan tesāse*. For two months the family had been living exclusively from millet, *enāle,* and some oil, *dilwil,* and they had to ration the former because the stocks were running low and the ass caravan that had left for the "Pays Dogon" to purchase millet had not yet returned. The mother of the two small children was pregnant again and had weaned the little boy, whose already poor condition had deteriorated steadily since then. When I arrived, both children were lying motionless in the sand, wasted to the bone, with bloated bellies beneath their ribs. They could barely open their eyes, a crust of henna – intended to draw the fever out of them – had dried on their heads, and flies swarmed around their etiolated bodies.

The mother had prepared *tabālāttāst*, cooked millet, but neither of the enervated children could tolerate it and regurgitated the food immediately. An *ālfāqqi* had come from a neighboring "campement" and together with his son sat in the tent with the sick children reciting the Koran to drive away with the holy words the *təšoṭṭ*, the evil eye, that according to the encampment inhabitants was responsible for the family's woes. I asked the children's father why he did not take them to the health center in Ber. He replied that, because this was a three-day camel ride away, "the children would die on the journey" – *"aratān*

Figure 3.34. *Malnutrition,* iba n-imənsiwān, *in an encampment at In Agozmi (April 2005).*

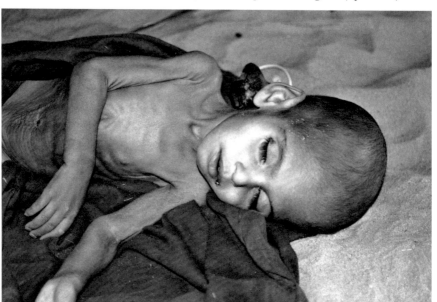

Figure 3.35. *and 3.36.*
Malnutrition in an encampment at In
Agozmi (March/April 2005).

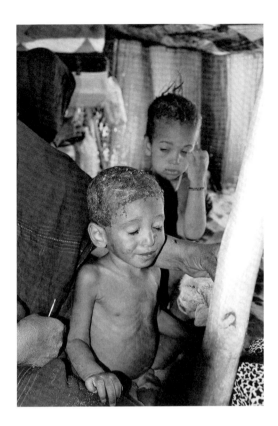

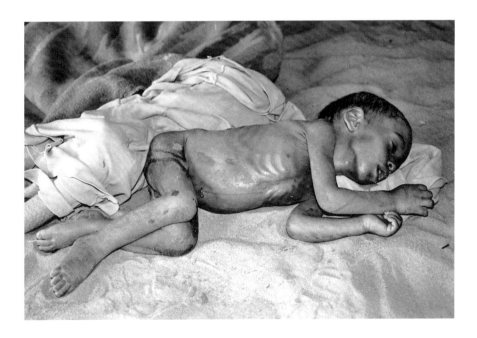

har ammutān dāy tabarāt". Furthermore, he could not just up and leave: while the majority of the men were on the ass caravan that had gone south to buy millet, those that remained behind had to tend the animals, collect water and protect the women and children. Two days later, the four-year-old girl died, and her brother followed shortly afterwards, leaving their kin to seek comfort in their knowledge that the souls of the children would go directly to paradise.

One month later, Médecins sans Frontières Luxembourg, MSF-L, based in Timbuktu, launched a "mission exploratoire" in the area around In Agozmi to evaluate the situation. During a three-day visit to 12 encampments, the doctors examined 42 children between 0 and 5 years of age. The results below are drawn from their report:[212]

Table 3.9.

Symptoms	Diarrhea	Coughing	Diarrhea, coughing
Number of cases	20	14	8

Diarrhea was recorded in 28 of the 42 examined children, and the MSF team also noted the deaths of 3 children who according to the population in the affected area had died within one week.

Table 3.10.

Diagnosis	Marasmus	Whooping cough	Bronchitis	Marasmus, bronchitis	Apparently normal
Number of cases	14	3	2	2	21

An upper arm circumference of less than 105 mm was measured in 14 of the 42 children examined (for MSF a circumference of <110 mm indicates undernourishment),[213] and *sāqqārnen*, whooping cough was diagnosed in 3 children.

Table 3.11.

Brachial circumference	<110 mm	=110 mm	>110 mm
Number of cases	16	3	23

212 Birama Diallo, "Rapport de la mission médicale, Aire d'Oudéika, Région de Tombouctou-Mali, 07 au 09 avril 2005", Programme Santé Nomade de MSF-L, Tombouctou (Mali), 2005.
213 In his health handbook, widely distributed in Mali, Werner's lower limits for malnutrition are less extreme than those of MSF: "Between the ages of 1 and 5 years, any child whose upper arm has a circumference of less than 14 cm is undernourished, however 'fat' the feet, hands and face appear to be. If the arm measures less than 12.5 cm, the child is seriously malnourished." David Werner, *Là où il n'y a pas de docteur* (Dakar: Enda Tiers-Monde, 2004) 167. On the diagnosis of malnutrition and the measurment of the brachial circumference see also Prudhon, *La malnutrition en situation de crise,* 33.

Nineteen of the children had an upper arm diameter of 110 mm or less, in 8 of whom it was only between 70 and 90 mm, a sign of severe malnutrition.

The study by MSF/L showed that at the end of March/beginning of April 2005, altogether 46% of the children examined were suffering from moderate to severe undernourishment.

About six weeks later, in May, Vétérinaires sans Frontières VSF Timbuktu and the national Centre de Santé de Référence in Timbuktu undertook another mission in the region in which the Kel Alhafra were living to launch a three-month food aid program and to provide medical assistance (although many families had no cash to pay for the medicines). A total of 314 children were examined during this mission, of whom 54.1% showed signs of undernourishment, 38.2% being diagnosed as suffering from severe and 15.9% from moderate malnutrition.[214] In the following months from May to July, the families with undernourished children received millet, enriched flour and oil to see them through to the approaching rainy season, but this emergency aid was just a drop in a bucket and the Kel Alhafra had no idea what lay ahead of them in the coming year, *"wār nəssan a wa imarān awātay wa imalān"*, whether enough rain would fall, whether the pastures would turn green and the haggard animals would recover and give birth to enough young to supply the humans with milk and meat, so that the children could fill their bellies once more with the foods imbued with *ālbarāka*, God's blessing.

3.5.5. Changes in food traditions – *tāmutait n-isudar*

"From August to May we used to live exclusively on milk, *axx,* butter, *udi,* meat, *isan,* and cheese, *tikāmmaren"*, the 74-year-old Zainbu recounted. "Life then was beautiful" – *"tamudre tāhuskāt dāγ awātay-dāγ"*, in the rainy season, *s-akāsa,* there was milk and meat, in the cold season of *tajrəst,* the milk was supplemented with some millet, while during the dry months of *ewelān,* although millet remained in the diet, there was always an adequate supply of milk from the camels and goats and a store of dried meat and cheese, and *ašədder* was drunk to quench the thirst. When food did go short, there were enough wild cereals such as *afāẓo* or *wāzzāj* to collect and cook.[215]

---

214 The report, however, provides no cutoff values for "moderate malnutrition" and "severe malnutrition", and a footnote simply remarks, that "the target children are those presenting with visual signs of malnutrition". See "Rapports de missions sur l'action d'urgence à Inagouzmi, Commune de Ber, Cercle de Tombouctou, Région de Tombouctou", mise en oeuvre: Vétérinaires Sans Frontières, Centre de Référence de Tombouctou, Financement: Coopération Suisse, PAM, Juillet 2005.

215 Interview at Intikewen with Faḍimatu Wālāt Muḥammad Attaher, Tin Albarāka Wālāt Muḥammad Ousmane, Amatu Wālāt Marušād, November 2005.

But the major droughts of 1967 (*awātay wa n-tamǝttānt ta n-iwān* – "the year in which the cows died"), 1973 (*awātay wa lābasān* – "the wicked year") and 1984 (*awātay wa n-manna wa išraynen* – "the year when the drought returned") have left their mark on Azawad. They killed off wild animals, decimated the herds, and the vegetation changed. Edible plants such as *afāẓo* (*Panicum turgidum* seeds), *asyāl* (fonio, *Panicum laetum*), *waẓẓāj* (also called *ayālas/tākane, Cenchrus biflorus*), *tejābārt* (*Echinochloa colona* seeds), *tašit* (*Eragrostis pilosa* seeds), *telājāṣt* (wild melon, *Citrullus lanatus*), *tamāssālt* (*Limeum indicum*), *ajǝruf* (*Tribulus terrestris*) and many others that were once collected and eaten by the Kel Alhafra during periods when food was scarce either no longer grow or are too rare to function as a significant alternative food source. The people rely on cereals such as millet, flour and rice, which have become the staples for some families. "We eat less meat than we used to" – *"wār nǝlla isan sund ihǝnnin"*, Zainabu told me, "rarely hunt wild animals now" – *"wār nǝtak ahoyy"*, "have less milk and butter" – *"wār nǝlla axx d-udi ajen"*, "and can no longer produce dried meat or cheese" – *"āba-s nādobed ǝmukān isan wi ǝqqornen d-tikāmmāren"*.[216] After the desolate months of *ewelān*, the dry season, in 2005, the subsequent rainy season, *akāsa*, was better than in the previous year, but the sheep and goats were still so weak that their offspring were small, and they did not produce enough milk. "The little milk that is available, is divided up in the encampment and usually drunk fresh immediately, before any butter can be made", Zainabu explained.[217]

"The heat during the dry season has also got worse, the sun burns more strongly and is more merciless than it used to be" – *"tāfukk tākus hullan s-ewelān fāll ihǝnnin"*, was the opinion of another woman in an encampment at Inkilla,[218] "many plants and trees no longer grow" – *"ihākšān ajotnān wār idawāl"*, such as *tasǝskārt* (*Dactyloctenium aegyptium*), *ilǝs n-tas* (*Polygala arenaria*), *tāfādofādot* (*Tragus berteronianus*), *ajāsāy* (*Gynandropsis gynandra*), *talǝggid* (*Cyperus jeminicus*), *efāyād* (*Blepharis linariifolia*), *ādārās* (*Commifora africana*) and *tadhānt* (*Boscia senegalensis* – which now only grows near the river). "The trees are dying" – *"ihākšān tamattnān"*, "and in many areas one has to go a long way to find enough wood for cooking" – *"dāy idāggān ajotnān ǝzzar atiljāwād ujǝj atajj isāyerān n-asǝŋ"*.[219] Many have begun to eat raw millet, which is very unhealthy, causing stomach ache, *teẓẓort n-tāsa*, and provoking fever, *tenāde*. Overall, the women were in agreement

---

216 Interview at Intikewen with Zainabu Wālāt Muḥammad ʿAli, November 2005.
217 Interview at Intikewen with Zainabu Wālāt Muḥammad ʿAli, November 2005.
218 Interview at Inkilla with Mariamma Wālāt Muḥammad, November 2005.
219 Ibid.

that these nutritional changes were in part responsible for the increasing incidence of certain diseases. "Even children today suffer from *tilāwayen* (rheumatism)" – *"ašal-i-dāy illan-t aratān ijrawān-t tilāwayen"*, formerly a disease
of old age, *torhənna n-imyārān*, said Faḍimāta, and young children suffer from
tedeje and all sorts of blisters and pimples that spread over the entire body:
"This is because we sometimes eat only cereals for the entire year" – *"a-wa-
s awātay fuk nətatt allon"*, she said. A 100-kg sack of millet used to last one
year, but today a family of five gets through such a sack in 15 days.[220]

The Kel Alhafra can only rarely live from the produce of their herds alone
these days and are forced to consume new foodstuffs that throw into total
confusion their familiar dietary system for sustaining the body's thermal equilibrium. These new foods are mostly classified as "hot", and since the Kel Alhafra often have no choice about what to eat, their bodies are permanently
overheated and they succumb to illnesses of a "hot" character. For the Kel Alhafra, new cereals include wheat, *ālkāma,* in the form of flour, *farin,* or cous-
cous, *kuskus*, maize, *māṣar ṣāba*, rice, *tafāyāt*, and pasta, *mākkāruni d-spa-
getti*, which, because of the shortage of butter, they prepare with oil, *dilwil,*
though this immediately transforms every dish into one with a "hot" character. Furthermore, the Kel Alhafra women say that although they have not been
using them for a long time, tinned tomato paste and dried onions, *tayfārt,* are
"hot" foods, *imənsiwān sund wadey fuk wi n-tākusse*, and provoke stomach
upsets, *ermās,* fever, *tenāde,* headaches, *tākmo n-eyāf,* arthritic pains, *tākmo
n-iyāssān,* malnutrition, *iba n-imənsiwān,* visual problems, *dāmbāraku,* and
a general loss of energy, *iba n-āṣṣahāt*. With the shortage of animal milk,
the women have also begun to feed their children powdered milk, *lahḍa,*
which is also classified as "hot", but it makes the children sick, and they suffer from diarrhea, *tufit,* vomiting, *ibsan,* and itching, *ukmāš*. Another alternative that used to be offered to children as a milk replacement, baobab powder,
tafəngora, and which is classified as "cold", is now very difficult to obtain.

Tea and sugar, *ātay d-əssukar*, are also classified as "hot", and although
they are not perceived as foods *per se*, they have established themselves as part
of everyday life and and no meal is complete without them. When the Kel Alhafra recite what is certainly their favorite adage, *"aman iman",* – "water is the
soul", *"axx isudar"* – "milk is nourishment", *"isan temḍe"* – "meat is tasty",
"əsink esāk" – "foods are the content of the stomach", they will often add with
a smile *"ātay tāhafnent"* – "tea is (provokes) the condition of *tāhafnent*".

One woman in an encampment at Buneyrub told me that "today the men
are always traveling to the city to buy tea, sugar and cereals, they are never in

---

220 Interview at Intikewen with Faḍimatu Wālāt Muḥammad Attaher, November 2005.

the encampment, and the women, children and their neighbors must care for the animals and supply themselves with water" – *"ašāl-i-dāɣ meddān təkken aɣrəm ālwāqq fuk ad išənšād ātay d-əssukār d-allon, wār ihan n-aməẓẓoɣ ālwāqq fuk, tiḍeḍen, aratān d-anhārājān ijəmmiyān i-irəzzejān d-israjān"*.[221] That their austere life has left its traces on them, on this point the Kel Alhafra are agreed, *"elām-nanāɣ ikāwāl"* – "our skin has become darker", they say with regret, and attribute this to the laborious daily fight for survival, to the lack of milk, *iba n-axx*, and the new "hot" foods, *isudar wi išraynen d-wi n-tākusse*. "Survival in the desert has become more difficult", especially for the women, who, in the absence of their husbands, in addition to their own tasks also have to perform those traditionally allocated to the men.

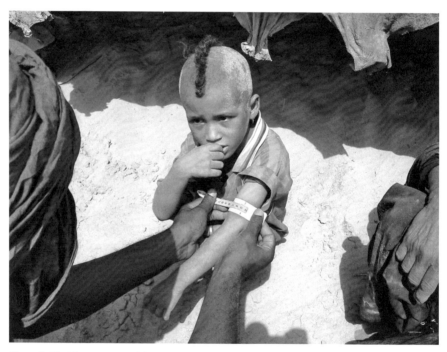

Figure 3.37. *Measurement of the upper arm circumference in an encampment at In Agozmi (June 2005).*

221 Interview at Buneyrub with Tiyāyya Wālāt Muttalāmīn, October 2005.

4. Cultural Interpretations of Illnesses

4.1. Disease categories and traditional therapies

The following disease categories, their descriptions, their perceived causes and the therapeutic options are all derived from the repertoire of the Kel Alhafra. Although it might be possible to extend and expand these categories, this repertoire corresponds to the information and knowledge mentioned and passed on to me by the Kel Alhafra during my research visits. I believe that those disease categories that are most significant for the Kel Alhafra are gathered in the following catalogue.

The Kel Alhafra usually discuss diseases without using any specific system or hierarchical ordering, although they will sometimes itemize them according to temperament, prevalance, season or the important elicitors such as *āmāyrəs*, an abrupt change in diet, or *iba n-imənsiwān*, malnutrition. I have therefore opted to list the disease types alphabetically. Only where there is an obviously equivalent medical term in English for the condition, and traditional healers have confirmed the indication, have I placed this name in italics in the heading. Otherwise, I have translated the Tamasheq term or the content provided by the Kel Alhafra.

ābiwəs (pl. ibiwəsān), Arabic: *ğarīḥ,* "wound"
Category: hot/cold
In the Kel Alhafra understanding, *ābiwəs* refers to an internal or external wound of any origin. More specificity is provided by applying modifiers to the term: *ābiwəs n-telāyt* describes a cut made by a small knife, *ābiwəs n-abṣar* refers to a cut made by a larger knife, *ābiwəs n-esāyer* indicates that the wound has been caused by a piece of wood, *ābiwəs n-təṭṭ* is a wound to the eye, *ābiwəs n-em* characterizes wounds inside the mouth, and *ibiwəsān n-tamāḍt* are birth-related wounds, as I have discussed in greater detail in chapter 3.4.3.
Causes: Any agent that can wound the body.
Therapy: For simple wounds, leaves of the *tāborāyt* (*Balanites aegyptiaca*) are placed on the site of the wound so that it dries out. A mixture of sugar, *əssukar,* and honey, *torawāt,* is also applied to assist the healing process. If a wound becomes infected, hot cow butter, *udi ikkusān n-tas,* is used to fight the infection, *ahəḍəḍu (atunjār).* For *ibiwəsān n-em,* wounds in the mouth, *aman n-ahəjjar,* a gargle of *Acacia nilotica/adansonii* seed capsules or leaves steeped in water is recommended.

adku, "abdominal pains/cramps"
CATEGORY: cold
adāka (pl. *idakān*) is the Tamasheq term for the human underbelly or pubic area; *adku,* or *teẓẓort n-adku,* refers to cramp-like pains in the abdominal region.
CAUSES: Kel Alhafra women identify abdominal pains as being gynecological in origin, *dāy əssəbab n-torhənnawen n-tideḏen*; in men, such pains are always attributed to a disease that is classified as cold, *torhənnawen n-təssəmḏe,* usually *tijdil āwas,* a bladder infection.
THERAPY: If the pains are bad, the patient takes a hip bath in luke-warm water containing leaves of the *ahəjjar* plant (Acacia adansonii).

adku wa n-tāyimit, "abdominal cramps while sitting" *(dysmenorrhea)*
CATEGORY: cold
Menstruating women often suffer from *adku,* in which case the cramps are referred to as *adku wa n-tāyimit* or *teẓẓort n-ārori,* "back pain".
CAUSES: *adku wa n-tāyimit* is gynecological in origin, *dāy əssəbab n-torhənnawen n-tideḏen,* according to the Kel Alhafra women.
THERAPY: A few days before menstruation, gently heated cow urine, *āwas n-tas ikkusān,* is mixed with butter, *udi,* and introduced into the vagina. If the pains are bad, the woman sits in the *ahəjjar* hip bath described above.

aḍkor, Arabic: *infāḥ,* "the filled being"
CATEGORY: hot
The belly is bloated, filled with water, eating anything causes discomfort and the internal organs are blocked. The Kel Alhafra say that *aḍkor* occurs mainly in the south, *s-ajuss,* around the river Niger. However, by taking care about what one eats, and not mixing foods inappropriately, this problem can be avoided.
CAUSES: *aḍkor* can be caused by the consumption of cold milk that has been left standing for too long, *axx sāmmeḏān* or by eating too much sugar, *əssukar,* or too much skimmed sour milk, *enedu.*
THERAPY: Having drunk an infusion of leaves of the *ājār* (*Maerua crassifolia*) in water, one eats a cathartic of millet porridge, *təllumt,* mixed with *ahārjəjəm* (*Cassia italica*), to empty the stomach, and finally some roasted sheep meat, *isan iknasnen wi n-tihātten.*

aḍu, Arabic: *ar-rīḥ,* "air"
CATEGORY: cold/hot
aḍu is air circulating in the organism, *dāy tayəssa,* in the belly, *dāy tāsa,* and thorax, *dāy tarāja,* that causes a congestion in bodily functions. The trapped

air makes noises inside the body, can become concentrated in a certain part and may cause stabbing pains, *tedeje*, flatulence and intestinal wind, *tixādasen*. If a birthing mother, *tenāmāẓẓort*, suffers from *aḍu*, it can block the contractions (see chapter 3.4.3.)

CAUSES: *aḍu* is caused by the overconsumption of foods classified as "cold", such as cold milk, *axx sāmmeḍān*, or *tafəngora,* mashed fruit of the baobab tree (*Adansonia digitata*).

THERAPY: Butter, *udi, ālmuxāynes* (*Cleome bradycarpa*), *ahārjəjəm* (*Cassia italica*), *āliswaḍ* (fine leaves of the *tebāremt* plant, *Cymbopogon schoenanthus*) and cow urine, *āwas n-tas,* are heated in water, and the resultant infusion is drunk for several days.

afugg (pl. ifuggān), Arabic: *fuġā'a,* "the torn muscle"
CATEGORY: cold
The symptoms are a strong cough, *tāsut*, fever, *tenāde*, headache, *tākmo n-eɣāf*, and a bronchial infection, *iḍmārān*. Physical overexertion in such a condition, such as carrying a heavy load while coughing, can exacerbate the illness and produce stabbing pains in the breast.

CAUSES: Physical exertion, especially carrying a heavy burden, while coughing.

THERAPY: The patient must rest, preferably in the tent, and bind the breast with a piece of cloth. He or she should eat lamb, *akrāwāt*, cooked with butter, *udi*, and drink an infusion of *tanust* (gum arabic), *ālmuxāynes* (*Cleome bradycarpa*), *tāhahist* (*Cadaba glandulosa*) and butter, *udi*.

aɣālab (pl. iɣālabān), "the dominated and vanquished being"
CATEGORY: hot/cold
Synonym for *təlleɣāf.*

ayəttus (pl. iɣəttusān), Arabic: *ḥarra,* "to faint" *(also epilepsy)*
CATEGORY: hot
The sufferer faints without warning; *ayəttus* is also used as a term to describe epilepsy.

CAUSE: *ayəttus* is always caused by the *kel tenere*, by spirits and demons.

THERAPY: No effective medication is known for *ayəttus*, but the Kel Alhafra are convinced that "maraboutage",[222] can drive the evil powers out of the sick person's body.

---

222 With the assistance of magic, the marabout can mobilize supernatural powers that have effects both in nature and in humans to drive an evil *ǧinn* out of the "possessed" person's body.

ahəḍəḍu **(pl. *ihəḍuḍutān)*,** "swelling, abscess" *(infection)*
CATEGORY: hot
Synonym for *atunjār* (see also the description in chapter 3.4.3.).

ahənnəj **(also *tākmo n-təṭṭāwen* or *ahḍəḍu n-təṭṭāwen)*,** Arabic: *al-'ainīn,*
"eye inflammation/infection", "eye pain" or "swelling of the eyes" *(conjunctivitis)*
CATEGORY: hot/cold
The symptoms of *ahənnəj* are red, weeping and burning eyes, which first thing
in the morning and at night are often glued shut. The illness is believed to be
highly contagious but responds to a 3– to 4-day treatment.
CAUSES: Lack of hygiene, *iba n-ašəšədaj.*
THERAPY: A child suffering from *ahənnəj* is given eyedrops of mother's milk,
while adults put *ikārkārān n-təšukmayent*, "that which is scraped out from inside a river mussel", or a small, black seed kernel, which they call *temājār
jāwāšt* and which has a cleansing effect, into the affected eye(s). More recently, families who live near Ber have also been purchasing on the Saturday
market a red juice from *Basella alba* fruits (Gambian spinach) that, used as
eyedrops, is credited as a cure for *ahənnəj*.

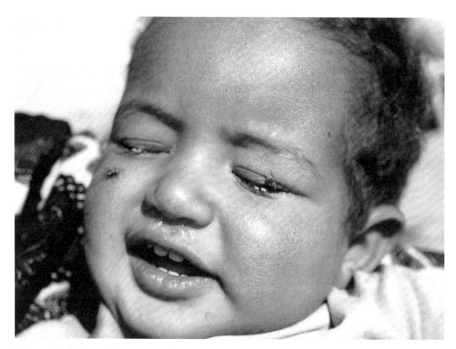

Figure 4.1. In the cold season, s-tajrəst, *small children especially suffer from eye inflammations,* ahənnəj, *as here in an encampment at Intikewen (November 2005).*

āhunšar, Arabic: *ru ʿāf,* "nose bleeds"

CATEGORY: hot

If excess heat accumulates in the body because "the inner organism is boiling over", *aswəs n-taγəssa,* it will result in headaches, *tākmo n-eγāf,* a heavy head, *eγāf āẓẓayān,* and heavy eyes, *tiəṭṭāwen āẓẓaynen,* and finally blood flowing from the nose to relieve this discomfort.

CAUSES: *issukās fuk,* everything that contains heat, such as the sun, *tāfukk,* "hot" foods, *išəkša ikkusnen,* etc. can cause *āhunšar.*

THERAPY: Red carnelian, *zākkāt,* is considered by the Kel Alhafra to have hemostatic properties and is hung around the neck as a remedy for *āhunšar.* To cool the body, cowpats, *timārγiten* (sing. *temārγit*), are placed on the head, leaves of the *təsuya* plant *(Picris asplenioides)* are stuffed into the nose or applied to the head, and clothes may be sprinkled with water.

ajmoḍ, "the rising up/emergence"

CATEGORY: hot

In *ajmoḍ,* a white-yellow spot develops on the cornea; it enlarges, itches and hurts, *ihee ukmāš d-teẓẓort,* and gradually causes blindness.

CAUSES: *ajmoḍ* can be caused by the consumption of too many foods classified as hot, *issukās,* or by a lack of hygiene, *iba n-ašəšədaj.*

THERAPY: Red pepper, *ižəkimba (Xylopia aethiopica),* is applied to the spot, which should then disappear.

ajnəwwi, "to have a digestive disturbance"

CATEGORY: hot

The symptoms are problems with digestion and belly pains, sometimes accompanied by vomiting, *ibsan,* fever, *tenāde,* headaches, *tākmo n-eγāf,* diarrhea, *tufit,* and sunken eyes.

CAUSES: According to the Kel Alhfra, *ajnewwi* is evoked by food incompatibilities.

THERAPY: The patient is given *aman n-ahəjjar,* water containing seed capsules of *Acacia nilotica.*

ākorkor, Arabic: *al-ǧarʿa,* "the scratching/scraping" *(dermatophytosis)*

CATEGORY: hot

ākorkor is the designation applied to a white, spreading, scab-like dermatosis on the head that destroys the hair.

CAUSES: The Kel Alhafra consider *ākorkor* to be hereditary, *etāri dāγ imārawān,* and as a sickness that affects entire families.

THERAPY: The Kel Alhafra are of the opinion that if the body of someone with *ākorkor* comes into contact with water, he or she will become seriously ill, and so those suffering from *ākorkor* often remain unwashed. Because *ākorkor* is classified as a "hot" disease, *isəssmaḍ*, a diet based on "cold" foods is advised. The Kel Alhafra also prepare a paste made from the roots of the *tāborāyt* tree *(Balanites aegyptiaca)*, which they mash, mix with cold water, *aman sāmmeḍān*, and apply to the head that has been shaved. An additional remedy is *bālāŋa*, shea butter,[223] which is rubbed into the affected areas of the skin

ālfaγ, Arabic: *aurāk* or *al-imra'*, "the explosion/detonation" *(thrombosis)*
CATEGORY: hot/cold
ālfaγ causes nausea, *tākmo n-ulh*, vomiting, *ibsan*, tiredness, *alāḍḍeš*, and pain in the thigh and lower leg, *təkm-e tayma-ənnes, elāγ-ənnes d-itəfrān-ənnes*. The Kel Alhafra recognize *ālfaγ* as an escalation of *tāhafnent*, in which the body feels cold even though the person concerned is sweating. Women who are overweight and have too little exercise are especially susceptible to *ālfaγ*, whose signs are yellow eyes, *tiəṭṭawen ti tāraγnen*, yellow gums, *tihayniwen ti tāraγnen*, a yellow skin, *elām āraγān*, and swollen feet.
CAUSES: The Kel Alhafra hold the view that *ālfaγ* is provoked by cold milk, *axx sammeḍ,* in particular fresh cow milk, but also by obesity and lack of exercise.
THERAPY: One therapy for *ālfaγ* is an infusion of the leaves of the *ājār* tree *(Maerua crassifolia)*. Lightly pounded whole millet, *tajārafjāraft n-enāle*, is another remedy which may be eaten alone or mixed with water, *aman*, and fresh milk, *axx kafayān*, and drunk three times a day. More exercise is advised, and dried meat, *tafārkit*, is also considered effective against *ālfaγ*.

ālšin/ušəḍ (also *torhənna ta n-tenere)*, Arabic: *ğunūn,* "insanity", "sickness of the emptiness, desire, loneliness"
The Kel Alhafra speak of insanity, *ālšin* (spirit, demon), or *ušəḍ,* mental disease (also *torhənna ta n-tenere*), when someone lives entirely in her or his own world, lacks reason, talks to her- or himself, does not participate in the social life of the group, and may sometimes have a malicious character and act violently toward others.
CAUSES: Spiritual errors, *anāfraγ n-tayətte*, moral guilt, *ābākkaḍ*, and apostasy, *ālžahil,* can result in possession, *ālšin*, by evil spirits and demons, *kel tenere* or *ifritān*.

---

223 Shea butter, *bālāŋa,* is made from the nut of *Vitellaria paradoxa*, and in a pure state can be kept for up to 4 years even at high temperatures. The Kel Alhafra buy *bālāŋa* on the Saturday market in Ber and use it, for example, to grease their goatskin water sacs, *iddidān*, and as a medication that is rubbed and massaged on painful parts of the body.

THERAPY: The Kel Alhafra view mental illnesseses (*torhənnawen ti n-tenere*) as curable by "maraboutage", in which the demons are driven out of the possessed body.

amādul n-iman, "begging for the soul"
CATEGORY: hot

In Tamasheq, *tamədilt* means "begging", and *amādul n-iman* designates the "beggar for the soul". *amādul n-iman* is a state that occurs shortly before death and has usually been preceded by an inflammation of the liver, *aɣrum*, or spleen, *amlāqqis*. Someone suffering from *amādul n-iman* can no longer sleep, may only be able to remain in a sitting position, and usually dies after a few days.

CAUSES: *amādul n-iman* is described as a progression of *tāhafnent*, for which the consumption of too many foods classified as "hot", *issukās* – such as sugar, *əssukar,* fresh milk, *axx kafayān*, fat, *tādhunt*, meat from the cow, *isan n-tas,* and the goat, *isan n-taɣāt* – is held responsible.

THERAPY: Crushed leaves of the *tājārt (Maerua crassifolia)* mixed with water. All therapies used for *tāhafnent* should also relieve the suffering of someone with *amādul n-iman.*

āmāɣras,[224] Arabic: *zuharī,* "that which cuts through the neck/that kills" *(syphilis)*[225]
CATEGORY: hot

The first symptoms of *āmāɣras* are *teẓẓort n-iɣāssān*, arthritic pains, fever, *tenāde*, intense itching, *ukmāš*, and small blisters on the skin, *timẓar.* In later stages of the disease, dark lesions appear on the skin, *tiforawen*, that itch, *təhee ukmāš.*

The Kel Alhafra are convinced that nothing can cure *āmāɣras* totally, not even the remedies offered by the *lāɣtortān*, the biomedically trained doctors in the health care centers. (Some people suffering from *āmāɣras* do go to the health care center in Ber, where they are given amoxicillin injections,[226] but as soon as they begin to recover, the therapy is usually broken off, and after a while the symptoms return.) The Kel Alhafra think that *āmāɣras* is particularly bad

224 *āmāɣras* (pl. *imāɣrasān*) is derived from the Tamasheq verb *əɣrəs*, which literally means "to cut the neck", "to kill", but also "to cut" and "to cross over".
225 The syphilis referred to here is the endemic, non-venereal syphilis (Bejel), which is usually contracted extragenitally during childhood and expresses symptoms on the skin, mucosa and bones exclusively in stages II and III. See *Roche Lexikon Medizin*, Hoffmann La Roche AG, 4th edition (Munich: Urban & Fischer, 1999).
226 *Amoxicillin* is a moderate-spectrum, bacteriolytic, β-lactam antibiotic.

during the dry season of *ewelān*, but that sufferers feel better during the rainy season, *s-akāsa*, when there is enough milk to drink.

CAUSES: According to the Kel Alhafra, *āmāγras* can be caused by *iba n-imənsiān*, malnutrition, *āmāγrəs,* a change in diet, as well as poor hygiene, *iba n-ašəšədaj,* and can be transmitted by fleas, *tilken,* and infected clothes.

THERAPY: The Kel Alhafra know of no effective treatment for *āmāγras.*

āmāγras wa māllān, "the white *āmāγras* (syphilis)" *(vitiligo)*
CATEGORY: hot

āmāγras wa māllān often begins with arthritic pain, *tākmo n-iγāssān,* and a white spot on the skin, *əsib wa māllān fāll elām,* that enlarges in size and spreads as white patches that eventually cover the entire body.

CAUSES: *āmāγras wa māllān* in the Kel Alhafra view is inherited, *etāri dāγ imārawān.*

THERAPY: No effective therapy is known.

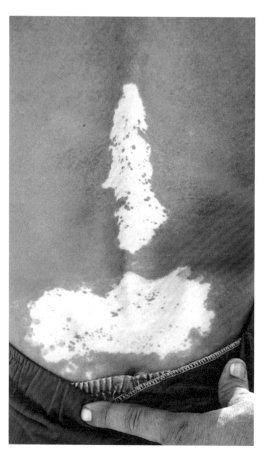

Figure 4.2. āmāγrās wa māllān
in an encampment at In Astilan (October 2005).

āmāɣras wa n-āfnoozān, *"āmāɣras",* (syphilis) that reduces *(leprosy)*
CATEGORY: hot
Synonym for *jəri,* leprosy.

āmāɣrəs, "traversing a difficult situation", "a change in diet"
CATEGORY: hot
āmāɣrəs is derived from the same root, *əɣrəs,* as *āmāɣras,* syphilis, but means here "traversing (a difficult situation, a difficult terrain)". *"ma təməɣrāsād?"* "What are you lacking?" is a common question during periods of dietary change; *"əməɣrāsāɣ i-axx",* the reply will often be: "I'm lacking milk". *āmāɣrəs* occurs when eating habits change, producing withdrawal and deficiency symptoms as well as causing a general debilitation of the organism, *tarəkkəm n-tayəssa,* a situation that encourages the development of diseases. This dietary switch, *āmāɣrəs,* is viewed by the Kel Alhafra as an illness in itself, *torhənna.* Faḍimatu, for example, told me that years ago, at time when there had been ample milk and butter in her encampment, she had visited her father in his encampment where there was a milk shortage, *iba n-axx.* From one day to the next, she had been forced onto a diet of just cereals, *allon,* and she had come out in black splotches all over her body, *tiforāwen tikāwālnen.*[227] Someone with *āmāɣrəs* suffers from headaches, *tākmo n-eɣāf,* vomiting, *ibsan,* fever, *tenāde,* and heavy eyes, *təṭṭāwen aẓẓaynen,* and the skin slowly turns darker, *elām ikāwāl.*
For the Kel Alhafra, *āmāɣrəs* is the most serious sickness because it can be the cause of all other illnesses. They also view it as the preliminary stage before *āmāɣras,* syphilis: *"āmāɣrəs əssəbab n-āmāɣras",* "*āmāɣrəs* is the cause of *āmāɣras".* *āmāɣrəs* can occur whenever there is a change in season or a change in diet; once established in the body it cannot be healed.
CAUSES: An inconsistent lifestyle, changes in eating habits, *tāmutāyt n-isudar.*
THERAPY: Although the Kel Alhafra are of the opinion that nothing can induce *āmāɣrəs* to disappear completely, foods classified as "cold", *isəssmaḍ,* are recommended, and *ālmuxāynes* (*Cleome bradycarpa*) in cold water should provide some relief.

āmāššār, Arabic: *ḥubūba al-funṭīya,* "the evil one", "the hard chancre" (*ulcus durum,* a primary effect of syphilis)
CATEGORY: hot
āmāššār is recognized by a blood-filled pimple that enlarges in size and suppurates if it is not treated. The Kel Alhafra say that *āmāššār* is a first

---

227 Interview at Intikewen with Faḍimatu Wālāt Muḥammad Attaher, November 2005.

sign of *āmāyras*, syphilis, but if the pimple is cut off, the affected person is healed.

CAUSES: Poor hyiene is considered to be a predominant cause of *āmāššār*.

THERAPY: The spot is cut away and then the wound site is cauterized with a hot iron, *taẓẓārt*.

āmaẓla (pl. imaẓlan), Arabic: *šəgīga,* "head cold" *(influenza, sinusitis)*
CATEGORY: hot/cold

"āmaẓla torhənna n-imyārān", the Kel Alhafra say "*āmaẓla* is a disease of old age". The first symptoms are an allergy, *tadihāt*, provoked by spending time with animals, which is followed by pains in parts of the face and head, *teẓẓort fāll idəm d-dāy-eyāf*, and a heavy cold, *əjjəburu*.

CAUSES: *āmaẓla* is elicited by an allergy, *tadihāt* (to dust, animals, etc.), or by damp, cold conditions, *təssəmḍe*.

THERAPY: If *āmaẓla* is not too serious, the Kel Alhafra put *asrāy*, a snuff, red pepper, *iẓəkimba (Xylopia aethiopica),* and *aḍutān*, essences, in the nose to loosen the mucus. If that remedy is not fully effective, the urine of a calf, *āwas n-āloki*, is mixed with butter, *udi*, and placed in the nose for a period of three days. If the illness persists, a ram, *ekrār*, is slaughtered, *ālmuxāynes (Cleome bradycarpa),* butter, *udi,* and *āhārjəjəm (Cassia italica)* are added to the meat, and the dish is eaten until the cold has worn off.

arāfāy, "small pimple on the skin"
CATEGORY: hot/cold

arāfāy is not a disease on its own, but the name given to a small, itchy skin blister or pustule that, like an allergy, *sund tadihāt*, can spread over the entire body.

CAUSES: *arāfāy* can be caused by strong heat, *tākusse*, rain, *ajənna*, but also poor hygiene, *iba n-ašəšədaj*, especially in overweight women who do not wash often.

THERAPY: The affected areas are washed with soap, *āṣṣabu*.

aslim (pl. isəlman), Arabic: *aslīm,* "muscle pain"
CATEGORY: hot/cold

aslim refers to muscular pain in a specified part of the body; the plural, *isəlman*, designates, instead, non-localized, general muscle pains.

CAUSES: *aslim* is caused by a type of *aḍu* that attacks the muscles, the cold, *təssəmḍe*, or strenuous physical work, *aššāyāl āṣṣohāt*.

THERAPY: Either the body is cleansed internally with a laxative, *isəssənkar,* and *āhārjəjəm (Cassia italica)* for three days, or the sick person washes her- or himself with a lotion made from leaves of the *tešāyt (Salvadora persica),* *tājārt (Maerua crassifolia)* and *tādhant (Boscia senegalensis),* and does not sleep under the open night sky, but in the protection of the tent. Sometimes the affected part of the body is percussed with a buttered gourd, or the sick person drinks an infusion of *ālmuxāynes* (*Cleome braḍycarpa*), and eats a lot of meat, *isan,* and butter, *udi.*

āssām (also essām), Arabic: *tasammum,* "poison", poisoning
CATEGORY: hot
"ihee āssām" – "he has been poisoned", the Kel Alhafra say of anyone who has been stung or bitten by a poisonous animal, has eaten spoilt food, *terk išəkša,* or an inedible plant, *terk tāẓoli,* drunk polluted water, *aman ikordātnen,* or has an infected wound (abscess), *atunjār (ahəḍəḍu),* that is poisoning the body internally (tetanus).
CAUSES: Snake poison, *āssām n-tāššālt,* scorpion poison, *āssām n-taẓārdemt,* dirty water, *aman ikordātnen,* spoilt food, *terk išəkša,* plant poisons, *āssām n-tāẓoli,* or an infected wound (abscess), *atunjār (ahəḍəḍu),* following an injury.
THERAPY: As an antidote to all forms of poisoning, the Kel Alhafra drink sour milk, *axx əssəlayān,* which should bind the poison within the body.
In the case of scorpion stings or snake bites, the Kel Alhafra slaughter an animal, empty the stomach of its contents and place the wounded body part (usually the foot) in the stomach until the pain has disappeared (the Kel Alhafra ascribe an extractive effect to the animal stomach). The poisoned individual is then fed butter, *udi,* as a cathartic, so that the vomiting, *ibsan,* clears the body of any remaining poison.
Sometimes, however, the bite is first cut to release the poison before the affected body part is placed in the animal stomach. A poison-extracting effect is also attributed to the "pierre noire",[228] *tāhunt ta n-asāfar,* which is placed on the bite.

asuntəl, Arabic: *lams,* "the contact"
asuntəl is not a disease as such but a gesture or touch, *isuntəl,* that reinfects a diseased body part (usually during inflammations, *itunjārān*).

---

228 *tāhunt ta n-asāfar,* "the black stone", is a specially treated piece of bone which is used as a treatment for snake bites, *assām n-tāššālt,* scorpion stings, *āssām n-taẓārdemt,* and abscesses, *ahəḍəḍu.*
According to an *enāsāfār,* a healer, *tāhunt ta n-asāfar* is prepared as follows: bones whose marrow has dried and from which the fat has been removed are cut into small pieces about 5 to 6 cm in length and about 3 cm in width, filed, and recleaned. The pieces are laid on glowing charcoal on a flat surface, with the bone cavity toward the ground, and then covered with more glowing charcoal. In this process, the color of the bones changes from white to black, after which they are dipped in luke-warm water until no more gas bubbles are released. To test the effectiveness of the "pierre noires", they can be pressed against the inside of the upper or lower lip: if they stick, the production has been successful. After use, the "pierre noire" can be regenerated by placing it for one hour in boiling water or for two years in milk.

ašyoḍ, Arabic: *ğarab,* "itches" *(scabies)*
CATEGORY: hot
The skin of those with *ašyoḍ* itches, *ihee ukmāš fāll-elām-ənnes,* and dries out, *elām iquurān,* and they may scratch themselves until they bleed. The Kel Alhafra view *ašyoḍ* as highly contagious, *ihee emāls.*
CAUSE: Poor hygiene, *iba n-ašəšədaj.*
THERAPY: The areas that itch are washed, and then either fat, *tādhunt,* or butter, *udi,* mixed with *tebāremt* (*Andropogon nadus*) is applied to the affected parts of the skin. However the Kel Alhafra also burn animal bones, *iγāssān n-irəzzejān,* filter out the black liquid and apply the clear filtrate to the infected areas of the skin.

atləb (pl. itəlban), "Medina or Guinea worm" *(dracunculiasis)*
CATEGORY: hot
itəlban or *ilənkānān* is the name the Kel Alhafra give to worms that live in water pools and can puncture humans in the feet causing a suppurating ulcer that often becomes infected and may develop into an abscess. *itəlban* occur on the banks of rivers and in the Gourma region, but the disease, the Kel Alhafra say, does not exist in Azawad.
CAUSE: Worms, *itəlban/ilənkānān,* puncture the soles of the feet of humans who enter water pools.
THERAPY: The Kel Alhafra say that with *atləb* one must wait until the ulcer bursts and the worm has found a way through the skin; then it can be removed with a needle.

āttaxma, "digestive disorder"
CATEGORY: hot
The Kel Alhafra use the term *āttaxma* to describe digestion problems in general, when the organs of digestion are not functioning properly. The sick person often experiences stabbing pain, *tedeje,* in the stomach region, loses his or her appetite, *wār irha imənsiwān,* and has a bloated belly.
CAUSES: *āttaxma* is caused by poorly digestible foods, incompatible food combinations and malnutrition, *iba n-imənsiwān.*
THERAPY: An attempt is made either to stimulate the digestive processes by drinking an infusion of *ālmuxāynes* (*Cleome bradycarpa*) in hot water, or to "cleanse" the digestive organs with a cathartic, *isəssənkar,* by ingesting every day three small balls of cow dung, or by placing a camel tail, *ašiwa n-amənis,* in water and finally drinking the liquid (this is used in general as an emetic and cathartic).

atunjār* (pl. *itunjārān;* also *ahəḍəḍu), Arabic: *'adwā,* "the flaring up/the relapse", "swelling, abscess" *(infection)*

CATEGORY: hot

The Kel Alhafra use the term *atunjār* (pl. *itunjārān*)[229] to describe such infections as a general infection of a wound, *atunjār n-ābiwəs,* a breast infection during breastfeeding, *atunjār n-ifáffān,* or an infection of birth wounds, *atunjār n-ābiwəs n-təršen hārāt* (also called *ahəḍəḍu,* "swelling", "abscess"), which are often accompanied by fever, *tenāde.*

CAUSE: Infections are caused by the consumption of too many foods classified as hot, *issukās,* and a surplus of heat in the body.

THERAPY: As therapy for general wound infections, *itunjārān,* the Kel Alhafra smear lukewarm cow butter, *udi n-tas,* on the infected site.

As a remedy for breast infections, *itunjārān n-ifáffān,* the women mix pepper, *ižəkimba (Xylopia aethiopica),* with water, *aman,* and massage this into the breast, or they prepare a compress of *ahəjjar (Acacia nilotica* seed capsules) mixed with goat or camel dung, *eyərrajān,* which they place on the infected site to withdraw the "heat", *tākusse.*

For birth wound infections, *itunjārān n-ābiwəs n-təršen hārāt,* a hip bath like that used to treat *ibiwəsān* is prepared, or camel dung, *eyərrajān* (sing. *ayərraj),* is burnt in a hole in the sand over which the woman sits so that the smoke can enter her body.

aẓāndi, Arabic: *bawāsīr,* "hemorrhoids"

CATEGORY: hot

Symptoms are feelings of heat and burning in the anus, and blood appears in the stools, *ihee ašni dāɣ asbəkki.*

CAUSES: For the Kel Alhafra, the major cause of *aẓāndi* is constipation, *tāɣārt n-tāsa* (literally, "the sealing of the stomach"), due to a monotonous diet, *atābatāt fáll-iyen amənsi,* or too much sitting in the saddle or in the tent. In addition, in advanced stages of pregnancy, the unborn child can press on the organs in the underbelly and provoke *aẓāndi* in the pregnant woman, *tālxamilt.*

THERAPY: Therapy comprises a laxative made from leaves of the *tāhahist (Cadaba glandulosa), ahārjəjəm (Cassia italica)* and *balāssa (Commelina for-skalei),* together with *ākāmen (Zornia glochidiata)* seeds. If this is not successful in removing the hemorrhoids, the Kel Alhafra cut them out and cauterize the wound (the exception being during pregnancy, when hemorrhoids should not be removed surgically).

---

229 *atunjār* is the verbal noun from *ənjər,* meaning "to fall ill again", "to flare up", "to suffer a relapse".

aẓəlmāẓ wi lābasnen, Arabic: *ḫānūq,* "the bad throat" *(diphtheria)*
CATEGORY: hot
aẓəlmāẓ wi lābasnen is characterized by difficulties in swallowing and white spots in the throat, *titbəqq timāllolnen.* Death usually occurs after five to six days.
CAUSES: *emāls,* infection, but also *issukās,* "hot" foods.
THERAPY: Remedies include: a gargle of water containing *tamākšwit,* a type of red earth, and leaves of the *torša (Calotropis procera);* a drink made from charcoaled *torša* dissolved in water; and pounded green thorns of the *tāborāyt (Balanites aegyptiaca)* placed on swollen parts of the neck.

dāmbāraku, Arabic: *'amā laylī,* "night blindness" *(nyctalopia)*
CATEGORY: hot
dāmbāraku is a visual impairment that becomes particularly noticeable at dusk and at night, *fənnəẓ n-ahānay hullan s-ehāḍ* (although vision is normal at full moon), but for which there are no other visible symptoms.
CAUSES: The Kel Alhafra attribute *dāmbāraku* to heritable causes, *etāri dāy imārawān-ənnes,* malnutrition, *iba n-imənsiwān,* anemia, *iba n-ašni,* and a lack of milk, *iba n-axx.*
THERAPY: Ample fresh milk, *axx kafayān,* and meat, *isan.*

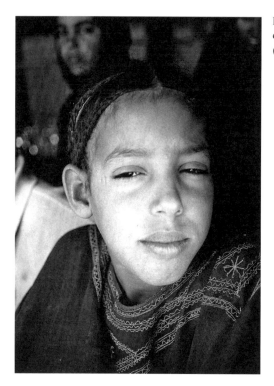

Figure 4.3. *A girl suffering from* dāmbāraku, *night blindness (Inkomen, November 2005).*

eɣāf wa lābasān, "the bad head"
CATEGORY: hot
Synonym for *tenāde ta n-afālla.*

eɣāf wa n-afālla, "the head from above"
CATEGORY: hot
Synonym for *tenāde ta n-afālla.*

eha, Arabic: *laysāra,* "miscarriage"
CATEGORY: hot
For a description of *eha* see chapter 3.4.3.
CAUSES: *tarəmməq* – a term in Tamasheq that encompasses moments of shock, being frightened and being anxious – can elicit a miscarriage, *eha,* as can *tārha* or *derhan,* a violent passion, an intense desire, *ejāḍāl,* a fall, *terk mājārād,* bad speech, *təšoṭṭ,* the evil eye, and *issukās,* foods with a "hot" character. (See also chapter 3.4.3.)
THERAPY: The women make pills from henna, *hālla* (*Lawsonia inermis*), mixed with butter, *udi,* which they swallow to stop the bleeding. They also drink henna powder, *ejel wa n-hālla,* dissolved in water.

ejāḍāl, Arabic: *'isqāṭ,* "fall"
ejāḍāl is the term used to describe any kind of fall, such as a fall from an animal like a donkey, *ejāḍāl n-ešāḍ,* or a camel, *ejāḍāl n-amənis,* or if a person stumbles and falls over somewhere. *ejāḍāl* can result in various injuries and fractures, and if a pregant woman, *tālxamilt,* falls, she may suffer *sāṭf n-tāsa,* "the emptying of the belly", i.e. a miscarriage.

ejāḍāl n-ehān, "the fall/collapse of the uterus" *(uterus inversion)*
ejāḍāl n-ehān, inversion of the uterus, occurs after a serious episode during pregnancy (for a more detailed discussion, see chapter 3.4.3.)
CAUSES: According to the Kel Alhafra, the uterus turns inside out, *ejāḍāl n-ehān,* when a birth has not gone well, when the mother is weakened by a succession of too many births, when a child is pulled forcibly out of the birth canal, or when, to expel an undetached placenta, too much pressure is applied to the uncontracted uterus and the umbilical cord.
THERAPY: The birth assistant immediately reverses the uterus, raises the mother's legs, binds them together, and leaves the *tenāmāẓẓort,* the birthing mother, lying on her back until the uterus has restabilized.

ejām, Arabic: *atāḥan,* "spleen" *(inflammation of the spleen)*
CATEGORY: hot
The Kel Alhafra use the term *ejām* for an inflammation of the spleen, *amlāqqis,* which as a consequence feels hard and enlarged and may cause pain.
CAUSE: The Kel Alhafra regard *ejām* as consequent to *tenāde tamāssāγarāt,* malaria.
THERAPY: The tail of a camel, *ašiwa n-amənis,* is placed in water that is subsequently drunk. In addition a laxative is prepared from *ahārjəjəm* (*Cassia italica*) and roots of the *tāborāγt* (*Balanites aegyptiaca*) to clean the body.

ermās, Arabic: *waǧa' al-ma'ida,* "upper stomach", "stomach pains" *(epigastralgia)*
CATEGORY: hot/cold
Pains in the upper abdomen, *ermās* (epigastrium), between the costal arch and the navel, which can be accompanied by nausea, *tākmo n-ulh.*
CAUSES: *ermās* is provoked either by too many "hot" foods, *isudar wi n-tākusse,* such as fatty meat, *isan wi ihan tādhunt,* oil, *dilwil,* pepper, *ižəkimba* (*Xylopia aethiopica*), or by too many "cold" foods, *isudar wi n-təssəmḍe,* such as the millet drink *ašədder,* or millet, *enāle,* itself.
THERAPY: The sick person eats a diet excluding all foods classified as "hot", such as fat, *tādhunt,* pepper, *ižəkimba* (*Xylopia aethiopica*) etc. and also drinks hot water mixed with *ahəjjar* (*Acacia nilotica* seed capsules), *tanust* (gum arabic), and *təllumt,* millet bran. When drunk before every meal, fresh milk, *axx kafayān,* with *ahəjjar* (*Acacia nilotica* seed capsuls), *tānafyāk, akāmen* (*Zornia glochidiata*) and *ālmuxāynes* (*Cleome bradycarpa*) should also provide some relief.

essām see ***assām***

ešer (pl. išerān), Arabic: *ḥadaš ḥafīf,* "the lightly wounded being", "scrape/ graze"
CATEGORY: hot/cold
The word *ešer* is derived from the verb *əšər,* meaning "to be lightly wounded", "to be scratched", "to be scraped". *"ma kāy išārān?"* the Kel Alhafra ask, "what has (lightly) injured you?" *"isāγerān",* the answer might be, "wood (that I was collecting)".
CAUSE: Any type of graze.
THERAPY: If the wound is very light, the Kel Alhafra are unlikely to treat it. If the scratch is deep, the therapy is similar to that used for other wounds (see *ābiwəs*) using leaves of the *tāborāγt* (*Balanites aegyptiaca*), a mixture of sugar, *əssukar,* and honey, *torawāt,* or hot cow butter, *udi ikkusān n-tas.*

əjjəburu, Arabic: *as-saḥāna,* "something enwrapped, packed", "common cold"
CATEGORY: hot/cold

On the basis of the symptoms, the Kel Alhafra use the word *əjjəburu* as a synonym for *āmaẓla,* but not when the cause is an allergy. The nose swells and becomes runny, the eyes are red and lacrimatory, and the person with *əjjəburu* has headaches and earaches and often develops a fever, *tenāde n-əjjəburu.*

CAUSES: *əjjəburu* can be elicited by a cold, *təssəmḍe,* by eating too much "cold" food, *issəmḍe,* but also too many hot foods, *issukās.*

THERAPY: *"iẓjə d-tāɣimit asāfar wa ofan n-əjjəburu",* the Kel Alhfra say, "being quiet and sitting still are the best remedies for a cold". One should lie down for three days and either drink an infusion of boiled *tādhant* leaves (*Boscia sengalensis*), or mix *tanust* (gum arabic) with *tāhahist* (*Cadaba glandulosa*) or *ālmuxāynes* (*Cleome bradycarpa*) and eat a handful, *iḍukāl,* three times a day.

əsib (pl. isibān), Arabic: *ḥabba* (pl. *ḥubūb*), "pimple, blister"
CATEGORY: hot

isibān is used by the Kel Alhafra as a general term for pimples, blisters and nodules.

əsib wa n-amākš, "the pimple that eats"
CATEGORY: hot

The initial symptom is a black papule on the skin, which is not at first painful. However, it suddenly begins to increase in size, becomes infected and destroys the skin around and below it, as far as the bone. The Kel Alhafra say that this spot, "eats the flesh to the bone", *"əsib wa n-amākš itatt isan har eɣās".*

CAUSE: The Kel Alhafra cannot identify the cause for *əsib wa n-amākš.*

THERAPY: *əsib wa n-amākš* cannot, according to the Kel Alhafra, be healed; the only recourse is to cut it out and cauterize the wound.

əsib wa n-āmmās (also *əsib wa n-tāsa),* "the spot that is found inside", "the stomach spot" *(ulcer)*
CATEGORY: hot

əsib wa n-āmmās is an internal ulcer that grows steadily and causes fever, *tenāde,* sleeplessness, *iba n-edes,* and exhaustion, *alāḍḍeš.* In bad cases, the ulcer becomes infected and forms an abscess, *ahəḍəḍu,* that opens inside, so that blood is seen in the feces; this stage often leads, the Kel Alhafra say, to death.

CAUSES: The Kel Alhafra cannot cite any cause for *əsib wa n-āmmās.*

THERAPY: A cold therapy with "cooling" items, *isəssmaḍ* (fresh milk, *axx kafayān,* millet, *enāle*) is followed by the attempt to cleanse the body with *isəssənkar,* a laxative (*ahārjəjəm, Cassia italica*).

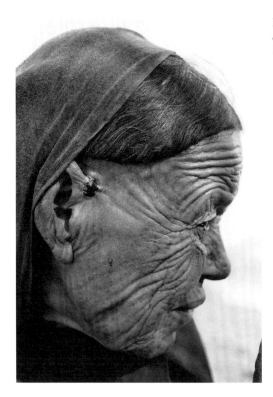

Figure 4.4. tamɣārt, *an old woman at Intikewen with* əsib wa n-amākš *(Intikewen, November 2005).*

əsib wa n-inākārāra, Arabic: *ṭu'lūl,* "wart", "corn"
CATEGORY: hot
isibān wi n-inākārāra is used by the Kel Alhafra to describe a small isolated "spot" on the sole of the foot or the hand, which has thorns that, "like the limbs of a tree", *sund iləktān n-emāyt,* send branches into the body.
CAUSES: People who go barefoot are susceptible to *isibān wi n-inākārāra.* Lack of hygiene, *iba n-ašəšədaj,* is an additional cause.
THERAPY: *isibān wi n-inākārāra* are cut off and the affected site is cauterized. Pounded thorns of the *tāborāyt* (*Balanites aegyptiaca*) are then applied to the wound to promote healing.

əsib wa n-tāmāɣrəyt,[230] "the pimple of those who have had a miscarriage"
CATEGORY: hot
əsib wa n-tāmāɣrəyt is an isolated pimple that appears anywhere on the body and develops over a period of two days. The area around the pimple is

---

230 *tāmāɣrəyt* is derived from the Tamasheq verb, *əɣrəy,* meaning "to have a miscarriage". It is possible that the origin of this term goes back to observations of animals with anthrax, *tanḍārt,* which often abort their fetuses.

inflamed and the person suffers from a high fever, *tenāde ta māqoorāt*. If the pimple appears on the head, *fāll eɣāf*, or the thorax, *fāll tarāja*, it is particularly dangerous and can be fatal.

CAUSE: Consumption of the meat of a *tanḍārt*, an animal infected with anthrax.

THERAPY: Leaves of the *ahākš* (*Acacia raddiana*) and the *torša* (*Calotropis procera*) are mixed with water and drunk. Then the Kel Alhafra place burnt *tājārt* (*Maerua crassifolia*) wood and *torša* (*Calotropis procera*) on the spot to heal it. Thorns of the *tāborāɣt* (*Balanites aegyptiaca*) are also pulverized and sprinkled on the wound to assist scarring. The Kel Alhafra never cut out *əsib wa n-tāmāɣrəyt*.

fāttas, Arabic: *fatīq,* "tissue breach" *(hernia)*
CATEGORY: cold
Something inside is torn, bulges softly outwards (usually in the underbelly), is painful and enlarges if it is touched, *asuntəl*, or when coughing, *tasut*.

CAUSES: According to the Kel Alhafra, *fāttas* develops either when someone has lifted a heavy weight, or during childbirth, when the labor efforts of the birthing mother have been particularly strenuous.

THERAPY: The Kel Alhafra do not know how to treat *fāttas*.

iba n-ašni, Arabic: *faqr ad-dam,* "lack of blood" *(anemia)*
CATEGORY: cold
Someone suffering from *iba n-ašni* has a pale skin, *elām-ənnes amšiši*, is often tired, *təlḍaš ālwāqq fuk*, and complains of headaches, *tākmo n-eɣāf*, and dizziness, *aɣālab*. The risks accompanying *iba n-ašni* are particularly high during pregnancy because the disease enfeebles the mother and she may die during labor if she loses too much blood.

CAUSES: Malnutrition, *iba n-imənsiwān*, or other diseases, *torhənnawen wiyādnen*, that enervate the body.

THERAPY: Consumption of meat, *isan,* and other "well-nourishing" foods, *išəkša wi olaɣnen*.

iba n-imənsiwān (also terk tamudre), "the lack of meals", "poor life" *(malnutrition)*
CATEGORY: hot
The Kel Alhafra call malnutrition *"iba n-imənsiwān"* – "a lack of meals", but also, *"terk tamudre"* – "a poor life". It manifests in situations in which the staple foods such as milk *axx,* meat, *isan,* butter, *udi,* or cereals, *allon,* are lacking. *iba n-imənsiwān* causes *āmāɣrəs*: those suffering from *iba n-imənsiwān* become emaciated, *əlbəkān*, and debilitated, *irəkkəmān*, they feel

tired, *ilḍašān*, and sick, *irhinān*, and may die from secondary diseases.
CAUSES: Drought, *mānna*, poverty, *talāqqāwt*, conflicts, *ikənnasān*, a
monotonous diet, *atābatāt fāll iyen amənsi*, a lack of knowledge, *iba n-tāmusne*,
etc. (see chapter 3.5.4.) are all identified as causes of *iba n-imənsiwān*.
THERAPY: Adequate, nutritious food, *išəkša wi olaynen d-inuflāynen*.

iba n-tārha n-imənsiwān, Arabic: *'adam aš-šahīya,* "the lack of desire for
meals", "loss of appetitie"
CATEGORY: hot/cold
Someone with *iba n-tārha n-imənsiwān* does not want to eat, *wār irha tetāte*, is
weak, *irəkkəm*, tired, *ilḍaš*, and has no energy, *wār ila āṣṣahāt*.
CAUSES: *iba n-imənsiwān,* malnutrition, *abārkot,* pregnancy, *torhənnawen*
diseases.
THERAPY: *təllumt,* millet porridge with water or milk, because *təllumt ar ulh,*
the Kel Alhafra say, "*təllumt* opens the heart" and restimulates the metabolism.

ibsan, Arabic: *qay',* "vomiting"
CATEGORY: hot
ibsan accompanies many diseases, especially those affecting the stomach and
the intestines, *torhənnawen n-ermās mey n-adānan.* If someone vomits for an
extended period of time, he or she can become seriously weakened.
CAUSES: Diseases of the stomach and intestinal tract, *torhənnawen n-ermās
d-ādānan,* headaches, *teẓẓort n-eyāf,* meningitis, *eyāf wa lābasān,* pregnancy,
abārkot.
THERAPY: Someone with *ibsan* should avoid foods that are classified as "hot",
issukās, and drink lukewarm water with *əššāyḥ (Artemisia santonica).*

iḍmārān, Arabic: *at-tihāb šu'abbī,* "heavy chronic cough" *(bronchitis)*
CATEGORY: hot/cold
iḍmārān describes a cough originating from deep in the breast and that has
persisted for a while, even if there is no accompanying disease.
CAUSES: The cold, *təssəmḍe,* the common cold, *əjjəburu,* influenza, *amāẓla,*
but also smoking, *silko.*
THERAPY: A drink comprising *tanust* (gum arabic), butter, *udi,* sugar, *əssukar,*
or honey, *torawāt,* in goat milk, *axx n-tayāt.* The meat of a lamb or kid,
isan n-akrāwāt mey isan n-eyāyd, and water containing *tāhahist (Cadaba
glandulosa), tānafyāk* or *ālmuxaynes (Cleome bradycarpa)* and red pepper,
iẓəkimba (Xylopia aethiopica), should also help against *iḍmārān.* Some Kel
Alhafra think that *taẓẓārt,* a plant used in tanning, can also be used to treat
iḍmārān.

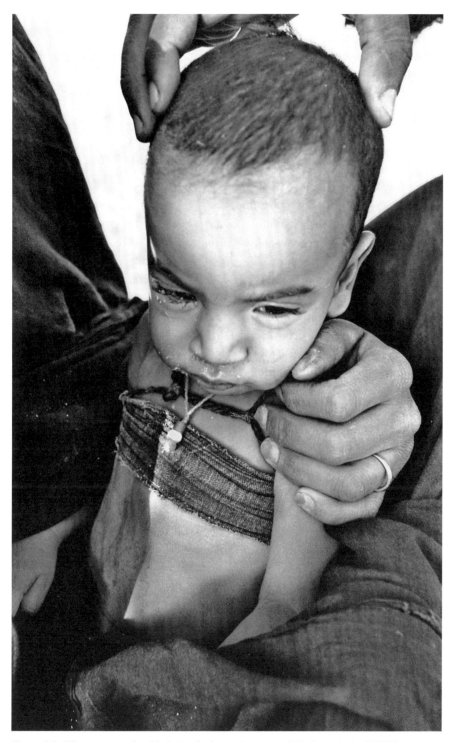

Figure 4.5. *When someone has* iḍmārān, *the breast is strapped (In Agozmi, April 2005).*

iḍmārān wi n-əjjəburu, "chronic cough with cold"
CATEGORY: hot/cold
iḍmārān wi n-əjjəburu is a strong cough accompanied by a cold, *əjjəburu*, and sometimes fever, *tenāde*.
CAUSES: The cold, *təssəmḍe*, common cold, *əjjəburu*, influenza, *amāẓla*.
THERAPY: As for *iḍmārān*.

iḍmārān wi lābasnen, Arabic: *al-gašuš al-ma'na*, "the bad, chronic cough" *(pneumonia)*
CATEGORY: hot
iḍmārān wi lābasnān begins with a heavy cough, *iḍmārān*, and yellow expectoration. Breathing is painful, *ikma asunfəs*, and the patient has a fever, *tenāde*, pains in the breast, *tākmo n-iḍmārān*, cannot lie on that part of the breast where there are *tedeje*, stabbing pains, and is in a generally very weak condition.
CAUSES: According to the Kela Alhafra, *iḍmārān wi lābasnen* is caused by the cold, *təssəmḍe*, during the cold season, *s-tajrəst*, but also by *afugg*, physical exertion while suffering from a strong cough.
THERAPY: A broth made from meat, *isan*, cooked in water. In another treatment, after drinking an infusion of *tadhānt (Boscia senegalensis)* leaves, which sometimes causes vomiting, a diet of sheep meat, *isan n-tihātten* and *tābālāttāst* is eaten until the symptoms subside. *tanust* (gum arabic) and *tāhahist (Cadaba glandulosa)* are also considerd to assist in curing *iḍmārān wi lābasnān*.

igādanāy (also bədi), Arabic: *ğudarī*, "smallpox"
CATEGORY: hot
Pimples, *isibān*, on the skin, that leave large scars. This disease no longer exists in nature.

ilənkānān, "Medina or Guinea worm" *(dracunculiasis)*
CATEGORY: hot
Synonym for *atləb* (pl. *itəlban*).

***imijlān* (sing. *emājāl*; also *tiwəkkawen n-tāsa*),** Arabic: *dūd*, "worms", "worms of the belly" *(intestinal parasites)*
CATEGORY: hot
imijlān are worms that live in the intestines, *dāy ādānan*, and can cause significant discomfort and pain.
CAUSES: The consumption of inadequately roasted meat or too much fresh milk, *axx kāfayān*, as well as poor hygiene, *iba n-ašəšədaj*.

THERAPY: Butter, *udi,* is mixed with cheese, *tikāmmāren taddāhnen, tāhahist (Cadaba glandulosa)* and red pepper, *ižəkimba (Xylopia aethiopica),* and eaten when the infested individual experiences pain.

inkəḍi,[231] "that which one hates"
CATEGORY: hot
Large pustules appear on the head, which heal when they have burst, but leave behind bad scars. Symptoms include fever, *tenāde,* headaches, *tākmo n-eɣāf,* and enlarged lymph nodes, *atunžār n-tifəɣen.* If the pustules become infected, the lymph nodes swell to such an extent that the disease can be fatal.
CAUSES: Too much food classified as "hot", *issukās.*
THERAPY: The pustules must be allowed to grow and burst. Then they are washed with soap and pounded thorns of the *tāborāyt (Balanites aegyptiaca)* are placed on the wound so that it dries out. The therapy is completed with a diet of goat meat, *isan n-tayāt,* or cow meat, *isan n-tas.*

išelal (also *tašləlt),* "opening which lets sunbeams through" (tree, tent riddled with holes etc.), "allergy to strong light"
CATEGORY: hot
If explosed to strong sunlight, someone with *išelal* has bad headaches, *teẓẓort n-eɣāf,* nausea, *tākmo n-ulh,* and can hardly open his or her eyes.
CAUSES: Sunlight, *ənnor n-tāfukk.*
THERAPY: Essences are placed in glowing charcoal and the fumes are inhaled.

jəri, Arabic: *baraṣ,* "leprosy"
CATEGORY: hot
The Kel Alhafra also call *jəri, āmāɣras wa āfnooẓān,* "the syphilis that reduces". The symptoms are strong sweating, exhaustion and nervosity. Scar-like streaks appear on the hand where the skin breaks and peels away to leave wounds that become infected and eat away the flesh until parts of the extremities fall off. *jəri* exists primarily near the river and the Kel Alhafra say that it does not occur in northern Azawad.
CAUSES: Hereditary transmission, *etāri dāɣ imārawān; jəri* usually afflicts entire families.
THERAPY: The Kel Alhafra know of no medication that is effective against *jəri.*

sāqqārnen, Arabic: *as-suʿāl ad-dīkī* also *al-ḥadd,* "whooping cough" *(pertussis)*
CATEGORY: hot/cold

---

231 The root *akəḍ* is to be found in *inkəḍi,* meaning "to hate", "to detest".

The Kel Alhafra report that epidemics of *sāqqārnen* are frequent, killing many children, but also adults. The disease usually lasts three months. The symtoms are swollen, dry eyes, vomiting, *ibsan*, and a chronic cough, *tāsut*, that sounds like a crowing cock. Children with *sāqqārnen* are not isolated by the Kel Alhafra (see chapter 3.3.4.).

CAUSES: *emāls*, contagion.

THERAPY: The patient is given ass milk, *axx n-tešāḍt*, the meat of a kid, *isan n-teɣse*, the meat of a hare, *isan n-timārwālen*, lamb meat, *isan n-akrāwāt*, fennek meat, *isan n-akorsi*, hedgehog meat, *isan n-tekānessit*, or fish, *imānan*. *"isan ɣās"*, "only meat", the Kel Alhafra say, is an effective treatment for *sāqqārnen*.

*šāggāɣ (*also *tamāḍrāyt n-tassididet)*, "the red one", "the small brother of measles" *(German measles, rubella)*

CATEGORY: hot

The Kel Alhafa sometimes call *šāggāɣ*, *"amāḍrāy n-tassididet"*, "the small brother of measles", because its course is less dangerous. The early symptoms resemble those of measles, *tassididet* – red eyes, headaches and red spots on the skin which feels hot. However, the symptoms usually subside after three to four days.

CAUSE: *tākusse*, excessive heat, and *emāls*, contagion.

THERAPY: As in the treatment of measles, *tassididet*, the initial therapies are those classified as "hot", and the patient is washed and wrapped up to encourage the body to sweat and bring the disease to the surface. This treatment is followed by medicaments and therapies classified as "cold", *isəssmaḍ*, to palliate the symptoms.

tābbašār, "to expose oneself to something"

CATEGORY: cold

"nayāɣ tābbašār" – "I rode without a saddle", the Kel Alhafra say for example, designating with *tābbašār* an action in which they have exposed their body to direct contact with something else, the consequences of which may be harmful. The skin of someone suffering from *tābbašār* itches, and he or she feels a fever between the skin and flesh. The skin does not feel hot to anyone else touching it, but the sick person feels an "inner fever" that can lead to paralysis within 24 hours.

CAUSES: *tābbašār* develops when one is surprised by a downpour and cannot dry the body immediately afterwards, or when one has walked too much and immediately afterward washes in a pool or river without first resting.

THERAPY: *issukās*, "hot" foods together with massage and manipulation of the joints. Then the Kel Alhafra burn *tebāremt (Andropogon nadus)* and mix the ashes with butter, *udi*, and smear this mixture on the feet.

tāddāryālt, Arabic: *'amā,* "blindness"
CATEGORY: hot/cold
The Kel Alhafra use the term *tāddāryālt* to describe a total loss of sight; a *emādderyəl,* a blind person, can no longer see.
CAUSES: Untreated conjunctivitis, *ahənnəj,* or a spot that develops inside the eye, *əsib wa n-ajmod,* and grows such that the eye can no longer be closed and becomes white and blind.
THERAPY: Treatments include placing the black seed kernels of *temājār jāwāst* in the eye to clean it, kohl *tazult* (antimony), and a subterranean desert stone that the Kel Alhafra call *mākkāra ta n-tuwāre,* which is crushed and rubbed into the eye. Ground cola nut, *goro,* and ground *tanust* (gum arabic) mixed with water and used as eye drops are also applied as remedies for *tāddāryālt.*

tādəmdəmt, Arabic: *ḫaras,* "muteness"
The Kel Alhafra use *adəmdam* to describe someone who cannot articulate with verbal language.
CAUSES: The Kel Alhafra view *tādəmdəmt* either as a condition that can be inherited or one that is provoked by the experience of a shock, *tarəmməq.*
THERAPY: *tādəmdəmt* can be cured by "maraboutage" if it is not inherited.

tadihāt, Arabic: *al-qarba,* "allergy"
CATEGORY: cold
tadihāt denotes an allergic reaction to dust, *aboqqāl,* animals, *irəzzejān,* aromas, *aḍutān,* and so on. Symptoms include coughing, sneezing, burning eyes and a running nose. *tadihāt* is often specified by an additional term: *tadihāt n-tiəṭṭāwen* describes an allergic reaction of the eyes, *tadihāt n-iḍmārān* is an allergy affecting respiratory passages, and *tadihāt n-azəlmaz* is an allergic reaction in the neck and throat.
CAUSES: Allergies can be elicited by camels, *imənas,* sheep, *tihātten,* goats, *ulli,* donkeys, *išāḍān,* dust, *aboqqāl,* aromas, *aḍutān,* and so on, but never by the cow.
THERAPY: *ālyonfārān* (cloves) are eaten or pounded and plugged into the nostrils. *tānyer,* a plant that grows on river banks, is burnt and the smoke inhaled.

tāfure (pl. *tiforawen),* Arabic: *al-amrāḍ al-ǧildīya,* "general term for dermatoses"
CATEGORY: hot
tāfure designates skin lesions in general, which often itch and spread over the body.
CAUSE: A lack of hygiene, *iba n-ašəšədaj.*
THERAPY: A diet with *isəssmaḍ,* cold foods. In addition, the Kel Alhafra prepare a paste from the roots of the *tāborāyt* tree, *ikewān n-tāborāyt (Balanites*

aegyptiaca), which they pound, mix with cold water, *aman sāmmeḍān,* and smear on the head. *bālāŋa,* shea butter rubbed into the affected skin areas, is another treatment.

tāfure n-āmāγras, "the dermatosis caused by *āmāγras*" *(syphylitic skin lesions)*
Category: hot
tāfure n-āmāγras designate small pimples and blisters on the skin or round skin lesions that turn black and are highly irritant.
Cause: *āmāγras,* syphilis.
Therapy: The Kel Alhafra know no effective remedy for *āmāγras.*

tāgarut, Arabic: *'aḍḍa,* "rabies"
Category: hot
The Kel Alhafra say that *tāgarut* is frequent. If someone is bitten by a possessed animal, the animal's *ǧinn* enters the victim's body, turning them mad so that they scream, foam at the mouth and eventually die. *tāgarut* is considered to be *torhənna ta n-tenere,* a mental disease.
Cause: The bite of a camel, donkey or dog possessed by a *ǧinn.*
Therapy: The Kel Alhafra know of no effective remedy for *tāgarut.* They go to a marabout for assistance and cauterize the bite with a glowing iron.

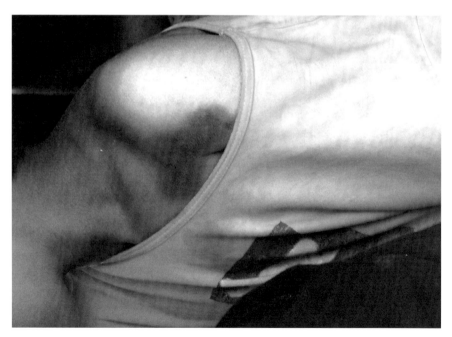

Figure 4.6. tāfure n-āmāγras, *skin lesions that turn black and itch severely (Buneyrub, March 2005).*

tāγārawiten (**sing.** *tāγārawit*),[232] Arabic: *nāsūr, pl. nawāsīr,* "those reduced to silence", "vaginal-perineal tear" *(fistulas)*
CATEGORY: hot/cold
In many women, but especially young mothers, the tissues around the vulva and the perineal area tear during birth or when the child is pulled with violence out of the birth canal. The Kel Alhafra do not sew these wounds, *ibiwəsān* (sing. *ābiwəs*), after the birth. A few Kel Alhafra women told me that sometimes the tears do not mend, resulting in incontinence, unpleasant odors and enormous inconvenience to the affected woman. *tāγārawiten,* "those reduced to silence", are borne with feelings of great shame and are rarely mentioned openly.
CAUSE: Birth wounds that do not mend properly.
THERAPY: The Kel Alhafra say that *tāγārawiten* cannot be cured.

*taγārt n-tāsa (*also *oγen),* Arabic: *imsāk,* "the sealing of the belly", "fastened/ tethered", "constipation"
CATEGORY: hot
Someone suffering from *taγārt n-tāsa* cannot defecate over a period of several days, is constipated, has flatulence and lacks energy.
CAUSES: Malnutrition, *iba n-imənsiwān,* a lack of exercise, *iba n-amrumər,* too much concentrated sour milk, *axx əssəlayān,* or too many "hot" foods, *issukās.*
THERAPY: Laxatives are prepared from leaves of the *tāhahist (Cadaba glandulosa),* from *ahārjəjəm (Cassia italica),* from leaves of the *balāssa (Commelina forskalei)* and from *akāmen* and drunk with water. For *taγārt n-tāsa,* the Kel Alhafra recommend in addition drinking fresh milk, *axx n-tas kafayān,* and in general taking in substantial quantities of liquid, although stagnant pool water, *aman n-iγārγārān,* should be avoided.

tāhafnent (**also known as** *tāhafnent māllāt,* "white" *tāhafnent*)
CATEGORY: hot/cold
For the Kel Alhafra, *tāhafnent* is not a disease as such but a condition of weakness, *arəkkəm,* and a loss of power, *iba n-āssahāt,* provoked by wastes from poorly digested foods that poison the organism internally. Symptoms are a loss of appetite, *iba n-tārha n-imənsiwān,* nausea, *tākmo n-ulh,* vomiting, *ibsan,* and a "fever between the skin and flesh", *tenāde jer elām d-isan,* whose heat cannot be felt by others touching the skin even though the person suffering from the condition feels overheated inside (as in *tābbašār). tāhafnent*

---

232 *tāγārawiten* (sing. *tāγārawit*) is derived from *γārāwwāt,* meaning "reduced to silence".

often accompanies other diseases such as *tenāde ta n-tamāssāyārāt, tenāde ti tākrayet* and *tawārāywārāy.*[233]

The Kel Alhafra say that people who get plenty of exercise, who are frequently on the move and have substantial physical strength rarely succumb to *tāhafnent*. It may however accompany *tenāde tamāssāyārāt* (malaria), and can even provoke this disease.

CAUSES: Everything sweet such as milk, *axx*, sugar, *ǝssukār,* fruits, *ilkāḍān,* or candy, *bonbontān,* can be responsible for *tāhafnent*. It can also be triggered by a sedentary lifestyle and obesity due to lack of exercise. If stagnant water from pools contains *tenāde tamāssāyārāt* (malaria), this in itself can precipitate *tāhafnent*.

THERAPY: *tāhafnent* is treated either with enemas or with medications that cause vomiting. For the enema, roots of the *tāborāyt (Balanites aegyptiaca)* are pounded, diluted with warm cow butter, *udi n-tas*, and water, and rectally injected. The emetic comprises, again, pounded *tāborāyt* roots with *ahārjǝjǝm (Cassia italica)* to cleanse the stomach. Subsequent treatment comprises a laxative made from *ahārjǝjǝm (Cassia italica)* with whole millet grains, *enāle,* cow urine, *āwas n-tas,* water, *aman,* and milk, *axx,* so that the *tāhafnent* leaves the body. This is followed by a meal of pounded *ahǝjjar (Acacia adansonii)* with *takrǝttit,* fresh butter, as well as advice and encouragement to get some exercise.

tāhafnent ta tāryāt, "*tāhafnent,* which is yellow"
CATEGORY: hot/cold

Some people also call this type of *tāhafnent,* "*tāhafnent tādalāt",* "*tāhafnent,* which is green/blue". The Kel Alhafra describe this form of *tāhafnent* as an escalation of the simple illness, with the same symptoms as *tāhafnent māllāt,* but the skin of the sick person taking on a yellow hue, *elām n-amarhin arayān.*

tāhafnent ti tākrayāt, "*tāhafnent,* which is fermented"
CATEGORY: hot/cold

tāhafnent ti tākrayāt designates the end stage of *tāhafnent* and is sometimes also referred to as "*tāhafnent tašāggāyāt",* "red *tāhafnent",* or "*tāhafnent ta kāwālāt",* "black *tāhafnent",* because the patient's vomit is laced with blood or takes on a black coloration. In *tāhafnent ti tākrayāt,* the body is no longer functioning properly, the circulation of the blood is blocked everywhere, and an inner "fermentation" process (similar to cheese making) takes place, leading to death.

---

233 For this reason, *tāhafnent* has been misidentified/mistranslated by various authors such as Sudlow (David Sudlow, *The Tamasheq of North-East Burkina Faso* [Cologne: Rüdiger Köppe, 2001]) and Heath (Jeffrey Heath, *Dictionnaire touareg du Mali* [Paris: Karthala, 2006]) as malaria, or by Hureiki (Jacques Hureiki, *Les médecines touarègues traditionnelles* [Paris: Karthala, 2000]) as jaundice.

***tāhayne* (pl. *tihayniwen)*, "gum inflammation"**
CATEGORY: hot
tāhayne is used as a term not only for the gums but also for a gum inflammation. The gums are red, *tāhayne tāšāggāyāt*, inflamed, *ihee ahəḍəḍu*, and bleed easily, *ihee ašni šik*.
CAUSES: Lack of oral hygiene, *iba n-ašəšədaj dāɣ em*, malnutrition, *iba n-imənsiwān*.
THERAPY: A mouthwash, *aman n-ahəjjar*, containing leaves or seed capsules of *Acacia nilotica*.

tājlifāt* (pl. *tājlifāten)*, "sensation of reluctance" *(nausea)
CATEGORY: hot/cold
Synonym for *tākmo n-ulh*.

***tākmo n-ārori / tezzort n-ārori*, "back pain"**
CATEGORY: cold
Synonym for *adku wa n-taɣimit*.

***tākmo n-asəjbas*, Arabic: *ālām fī mustadaqq*, "backache"**
CATEGORY: cold
In *tākmo n-asəjbas*, pain is felt in the entire lower back region including the sites of attachment for the long back muscles and the lumbar muscles.
CAUSES: The Kel Alhafra women regard the primary causes of *tākmo n-asəjbas* as gynecological in origin, such as the sequelae to a difficult birth, or during dysmenorrhea, but carrying heavy objects or malnutrition, *iba n-imənsiwān*, are also recognized as triggers for back pain.
THERAPY: The painful area is washed with a solution containing leaves of the *tešāɣt (Salvadora persica), tājārt (Maerua crassifolia)* and *tādhant (Boscia senegalensis),* and rubbed with butter. A diet with foods classified as "hot" is recommended.

***tākmo n- azəlmāz*, Arabic: *ālām az-zaur*, "sore throat"**
CATEGORY: hot/cold
Someone suffering from *tākmo n-azəlmāz* has a sore throat and difficulties swallowing, and there may be red points visible in the pharynx. The voice sounds hoarse.
CAUSES: The consumption of *issukās*, too much hot food, but also the cold, *təssəmḍe*.
THERAPY: If the *tākmo n- azəlmāz* is due to the overconsumption of "hot" foods, the remedy is to reduce the "heat in the throat", *tākusse dāɣ azəlmāz*,

with *isəssmaḍ*, "cold" foods. If on the other hand, it is due to catching cold, *təssəmḍe*, the body is warmed, and the sick person drinks an infusion of *tādhant (Boscia senegalensis)* leaves, water and *tanust* (gum arabic).

tākmo n-eɣāf, Arabic: *ṣudāʿ*, "headaches"

CATEGORY: hot

tākmo n-eɣāf designates headaches that can escalate to *eɣāf wa lābasān*, meningitis; the pain is sometimes accompanied by vomiting, *ibsan*.

CAUSES: Heat, *tākusse,* too much sun, *tāfukk,* foods classified as "hot", *issukās*, constipation, *tayārt n-tāsa*, and meningitis, *tenāde ta n-afālla*.

THERAPY: To cool it down, moistened *tāborāɣt (Balanites aegyptiaca)* leaves are placed on the head, camel urine, *āwas n-amənis*, is poured over the head, soap is rubbed on the head, and wet sand or henna are applied to the head.

If the pain is particularly bad, the Kel Alhafra sometimes cut the sick person's forehead to release the overheated blood, a procedure they call *ukəs n-ašni*, "the taking out of the blood". This should afford the sufferer some relief from the pain.

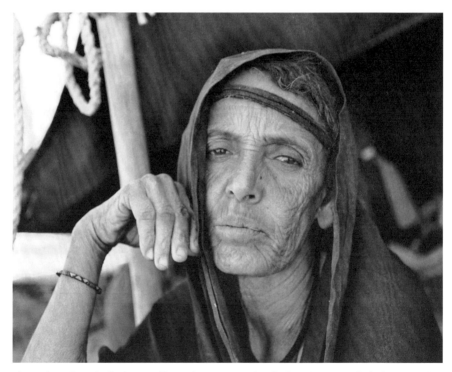

Figure 4.7. *If a Kel Alhafra is suffering from a strong headache,* tākmo n-eɣāf, *the head may be bound with a strip of material (Tin Timāɣayān 2005).*

tākmo n-iɣāssān, Arabic*: ālām al-ʿaẓm,* "bone pains", "joint pains"
CATEGORY: hot/cold
Nearly every Kel Alhafra complains of *tākmo n-iɣāssān*, poorly localizable
pains in the bones. The Kel Alhafra claim that this problem has become more
widespread during the recent past; once "a disease of the elderly", *torhənna ta
n-imɣārān*, today children suffer from it too.
CAUSES: The Kel Alhafra cite several causes for *tākmo n-iɣāssān*: *issukās*, too
many "hot" foods, *iba n-imənsiwān*, malnutrition, but also hard physical labor
and an arduous life.
THERAPY: To relieve *tākmo n-iɣāssān*, the Kel Alhafra set fire to seven balls
of camel dung place resin from the *ādārās* tree *(Commifora africana)* on top,
and, lying down, inhale the aromatic smoke.

tākmo n-iləs, "the pain of the tongue" *(aphtha)*
CATEGORY: hot
tākmo n-iləs describes small white ulcers, *isibān wi māllolnen*, on the tongue,
fāll iləs, that burn and are painful when they are touched.
CAUSES: Lack of oral hygiene, *iba n-ašəšədaj dāɣ em*.
THERAPY: A mouth rinse, *aman n-ahəjjar*, containing *Acacia nilotica* leaves or
seed capsules.

tākmo n-timāẓẓujen, Arabic: *waǧaʿ al-āḍān,* "earache", "ear infection"
CATEGORY: hot
tākmo n-timāẓẓujen designates an ear infection with pain in the inner ear,
sometimes with pus oozing from the ear, which hurts when pressure is put on
it. The Kel Alhafra say that *tākmo n-timāẓẓujen* will lead to deafness, *tāməẓẓəj*,
if the infection is not successfully treated. They also report that ear infections
occur most frequently during the cold season, *s-tajrəst*.
CAUSES: The cold, *təssəmḍe,* a cold wind, *aḍu sāmmeḍān*, meningitis, *eɣāf wa
n-afālla,* "hot" foods, *issukās*.
THERAPY: If a small child is suffering from an ear infection, drops of mother's
milk, *axxfəf*, or juice from *tājārt (Maerua crassifolia)* leaves are administered
to the ear. If a cold, *wa n-təssəmḍe*, is responsible for *tākmo n-timāẓẓujen*,
drops of lukewarm butter, *udi*, are used. Some women claim that pounded and
heated roots of the *tāborāɣt (Balanites aegyptiaca)* sprinkled into the ear are
also helpful.

tākmo n-ulh* (also *tājlifāt,* pl. *tājlifāten), Arabic: *ǧašīyān,* "pain of the heart",
"the feeling of reluctance", "nausea" *(hypotonia, hypertonia, bradycardia,
tachycardia)*

CATEGORY: hot/cold

For the Kel Alhafra, *tākmo n-ulh* describes a state of emotional pain like grief or anxiety, but also physical indispositions such as nausea, hypotonia (low blood pressure), hypertonia (high blood pressure), bradycardia (slow pulse rate) or tachycardia (high pulse rate). *tākmo n-ulh* can be accompanied by vomiting, *ibsan*, an irregular pulse, *ulhawān*, swollen feet, breathing difficulties and problems during physical exertion, and pain in the breast, shoulder or left arm.

CAUSES: *tākmo n-ulh* can be provoked by pregnancy, obesity, food incompatibilities or strong physical exertion.

THERAPY: Physical activity is to be avoided, and the patient should rest. If the symptoms are particularly bad, he or she should lie down for seven days. An infusion of roots of the *tāborāyt (Balanites aegyptiaca)* in water is used as an emetic, or *ahārjəjəm (Cassia italica)* is mixed with whole millet grains and fresh butter, *takrəttit*, as a laxative.

tamǝlle n-tǝṭṭ, "the white of the eye"

CATEGORY: hot

In *tamǝlle n-tǝṭṭ*, a white skin, *tamǝlle n-tǝṭṭ*, gradually spreads over the eye until it is completely covered. The Kel Alhafra say that *tamǝlle n-tǝṭṭ* is common but curable.

CAUSES: Excess heat in the body due to the overconsumption of foods classified as hot, *issukās*.

THERAPY: The remedy preferred by the Kel Alhafra for *tamǝlle n-tǝṭṭ* are eye drops of mother's milk, *axxfəf*. Alternative remedies are as for other eye conditions: black seeds of the *temājār jāwāst* placed in the eye to clean it; kohl, *taẓult* (antimony); a subterranean desert stone that the Kel Alhafra call *mākkāra ta n-tuwāre* that is crushed and sprinkled in the eye; eye drops of ground cola nut, *goro*, and ground *tanust* (gum arabic) mixed with water.

tāmǝẓẓəj, Arabic: *ṭaraš,* "deafness"

CATEGORY: hot/cold

The Kel Alhafra consider *tāmǝẓẓəj*, deafness, to be incurable; it is also not heritable.

CAUSES: Deafness ensues if one spends too long in the river with one's head underwater; if one receives a *tāzuget*, a heavy blow to the neck; or if an ear infection has not been cured.

THERAPY: "There is no medication for *tāmǝẓẓəj*", the Kel Alhafra say, *"wār ihee asāfar n- tāmǝẓẓəj"*.

tanābdānt (*also *bəddən), Arabic: *azḥāf al-ʿaib,* "the lamed, crippled being"
CATEGORY: hot/cold
By *tanābdānt,* the Kel Alhafra mean physical damage to the structures of support and movement, or of individual organs, which impair a person's physical performance.
CAUSES: Inheritance, *etāri dāy imārawān,* or as residual damage of a serious disease such as meningitis, *tenāde ta n-afālla,* malaria, *tenāde tamāssāyarāt,* or *tābbašār.*
THERAPY: The Kel Alhafra say that there is no effective remedy for *tanābdānt.*

tanānnāyāt, Arabic: *layya,* "the severe chafing and pressing"
CATEGORY: hot/cold
In Tamasheq, *nānnāyāt* means "strong chafing and pushing with great force". The Kel Alhafra compare *tanānnāyāt* with a screw turning forcefully into the body and causing intense pain. Symptoms include bad abdominal pains, a strong urgency to defecate, without diarrhea but with mucus and blood in the stools.
CAUSES: Following overconsumption of "hot" or "cold" foods, the digestion cannot function properly, *tarəkkəmt n-tāsa,* due to *aḍu,* air trapped in the body.
THERAPY: If the *tanānnāyāt ta n-tākusse* has a "hot" cause, water is mixed with cheese, *aman n-takāmmārt,* and drunk, but water containing *ālmuxāynes (Cleome bradycarpa),* together with butter, *udi,* and *ālišwaḍ* (fine *tebāremt, Cymbopogon schoenanthus,* leaves) should also help against *tanānnāyāt ta n-tākusse.*
For *tanānnāyāt* of a "cold" origin, *ta n-təssəmḍe,* however, cheese, *takāmmārt,* is grilled over a fire, pounded, mixed with butter, *udi,* and eaten. Also recommended, however, are goat meat, *isan n-tayāt,* hot butter, *udi ikkusān,* coffee, *ālqāhwa,* and hot milk, *axx ikkusān.*

taqāst, Arabic: *aḍ-ḍars,* "toothache"
CATEGORY: hot/cold
The Kel Alhafra use *taqāst* to designate toothache and tooth infections.
CAUSE: Lack of oral hygiene.
THERAPY: Tobacco, *tāba,* tea leaves, *āla,* or fat, *tādhunt,* are stuffed in the carious hole and heated with a glowing iron, or the infected area of the tooth is cauterized.

tassididet, Arabic: *al-ḥaymar,* "measles"
CATEGORY: hot
In *tassididet,* small, red spots, *titbəqq tišāggāynen,* first only detectable under the skin, break out all over the body. The sick person suffers from

cold symptoms, *əjjəburu*, headaches, *tākmo n-eɣāf*, and a high fever, *tenāde māqoorāt*. The Kel Alhafra view *tassididet* as highly contagious and they dread it because it can be fatal or lead to blindness.

CAUSE: *emāls*, infectious transmission; the Kel Alhafra say that people from outside bring the disease into the encampments. Those suffering from *tassididet* are not isolated (see chapter 3.3.4.).

THERAPY: The Kel Alhafra say that they have no effective therapy for *tassididet*. Someone with the disease is always first treated with *issukās*, "hot" therapies: he or she is washed, wrapped up and warmed so that sweating brings the spots to the surface. Sand is sprinkled in the eyes to disperse the spots there and to prevent blindness. Once the spots have appeared on the skin, medication and therapies classified as "cold", *isəssmaḍ*, are used.

***tāsut (*pl. *tisuten), Arabic: *al-quḥḥa*, general term for "coughing"
CATEGORY: hot/cold
The Kel Alhafra use the term *tāsut* to describe a cough in general, whether it accompanies a cold, *əjjəburu*, bronchitis, *iḍmārān*, asthma, *təssah*, or an allergy, *tadihāt*, or has been provoked by smoking. To treat a cough, the Kel Alhafra apply the remedy appropriate for the specific cause.

tāsut ta n-iḍmārān – "coughing of the bronchial tubes" *(bronchitis)*
CATEGORY: hot/cold
Coughing accompanied by pain in the chest, *tezzort n-iḍmārān*.
CAUSES: *təssəmḍe*, the cold, colds, usually at the beginning of *tajrəst*, the cold season, but also excessively strong sunlight, *tāfukk*, wind, *aḍu*, and sleeping in the open air, *tenāsedāy jelele*.
THERAPY: As cough cures, the Kel Alhafra drink water with *tanust* (gum arabic), *tāhahist (Cadaba glandulosa), tānafyāk*, or cooked goat milk with red pepper *(Xylopia aethiopiaca), axx n-tayāt ikkusān d-ižəkimba*.

***tāsut talābasāt,* Arabic: *al-quḥḥa al-funṭīya,* "the bad cough" *(tuberculosis)*
CATEGORY: hot
tāsut talābasāt manifests with a nocturnal fever that sets in at dusk and disappears by dawn. The coughing and *iḍmārān* gradually get worse, especially at night, and the sick person loses his or her appetite, loses weight and becomes weak, has pains in the chest or the back, and the bones may become distorted.
CAUSES: The Kel Alhafra view *tāsut talābasāt* as a hereditary disease that afflicts entire families, although sometimes it can develop from *iḍmārān*, bronchitis, *iba n-imənsiwān*, malnutrition, excessively strong sunlight, or hard living conditions.

THERAPY: The Kel Alhafra say that not only do they have no effective therapy for *tāsut talābasāt*, the modern medications available in the city are also powerless against the disease.

A woman with tuberculosis who had received treatment at the hospital in Timbuktu told me that at night, when the coughing fits prevented her from sleeping, drinking cold coffee, *inebhān ālqāhwa*, brought her some relief.

(However, an *enāsāfar*, a healer, from Ber maintained that the *imγad* among the Kel Serere in the Gourma region know a remedy for *tāsut talābasāt*: following an emetic of the *tādhant* plant in water, the patient undertakes a 40-day diet with sheep meat, *isan n-tihātten*, milk, *axx*, and plenty of water, *aman ajootnen*.)

tawārāγwārāγ, "that which colors the skin yellow"
CATEGORY: hot
wārāγwārāγ in Tamasheq means "to spin and look in all directions", a movement which brings the body to a condition of dizziness, *aγālab*, nausea, *tākmo n-ulh*, and causes a yellowing of the skin, *elām ārāγān*. Such symptoms are especially common during the sixth to ninth months of pregnancy, *γor talxāmilt dāγ iγor wa n- sāḍis har iγor wa n- tāẓa*.
CAUSES: Lack of exercise, *iba n-imərumorān*, a sedentary state, *azuzəγ*, malnutrition, *iba n-imənsiwān*.
THERAPY: First a laxative made from *ahārjəjəm (Cassia italica),* whole millet grains, *enāle,* cow urine, *āwas n-tas,* water, *aman,* and milk, *axx,* followed by a diet of pounded *ahəjjar (Acacia adansonii)* leaves with *takrəttit,* fresh butter, and the recommendation to take more exercise.

tedeje, Arabic: *daqqat al-ǧašuš,* "the stabbing"
CATEGORY: hot/cold
The root, *ədəj*, "to stab", is present in *tedeje*, a stabbing pain in the lungs, abdomen or chest elicited by a disease. (For *tedeje* as a symptom accompanying *iḍmārān wa lābasān*, pneumonia, see *tedeje ta n-iḍmārān*.)
CAUSES: *tedeje* can be caused by a common cold and cold air, *aḍu sāmmeḍān*, but also by *aḍu*, air circulating in the body that becomes dammed up and causes stabbing pains (see *tedeje ta n-aḍu*).
THERAPY: The Kel Alhafra employ foods and therapies classified as "hot", *issukās*.

tedeje ta n-aḍu, Arabic: *daqqat ar-rīḥ,* "the stab of the air"
CATEGORY: hot/cold
tedeje ta n-aḍu designates a stabbing pain at a specific point inside the body.

CAUSES: Either an inappropriate movement, or the build-up of *aḍu* in the body due to the consumption of indigestible foods.

THERAPY: To drive the accumulated air out of the body, a drink comprising *ālmuxyānes (Cleome bradycarpa)* and *ālišwaḍ* (fine leaves of the *tebāremt, Andropogon nadus*) in hot water mixed with butter.

tedeje ta n-iḍmārān, Arabic: *daqqat aṣ-ṣadr,* "the stabbing in the breast"
CATEGORY: hot/cold

tedeje ta n-iḍmārān designates a stabbing pain in the chest, usually accompanying *iḍmārān wa lābasān*.

CAUSE: Bronchitis, *iḍmārān*, that has already lasted two or three weeks.

THERAPY: *tanust* (gum arabic), red pepper, *ižəkimba (Xylopia aethiopica)* and *ālmuxāynes (Cleome bradycarpa)* are drunk in hot water. Foods classified as "hot", *issukās*, are also used as a remedy for *tedeje ta n-iḍmārān*.

temāslāγt, Arabic: *ar-rabw,* "suffocation" *(dyspnea)*
CATEGORY: hot/cold

An acute coughing attack provoked either by an allergy or if something gets stuck in the throat while eating.

CAUSE: Allergy, *tadihāt*, or choking on food.

THERAPY: If the coughing attack is due to an allergy, the Kel Alhafra apply the same therapies that they use for *təssah*, asthma.

tenāde (pl. tinədd), Arabic: *al-ḥumma,* general term for "fever"
CATEGORY: hot

tenāde accompanies many diseases: the sick person suffers from an overheated body, has headaches and sweats.

CAUSE: Dependent on the type of fever.

THERAPY: In general, "cooling" therapies, such as *tikāmmāren dāγ aman d-ālmuxaynes,* cheese in water with *ālmuxaynes (Cleome bradycarpa),* are applied to reset the body's thermal equilibrium. A person with fever should drink a lot of water and may chew green twigs of the *tāborāγt (Balanites aegyptiaca), tilifāwt n-tāborāγt*. In addition, a laxative made from *ahārjəjəm (Cassia italica)* and an emetic, *ikewān n-tāborāγt,* roots of the *tāborāγt,* are used to cleanse the body.

tenāde talābasāt, "the bad fever"
CATEGORY: hot

tenāde talābasāt is used both as a synonym for *tenāde ta n-afālla,* meningitis, but also to describe a fever that begins like influenza, *sund əjjəburu,* but is then accompanied by vomiting, *ibsan*, and in severe cases may lead to paralysis.[234]

CAUSES: Heat, *tākusse*, sun, *tāfukk*, and an excess of foods classified as "hot", *issukās*.

THERAPY: As for *tenāde ta n-afālla*.

tenāde ta n-afālla, Arabic: *al-ḥumma al-funṭīya,* "the fever from above/of the head", "the sickness from above". Also *tenāde ta n-eyaf* , "the fever of the head"; *tenāde talābasāt,* "the bad fever"; *eyāf wa n-afālla,* "the head from above"; *eyāf wa lābasān,* "the bad head"; *torhənna ta n-afālla,* "the sickness from above" and *torhənna ta n-tāfukk,* "the sickness of the sun" *(meningitis)*

CATEGORY: hot

tenāde ta n-eyāf, "the fever of the head", afflicts the uppermost part of the body, hence the designations modified by *"ta n-afālla",* "from above". The Kel Alhafra say that *torhənna ta n-afālla* is common and affects both children and adults. The symptoms are a strong headache, *tezzort n-eyāf,* and fever, *tenāde,* and after a few days the head becomes locked, the neck stiff, and the eyes stare upwards. The patient's sweat has an acrid smell, and after a few days he or she may show extensive signs of paralysis.

CAUSES: *tenāde ta n-eyāf* is attributed either to over-exposure to the sun or to foods classified as "hot", such as goat meat with butter, *isan n-tayāt d-udi,* sheep milk with cooked goat meat, *axx n-tihātten d-isan n-tayāt saŋŋān,* or just milk, *axx,* alone.

THERAPY: In addition to giving the sick person a lot of cold water to drink, the hot body is washed in a solution of water containing *ājār* and *tešāyt (Maerua crassifolia and Salvadora persica)* leaves. To bring the fever down, henna, *hālla (Lawsonia inermis)* is applied to the head, or a mixture of leaves of the *tājārt (Maerua crassifolia)* and camel urine, *āwas n-amənis,* is placed on the head.

tenāde ta n-āmāɣrəs, "the fever of the change in diet"

CATEGORY: hot

The fever of *āmāɣrəs* is one of the "withdrawal symptoms" that occur when dietary habits change, particularly at seasonal transitions. It may also accompany malnutrition.

CAUSES: *iba n-imənsiwān,* malnutrition, and *āmāɣrəs,* the absence of a dietary custom.

---

234 The Kel Alhafra have no explicit term to describe polio, but view *tenāde talābasāt* as a condition that can lead to paralysis, especially in children.

THERAPY: The Kel Alhafra recommend a diet based on foods classified as cold, *isəssmaḍ*, but *ālmuxāynes (Cleome bradycarpa)* with cold water, *aman sammeḍān*, may also relieve *tenāde ta n- āmāyrəs*.

tenāde ta n-ehāḍ, Arabic: *ḥumma al-lail,* "the fever of the night"
CATEGORY: hot
tenāde ta n-ehāḍ describes a nocturnal fever that causes sweats and occurs during *tāsut talābasāt,* tuberculosis.
CAUSE: *tāsut talābasāt,* tuberculosis.
THERAPY: The Kel Alhafra regard *tāsut talābassāt* as incurable.

tenāde ta n-əjjəburu, Arabic: *ḥumma as-saḥāna,* "the fever of the common cold"
CATEGORY: hot
tenāde ta n-ejjəburu is a fever that accompanies a heavy cold, *əjjəburu māqoorāt.*
CAUSES: The cold, *təssəmḍe,* too much "cold" food, *isəssmaḍ,* but also too many "hot" foodstuffs.
THERAPY: As for *əjjəburu.*

tenāde ta n-iḍmārān, Arabic: *ḥumma at-tihāb šu'abbī,* "the fever of the bronchial tubes"
CATEGORY: hot
tenāde ta n-iḍmārān designates the fever that accompanies a severe bronchitis, *iḍmārān.*
CAUSE: *iḍmārān,* bronchitis.
THERAPY: As for bronchitis, *iḍmārān.*

tenāde ta n-tamāssāyarāt (*also *tenāde tamāssāyarāt/tenāde ta tāšrayāt), "the fever at the end of the rainy season", "the new fever" *(malaria)*
CATEGORY: hot
tenāde ta n-tamāssāyarāt designates a fever that, according to the Kel Alhafra, is becoming increasingly more common at the end of the rainy season, *s-yārāt.* The symptoms are fever, *tenāde,* headaches, *tākmo n-eyāf,* and shivering, *tisas,* followed by sweats, *tide,* and vomiting, *ibsan.*
CAUSES: The Kel Alhafra attribute *tenāde ta n-tamāssāyarāt* to the consumption of milk at the end of the rainy season, *axx s-yārāt, amāyrəs,* or strong solar radiation, *tāfukk.*
THERAPY: *isəssmaḍ,* cold therapies, such as drinking plenty of water, and chewing *tilifāwt n-tāborāyt,* fresh, green *tāborāyt (Balanites aegyptiaca)*

twigs. The body may be cleansed using either a laxative, *isəssənkār,* (e.g. *ahārjəjəm, Cassia italica*), or an emetic, such as pounded *tāborāyt* roots drunk with water.

tenāde ta n-təssəmḍe, "the cold fever"
CATEGORY: cold
tenāde ta n-təssəmḍe is a specifically "cold" form of fever in which the body feels cold to the touch but the sick person experiences an inner fever. *tenāde ta n-təssəmḍe* is considered by the Kel Alhafra to be more serious than the fevers categorized as "hot" because it lasts a long time, may become chronic and is difficult to cure. *tenāde ta n-təssəmḍe* is always accompanied by *ermās,* stomach discomfort.
CAUSES: The cold, *təssəmḍe, tābbašār,* "exposure to something" and *tāhafnent.*
THERAPY: Butter, *udi,* fresh milk, *axx kāfayān,* and *tānafyāk.*

tenāde ta tāšrayāt, Arabic: *al-ḥumma al-ğadīda,* "the new fever"
CATEGORY: hot
The Kel Alhafra use the term *tenāde tāšrayāt* to describe a fever that has only appeared in the last ten years. Their descriptions of the symptoms correspond to those for *tenāde ta n-tamāssāyarāt,* but *tenāde tāšrayāt* is not associated with any particular region (for example proximity to rivers) and today occurs everywhere in Azawad.
(For the causes and therapy, see *tenāde ta n-tamāssāyarāt*).

tenāde ti tākrayet, "the fever of fermentation"
CATEGORY: hot
In the "fermenting fever", *tenāde ti tākrayet,* the body is in a condition resembling that of *axx ikāray,* fermented sour milk, or milk that has been curdled to make cheese: the entire body has a yellow coloration, the white of the eye is also yellow, and the disease is usually fatal after a few days.
CAUSES: *tenāde ti tākrayet* sets in when the liver is no longer functioning properly, but can also be provoked by malaria.
THERAPY: Milk with leaves of the *tājārt (Maerua crassifolia)* and millet por- ridge, *təllumt. təllumt* should open the heart, *ar ulh,* to restimulate the dam- aged organism.

tenāde ti n-kāraḍ, "the three-day fever" *(chronic malaria)*
CATEGORY: hot
tenāde ti n-kāraḍ is used by the Kel Alhafra to describe a three-day, chronic fever with symptoms resembling those of *tenāde ta n-tamāssāyarāt.*

CAUSE: *tenāde ta n-tamāssāyarāt*, chronic malaria that has not been cured.
THERAPY: A diet rich in meat is recommended, together with milk, *axx*, leaves of the *tājārt (Maerua crassifolia)* and *təllumt*, millet porridge.

***təlleyāf* (pl. *təlleyāfen*; also *ayālab*, pl. *iyālabān)*,** Arabic: *dauḥa,* "the bouncing of the head", "the dominated and besieged being" *(vertigo)*
CATEGORY: hot/cold
təlleyāf causes feelings of dizziness and loss of balance and may lead to an impairment of the circulation, *arəkkəm n-tayəssa*, and fainting, *ayəttus*.
CAUSES: Pregnancy, *abārkot*, anemia, *iba n-ašni*, heart problems/nausea, *tākmo n-ulh,* but also strong headaches, *tezzort n-eyāf*, *tawārāywārāy*, hunger, *jələk*, or thirst, *fad*.
THERAPY: Avoidance of bending over too quickly and heavy, physical exertion. If someone's symptoms are bad, they are recommended to lie down.

***təssāh*,** Arabic: *ar-rabw*, "shortness of breath" *(asthma)*
CATEGORY: hot/cold
The signs of *təssāh* are breathlessness, with the lips and fingernails turning blue, while the veins in the neck swell. The Kel Alhafra view *təssāh* as hereditary and it can also provoke bronchitis, *iḍmārān*.
CAUSES: *təssāh* is elicited either by allergies, *tadihāten* (to dust, animals etc.), or by the consumption of food left uncovered overnight and thus exposed to the *kel tenere*, which, having "contaminated" the food, gain entry into the body of anyone eating it.
THERAPY: *təssāh* can be cured by drinking a mixture of pounded *tāborāyt (Balanites aegyptiaca)* roots mixed with butter, *udi*, and water, *aman*.

***tibiay* (also *ahəḍəḍu n-tākorsāyt d-tifəyen)*,** "the swelling of Adam's apple and the lymph nodes in the neck"
CATEGORY: hot
The symptoms of *tibiay* are fever and small red spots in the throat, *titbəqq tišāggāynen*, that turn yellow when they have healed. The Kel Alhafra say that *tibiay* is highly contagious and can be fatal if it is not treated properly because it closes the throat, preventing speech and swallowing.[235]
CAUSES: Foods classified as "hot" such as fat, *tādhunt*, salt, *tesəmt,* and pepper, *ižəkimba (Xylopia aethiopica),* but also bitter substances.

---

235 Ousman describes *tibiay* as "amygdalite", tonsilitis or "lymphadénite cervicale", inflammation of the neck lymph nodes. See Mohamed Ousman, *La médecine traditionnelle tamachèque en milieu malien* (Bamako 1981) 26.

THERAPY: People affected with *tibiay* gargle with an infusion of *akārkāra*, a plant that grows near the river Niger, and suck on *umm ālxer*, resin of the *ādārās* tree *(Commifora africana)*.

tijdil āwas, Arabic: *al-ʿaṣr,* "the urine refusal"
CATEGORY: hot/cold
tijdil āwas is derived in part from the verb *əjdəl*, meaning "to forbid", "to prevent something". On the one hand, the Kel Alhafra use *tijdil āwas* to describe any complaint associated with the bladder or the abdomen in a very general sense and without any further precision. However, *tijdil āwas* can also be used quite explicitly for a bladder infection (frequent urges to urinate, pain urinating, pain in the flanks, and in bad cases, blood in the urine and fever) or, in men, prostate troubles (urge to urinate but inability to do so, sometimes accompanied by fever). (When I asked one woman if she could describe her *tijdil āwas* in more detail, she told me she was suffering from *tākmo n-lutan*, pain in the region of her ovaries, and that she could not retain her urine, another symptom she subsumed under the collective term *tijdil āwas*.)[236]
CAUSES: Too much sun, *tāfukk tajət*, hot sand, *ešəš,* but also the cold, *təssəmḍe*.
THERAPY: For *tijdil āwas*, the Kel Alhafra recommend drinking a lot and then, depending on whether the cause is of a "hot" or a "cold" character, *isəssmaḍ,* "cold" therapies (such as sitting in the river), or *issukās*, "hot" therapies (e.g. the consumption of fresh milk, *axx kafayān*) are applied. In addition, anyone suffering from *tijdil āwas* should not work in the sun, *wār təššāyālād dāy tāfukk*, or walk on hot sand, *wār təkked fāll ešəš*.
If a woman is suffering from a bladder infection, *tijdil āwas* – which, according to the Kel Alhafra women, can happen frequently during the cold season, *s-tajəst* – she will dig a hole in the sand and heat charcoal in it. She then places essences, *aḍutān*, on the glowing charcoal and sits over it to let the smoke penetrate her body. She will also try to consume as much meat, *isan*, and butter, *udi*, as possible.

tijdil āwas təssāryāt ihee ašni, "urine accumulation that burns and contains blood" *(schistosomiasis)*
CATEGORY: hot
The symptoms are pains in the abdomen and between the legs, especially after urinating. Blood is found in the urine, *ihee ašni dāy āwas*. The Kel Alhafra view *tijdil āwas təssāryāt ihee ašni* as an escalation of *tijdil āwas*.

236 Interview at Inkilla with Faḍimata Wālāt Alyāḍ, November 2005.

CAUSES: As for *tijdil āwas*: too much sun, *tāfukk tajət*, hot sand, *ešəš,* and the cold, *təssəmḍe.*
THERAPY: As for *tijdil āwas.*

tilāwayen, "joint pains" *(rheumatism)*
CATEGORY: hot/cold
The Kel Alhafra use the term *tilāwayen* for joint pains that can develop into swollen, red joints and infections. They report that both adults and children suffer from this complaint.
CAUSES: Too many foods classified as "hot", *issukās,* but also the cold, *təssəmḍe,* and malnutrition, *iba n-imənsiwān.*
THERAPY: A drink made from *tanust* (gum arabic) with butter, *udi,* sugar, *əssukar,* or honey, *torawāt,* and goat milk, *axx n-tayāt.* Other remedies include: the meat of a lamb or kid *(akrāwāt* or *eγāyd),* or water containing *tāhahist (Cadaba glandulosa), tānafyāk* or *ālmuxaynes (Cleome bradycarpa)* and *ižəkimba (Xylopia aethiopica).* Some people also mix *tazzārt,* a plant used for tanning, with butter, *udi,* and spread this on the painful parts of the body.

timāẓẓujen, "ear pain", "ear infection"
CATEGORY: hot
See *tākmo n-timāẓẓujen.*

timennāḍ, "the squirming with pain", "digestive disorder"
CATEGORY: hot/cold
timennāḍ is used by the Kel Alhafra for stomach colics that are sometimes accompanied by fever, *tenāde.* The symptoms include the urge to defecate, *oḍan tenere,* but difficulty doing so, and the feces contain mucus, *ihee ašānyaman dāγ isbəkkitān.* It should be noted, however, that *timennāḍ n-tiḍeḍen,* "women's cramps", and *timennāḍ n-təršen hārāt,* "cramps during the attempt to have something", are used to designate labor pains.
CAUSES: Too many foods classified as "hot", dirty water, *aman ikordatnen,* but also malnutrition, *iba n-imənsiwān.*
THERAPY: *timennāḍ* due to *issukās,* "hot" foods, is treated with the drink, *aman n-ahəjjar,* water containing seed capsules from *Acacia nilotica,* and rice porridge, *iləwa n-tafāyāt,* with butter. For *timennāḍ* with a "cold" cause, treatments are: sweetened sour milk, *axx əsəlayān d-əssukār,* to which crumbled cheese, *tikāmmāren taddāhnen,* has been added; rice with *akāmen (Zornia glochidiata)* seeds and seven seeds from the fruits of the *tālšušāt (Aframomum melegueta);* an infusion of *ālmuxāynes,* water and fresh butter, *takrəttit.*

***tiwəkkawen* (sing.** *tawəkke n-tāsa),* "worms" *(intestinal parasites)*
CATEGORY: "hot"
Synonym for *imijlān*.

torhənna ta n-afālla, "the disease from above/the north" *(meningitis)*
CATEGORY: hot
See tenāde *ta n-afālla.*

torhənna ta n-tiksənna, "the disease in which one is carved" *(peritonitis)*
CATEGORY: hot
The Kel Alhafra report that *torhənna ta n-tiksənna* was particularly frequent
during the drought year of 1984. The abdominal skin is inflamed, and there is
pain in the region of the stomach and below the ribs.
CAUSE: Poorly cooked meat.
THERAPY: An incision is made into the inflamed and swollen site on the abdomen and salt is sprinkled into the incision; this should pull the disease out of
the body. The Kel Alhafra say, however, that in advanced stages of the disease,
there is no cure, and the disease is then often fatal.

torhənna ta n-tāfukk, "the disease of the sun" *(meningitis)*
CATEGORY: hot
Synonym for *tenāde ta n-afālla*, meningitis

torhənna ta n-tenere, "the disease of the vastness/emptiness/desire/wilder-
ness" *(mental illness)*
Synonym for *alšin/ušed*.

tufit, Arabic: *ishāl,* "diarrhea"
CATEGORY: hot/cold
tufit is the general term for any kind of diarrhea. According to the Kel Alhafra
it is not transmissible between individuals.
CAUSE: Unhygienic foods, *išəkša wi wār šādij.*
THERAPY: Remedies for diarrhea are: a drink of *ahəjjar (Acacia nilotica* seed
capsules) and *tafəngora,* pulverized fruit of the baobab tree *(Adansonia digitata),* in water; crumbled cheese, *tikāmmāren taddāhnen*; rice, *tafāyāt.*

tufit ta n-tākusse, "diarrhea of the heat"
CATEGORY: hot
tufit ta n-tākusse has a bad smell, occurs less often that diarrhea with a "cold"
cause, and the feces contain mucus, *tafāyāt.*

CAUSE: As the name implies, *tufit ta n-tākusse* is caused by the overconsumption of *issukās* foods classified as "hot", *issukās*.

THERAPY: A diet of rice, *tafāyāt*, cooked with a lot of water and sweetened with sugar, *əssukar*, together with coffee, *ālqāhwa*, and *aharjəjəm (Cassia italica)* with cold water, or *tafəngora*, pulverized fruit of the baobab *(Adansonia digitata)*, with cold milk, *axx sāmmeḍān*.

tufit ta n-təssəmḍe, "diarrhea of the cold"

CATEGORY: cold

In contrast to diarrhea classified as "hot", "diarrhea of the cold", *tufit ta n-təssəmḍe*, is odorless, flows continuously, but also contains mucus, *əšānyaman*.

CAUSE: Foods classified as "cold", *isəssmaḍ*.

THERAPY: Rice, *tafāyāt*, with a lot of butter, *udi*, and in addition, coffee with hot butter, *ālqāhwa d-udi*, to prevent dehydration.

tufit tādiwāt ta n-timennāḍ, Arabic: *layya*, "diarrhea accompanied by cramps"

CATEGORY: hot/cold

The disease picture in *tufit tādiwāt ta n-tamennāt* is similar to that for *tanānnāyāt*: diarrhea with blood, *ašni*, and mucus, *təšānyəšt*, and strong colic. If such a diarrhea has a "cold" origin, *wa n-təssəmḍe*, it is considered by the Kel Alhafra to be far more serious than when the cause is "hot", *wa n-tākusse*.

CAUSES: Unhygienic foods, *išəkša wā šādijnen*, and dirty water, but also *aḍu*, air circulating in the body.

THERAPY: A drink made from *ahəjjar (Acacia nilotica* seed capsules) mixed with *tafəngora* (pulverized baobab, *Adansonia digitata*, fruit) and crumbled cheese, *tikāmmāren taddāhnen*, in cold water, *aman sāmmeḍnen*, or goat milk, *axx n-tayāt*, depending on the cause. Rice dishes, *əsink n-tafāyāt* are also recommended, as is chewing fresh, green twigs of the *tājārt (Maerua crassifolia)*.

tufit ta n-lāho, "diarrhea caused by the milk of a pregnant mother"

CATEGORY: hot

tufit ta n-lāho refers to diarrhea in small children who have not yet been weaned but whose mother is already pregnant again. The Kel Alhafra are convinced that the milk of a pregnant woman, *lāho*, causes chronic diarrhea in the child she is breastfeeding. The baby ejects the nourishment undigested, its belly is bloated and it becomes weak and sickly.

CAUSE: Breastfeeding with *lāho*, the milk of a pregnant woman.

THERAPY: The infant is given *isəssmaḍ*, "cold" foods, especially cooked rice, *tafāyāt*, together with water containing *ahəjjar (Acacia adansonii), tafəngora*, pulverized fruit of the baobab *(Adansonia digitata)*, and crumbled cheese, *tikāmmāren taddāhnen*.

ubšej, Arabic: *nukāf,* "chickenpox" *(varicella)*
CATEGORY: hot
In the beginning, the disease resembles *igādanāy*, "smallpox". Blisters appear first on the upper body then on the face, hands and feet. Fever, *tenāde*, is also possible in the early stages of the disease. *ubšej* is considered to be highly contagious. The Kel Alhafra say that it is common, afflicts children as well as adults, lasts for three to four weeks, but occurs only once in a person's lifetime. If the individual is not strong enough to bring the disease to the surface, it can turn inwards and may be fatal.
CAUSE: The Kel Alhafa say that *ubšej* is transmitted by the wind, *aḍu*.
THERAPY: Someone with *ubšej* is wrapped up and warmed, so that the blisters emerge. He or she is then given *aman n-tešāyt*, water with *Salvadora persica* leaves, and *aman n-tājārt,* water with *Maerua crassifolia* leaves, to drink. It is important that the patient stays out of the wind and does not sleep in the open air.

ukbəẓẓān, "that which clenches the fist" *(mumps/epidemic parotitis)*
CATEGORY: hot
In Tamasheq, *kəbəẓẓət* means "to squeeze in the hand", "to clench the fist", "to close up the hand". Someone with *ukbəẓẓān* has a high fever, *tenāde*, for five to seven days, headaches, *tākmo n-eyāf*, earache, *tākmo n-timāẓẓujen*, the lymph nodes in the neck are swollen, *tākmo n-timāẓẓujen*, and it is difficult to swallow. The Kel Alhafra say that *ukbəẓẓān* is highly contagious, and that it sometimes breaks out twice a year in their encampments.
CAUSE: Foods classified as "hot", *issukās*.
THERAPY: "Cooling" therapies, *isəssmaḍ*, that is drinks such as: *ālmuxāynes (Cleome bradycarpa)* in cold water; *aman n-ahəjjar*, water with *Acacia nilotica* seed capsules; *tafrənka n-akārkāra*, leaves of a tree from the Gourma region in water; *tamākšwit*, a red earth mixed with water; *tafəngora*, pulverized baobab *(Adansonia digitata)* fruit mixed with water or cold milk.

ukəs n-ašni, Arabic: *dam,* "the removal of the blood"
In cases of strong headaches, *tezzort n-eyāf*, dizziness, *təlleyāf*, if the eyes are red and painful, *tākmo n-təṭṭāwen*, or when blood begins to accumulate in the head, *ahunšar,* the Kel Alhafra talk of *ukəs n-ašni*, which is not a disease classification as such, but a therapeutic method.
CAUSE: Excessive heat in the body due to excessive exposure to anything classified as *issukās*, "hot:" food *išəkša*, sun, *tāfukk*, the river, *ejreu,* etc.
THERAPY: To provide relief, an incision is made in the forehead with a razorblade so that the overheated blood can leave the body. Leaves of the *tāborāyt (Balanites aegyptiaca)* are then placed on the head.

4.2. Disease classifications

Diseases and their inherent characters

As has already been discussed, the Kel Alhafra view the human body as inter-
nalizing a hot and a cold life principle whose equilibrium depends on a balance in the individual's everyday world. The natural environment, a person's
living conditions, food intake and diseases all have an influence on this balance. In a healthy body, in which the well-adjusted interaction of these complementary forces reflects the Kel Alhafra conception of the universe, the circulation, *ibardān n-ašni*, and respiration, *aššāyāl n-unfas* (which pumps the blood
through the veins), driven by the heart, *ulh*, are responsible for the appropriate
functioning of the organs and thus, for the body's thermal equilibrium. If even
the tiniest part of this harmonic totality is disturbed, the interdependent system risks losing its stability. It can become deformed and enter a state of disso-
nance, express itself as a disease. If, for example, the human organism takes in
too much heat, *tākusse*, it overcooks and the blood coagulates, *aswas d-kārāt
n-ašni*, giving rise to diseases of a "hot" character. If, on the other hand, the
body is influenced by too much cold, *tassamde*, the blood cools down, *isassmad
n-ašni*, resulting in inadequately functioning organs, *tarakkam n-isakwān*, and
the appearance of diseases classified as "cold", *torhannawen n-tassamde*.

According to the symptoms, the Kel Alhafra assign disease to the category of hot or cold. "Hot" diseases, *torhannawen n-tākusse*, are always acute:
the signs appear suddenly and the course of the disease is brief and severe. In
the case of diseases that are potentially fatal, death can occur rapidly in the absence of therapeutic intervention. Diseases of a "hot" character are usually visible on the surface of the body and manifest as inflammations, flatulence, congestion, secretions or bloody excreta from within the body. Fever, *tenāde*, that
can be felt on the overheated body, is always an indication of a disease in the
"hot" category. All externally visible skin diseases and diseases that originate
from the river or water pools, for example intestinal parasites, *imijlān*, or the
Guinea worm, *atlab*, are classified as "hot". However, the end stage of certain
diseases, such as *tāhafnent* or *idmārān wi lābasnen* (pneumonia), whose onset
was not necessarily due to "hot" causes, can also in serious cases turn into an
acute, life-threatening "hot" condition. In general, "hot" diseases may cause a
great deal of suffering for a fairly short period of time, but with the appropriate therapy they can disappear as quickly as they emerged. "Cold" diseases,
torhannawen n-tassamde, on the other hand are chronic. They hide in the body
over a period of time before they become apparent, and when they do, the disease may already have reached a well-advanced stage. Because someone with
a "cold" disease often ignores or does not notice it for a long time, the disease

settles within the body, is difficult to cure, and the disease course is described by the Kel Alhafra as sluggish and protracted.[237]

The Kel Alhafra identify, in general, *issukās*, things (e.g. food, nature etc.) that have a "warming" effect on the body as the cause of "hot" diseases, while *isəssmaḍ*, things that have a "cooling" impact on the organism are answerable for "cold" diseases (see section 4.2.). Diseases of a "hot" charachter, *torhənnawen ti n-tākusse*, are always treated with *isəssmaḍ*, therapies that have a cooling effect on the overheated organism. Likewise, following this theory of opposite curing opposite (*contraria contrariis*[238]), "cold" diseases are given a warming treatment, *issukās*. Some diseases though have, according to the Kel Alhafra, a hybrid temperament: they can be provoked by either *issukās* or *isəssmaḍ*, or during the course of the disease its thermal character can switch; in both cases, the treatment must be appropriate to the disease character.

The Kel Alhafra do not subdivide diseases according to certain shared features – e.g. infectious diseases or hereditary diseases – but according to their "hot", "cold" or "hybrid" temperament. The table below illustrates this subdivision of their disease repertoire.[239]

Table 4.1. *Classification of diseases according to their "hot", "hybrid" or "cold" character*

torhənnawen n-tākusse diseases of a "hot" character	*torhənnawen ti n-tākusse hakəd ti n-təssəmḍe* diseases that can be of a "hot" as well as a "cold" character	*torhənnawen n-təssəmḍe* diseases of a "cold" character
aḍkor – bloating *aɣəttus* – to faint/epilepsy *ahəḍəḍu* – swelling/abscess *āhunšar* – nose bleed *ajmoḍ* – spot in the eye *ajnəwwi* – digestive disturbance *ākorkor* – dermatophytosis *amādul n-iman* – "begging for the soul" *āmāɣras* – syphilis *āmāɣras wa māllān* – vitiligo *āmāɣras wa āfnoozān* – leprosy *āmāɣras* – dietary change *āmāššār* – ulcus durum	*ābiwəs* – wound *aḍu* – air *aɣālab* – dizziness *ahənnəj* – conjunctivitis *ālfaɣ* – thromboses *āmazla* – common cold *arāfāɣ* – small pimple on the skin *aslim* – muscular pain *ermās* – stomach pain *ešer* – scrape *əjjəburu* – common cold *iba n-tārha n-imənsiwān* – loss of appetite *iḍmārān* – bronchitis	*adku* – abdominal pains/cramps *adku wa n-tāɣimit* – dysmennorhea *afugg* – "the torn muscle" *fāttas* – hernia *iba n-ašni* – anemia *tābbašār* – "to expose oneself to something" *tadihāt* – allergy *tākmo n-asəjbas* – backache *tenāde ta n-təssəmḍe* "the fever of the cold" *tufit ta n-təssəmḍe* – diarrhea of the cold

237 The traditional healer Walett Faqqi in the text "isefran" defines "cold" and "hot" much as they are characterized by the Kel Alhafra: "In general, 'hot' diseases develop quickly, in one direction or the other; 'cold' maladies develop so slowly that they are not perceptible until an advanced and dangerous stage." Walett Faqqi, *Isefran*, 12.

238 The theory that every dyscrasis can be treated with its opposite is found in Galen: *"yanbaġī an tu'āliġa kulla mizāǧin bi-diḍḍihi"* – "you must treat every temperament with its opposite". Max Meyerhof, *Ḥunain ibn Isḥāq* (Cairo: Government Press, 1928) 179, 15.

239 The criteria of disease classification studied by Laderman in Malaysia are similar to those used by the Kel Alhafra (which could again point to the influence of Arabic medicine during the Islamization of South East Asia). See Carol Laderman, "Symbolic and Empirical Reality: A New Approach to the Analysis of Food Avoidances", *American Ethnologist* 8.3 (1981): 468–493.

torhənnawen n-tākusse diseases of a "hot" character	*torhənnawen ti n-tākusse hakəd ti n-təssəmḍe* diseases that can be of a "hot" as well as a "cold" character
āssām – poisoning *ašyoḍ* – scabies *atləb* – Medina or Guinea worm *āttāxma* – digestive disorder *atunjār* – infection *azāndi* – hemarrhoids *azəlmaẓ wi lābasnen* diphtheria *dāmbāraku* – night blindness *eɣāf wa lābasān/eɣāf wa n-afālla* – meningitis *eha* – miscarriage *ejām* – inflammation of the spleen *əsib* – pimple, blister *əsib wa n-amākš* – "the pimple that eats" *əsib wa n-āmmās* – internal ulcer *əsib wa n-inākārāra* – wart *əsib wa n-tāmāɣrəyt* – "the pimple of those who have had a miscarriage" *iba n-imənsiwān* – malnutrition *ibsan* – vomiting *iḍmārān wi lābasnen* – pneumonia *igādanāɣ* – smallpox *imijlān (sing. emājāl)* – worms *inkəḍi* – "that which one hates" *išelal* – allergy to strong light *jəri* – leprosy *šāggāɣ* – German measles (rubella) *tāfure (pl. tiforawen)* – dermatosis *tāfure ta n-āmāɣras* – syphilitic skin lesions *tāgarut* – rabies *taɣārt n-tāsa* – constipation *tāhayne* – gum inflammation *tājlifāt* – nausea *tākmo n-eɣāf* – headaches *tākmo n-iləs* – aphtha *tākmo n-timāẓẓujen* – ear inflammation *taməlle n-təṭṭ* – "the white of the eye" *tassididet* – measles *tāsut talābassāt* – tuberculosis *tāwārāɣwārāɣ* – "that which colors the skin yellow" *tenāde* – fever *tenāde talābasāt* – "the bad fever" *tenāde ta n-afālla* – meningitis *tenāde ta n-āmāɣrəs* – fever due to dietary change *tenāde ta n-ehāḍ* – "fever of the night" *temāde ta n-əjjəburu* – "fever of the common cold" *tenāde ta n-iḍmārān* – "fever of bronchitis" *tenāde ta n-tamāssāɣarāt* – "the fever at the end of the rainy season" *tenāde ta tāšrayāt* – "the new fever" *tenāde ti tākrayet* – "the fever of fermentation" *tenāde ti n-kāraḍ* – "the 3-day fever" *tibiaɣ* – "the swelling of the lymph nodes in the neck" *tijdil āwas təssārɣāt ihee ašni* – "urine accumulation that burns and contains blood" (schistosomiasis) *torhənna ta n-tiksənna* – "the disease in which one is carved" *tufit ta n-lāho* – diarrhea caused by a pregnant woman's milk *tufit ta n-tākusse* – diarrhea of the heat *ubšej* – chickenpox *ukbəẓẓān* – mumps	*iḍmārān wi n-əjjəburu* – cold-associated bronchitis *sāqqārnen* – whooping cough *tāddārɣālt* – blindness *tāɣārawiten (sing. tāɣārawit)* – vaginal-perineal tears, fistulas *tāhafnent* (no Western equivalent) *tākmo n-azəlmaẓ* – neck pain *tākmo n-iɣāssān* – bone pains *tākmo n-ulh* – heart troubles/nausea *tāməẓẓəj* – deafness *tanābdānt* – the lamed, crippled being *tanānnāɣāt* – severe stomach pain *taqāst* – toothache *tāsut* – coughing *tāsut ta n-iḍmārān* – bronchitis *tedeje ta n-aḍu* – "the stab of the air" *tedeje ta n-iḍmārān* – "the stabbing in the breast" *təlleɣāf* – dizziness *temāslāɣt* – coughing/suffocation *təssāh* – suffocation/asthma *tijdil āwas* – "the urine refusal" *tilāwayen* – rheumatism *timennāḍ* – digestive disorder *tufit* – diarrhea *tufit tādiwāt ta n-timennāḍ* – "diarrhea accompanied by cramps"

afālla āṣṣahāt, ajuss torhənna – **"vigor dominates in the north, sickness in the south"**

In the above table, there is quite clearly a preponderance of diseases classified as "hot" over those of a "cold" or hybrid character. When I asked the Kel Alhafra for the reasons behind this imbalance, they replied that many of the "hot" diseases have only appeared in recent years, along with the major droughts and the changes in their habits.

Figure 4.8. *Frequency of the diseases characterized as "hot", "hybrid", and "cold".*

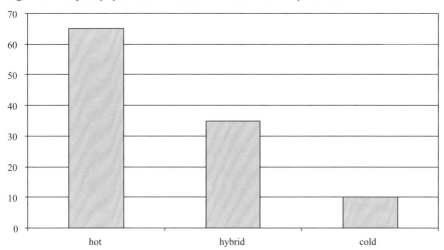

"Today there are many diseases that we do not recognize" – *"ašāl-i təhee torhənnawen tājotnen wār nəzzej"*, said Ninde, an unmarried woman aged about 70 in an encampment at Inkomen.[240] The dietary changes have brought with them *amāyrəs*, a condition of general debilitation, she continued, and the new foods, mainly classified as "hot", *isudar wi išraynen ikusnen*, together with the shortage of milk, *iba n-axx*, and malnutrition, *iba n-iмənsiwān*, also encourage the development of "hot" diseases, especially skin diseases, blisters and pimples, *isibān*. In addition, the failure of the rains, *iba n-ajənna*, has forced many to move further south, *ebre n-ajuss*, in the direction of the river, *ebre n-ejreu*, to the cities, *ebre n-eyārman*, and temporary jobs, *əššāyāl wa n-āfus*, but also into becoming settled, either totally or in part. When the rains fail and there is insufficient pasture in Azawad, the Kel Alhafra must move toward the riverine zone to obtain sufficient water and fodder for their

240 Discussion at Inkomen with Khadījatu Wālāt Muḥammad, Asiātu Wālāt Ḥāmmadu, Faḍimāta Wālāt Amnuḥen, Faḍimāta Wālāt Almunser, November 2005.

herds. However, they describe the southern regions of their nomadic territory as "unhealthy", *wār ihee āṣṣahāt*, and attribute to them diseases of a "hot" character. *"ajuss išakšāl tiɣārrās"*, Ninde said, "the south shortens the life-span". Furthermore, she continued, "in the south we succumb to fever diseases, *torhənnawen ti n-tenāde*, flatulence, *aḍkor*, *ilənkənān* (dracunculiasis) and *ti-jdil āwas təssāryāt ihee ašni*, 'urine accumulation that burns and contains blood'". The south is also unnourishing, the foods contain no *ālbarāka*, they are worthless, *iba n-ālbarāka dāy isudar*, and the animals are also never sati-ated by the pastures in the south. "In the south one has to eat all the time for the body to retain its strength", another woman complained, *"s-ajuss ihuššāl i-āwadəm a-itatt dāy ālwāqq fuk a-ittat āṣṣahāt-ənnes"*. "That makes one sick" – *"itārhan"*, and she underlined her statements with a saying: *"afālla āṣṣahāt ajuss torhənna"*, – "vigor dominates in the north, sickness in the south".[241] The Kel Alhafra are convinced that they are not made to tolerate the climate in the south and even go so far as to claim that Tamasheq fractions that marry in the south and settle there will gradually die out (as an exam-ple they cite the *išerifān*[242] who as *imilalān*, "whites", have practically disap-peared in the Gourma region south of the Niger – just three families remain). "If we want to live in the climate of the south, we must marry the people there, *āddināt wi kāwwalnen*, with the blacks, and mix the blood so that we are not carried off by 'hot' diseases and the prevailing climate", a middle-aged Kel Al-hafra man chipped in, fueling a further debate about the perpetuation of tradi-tions and the widely discussed questions of identity. Nevertheless, the Kel Al-hafra are unanimous: *"tikusu wār təjəs sunnāt"* – "the heritage will not move to the south".[243]

Unlike the "hot" south, northern Azawad is viewed by the Kel Alhafra as a region of the cold, *ākall n-azāwad n-təssəmḍe*, and of "cold", chronic sick-nesses, *"torhənnawen ti tāggorātnen dāy nānāy"* – "the diseases that hide in us". However, these are fewer in number and less frequent than the "hot" diseases. Furthermore, the north is blessed with *ālbarāka*, the divine power that bestows on even the smallest plant a higher nutritional value and heal-ing potency than is found in the southern vegetation. *"s-afālla āddināt fuk*

---

241 Discussion at Inkomen with Khadījatu Wālāt Muḥammad, Asiātu Wālāt Ḥāmmadu, Faḍimāta Wālāt Amnuḥen, Faḍimāta Wālāt Almunser, November 2005.

242 The Tamasheq fractions of the *išerifān* identify themselves as direct descendants of the prophet Mohammed and live in the regions of Méma, Kita, Niya, Timbuktu and Gao (on the *išerifān* see Charles Grémont, André Marty, Rhissa ag Mossa, Younoussa H. Touré, *Les liens sociaux au Nord-Mali. Entre fleuve et dunes* (Paris: IRAM/Karthala, 2004); Jacques Hureiki, *Essai sur les origines des Touaregs* (Paris: Karthala, 2003).

243 Discussion at Inkomen with Khadījatu Wālāt Muḥammad, Asiātu Wālāt Ḥāmmadu, Faḍimāta Wālāt Amnuḥen, Faḍimāta Wālāt Almunser, November 2005.

ādoobān tamudre" – "everyone can live in the north", the Kel Alhafra say, *āddināt wi n-arābānda day*, "even the people from the south", *"mušan wār ādoobān tāẓidert n-aẓāmanān wa n-təssəmḍe d-tajāsān təssəmḍe a hānāy wa ti nākkāneḍ"* – "although they have more problems in the cold season than we do and are more susceptible to 'cold' diseases". The Kel Alhafra consider themselves to be metabolically fit for the northern climate of Azawad and much more tolerant of its cold than the heat of the south. However, they have observed great changes in the region in the last few decades: the climate has generally become warmer, rain is less frequent, the desert is spreading, many plants and animals have disappeared, and all of these changes have brought with them new diseases, the majority of a "hot" character.

Seasonal frequency of diseases

Table 4.2. *Seasonal frequency of "hot" and "cold" diseases*

Season	Month											
	Jan	Feb	Mar	Apr	May	Jun	Jul	Aug	Sep	Oct	Nov	Dec
akāsa						▒	▒	▒	▒			
γarat									█	█	█	█
tajrəst	█	█										█
ewelān				█	█	█						

▒ *"cold" diseases* – torhənnawen ti n- təssəmḍe

█ *"hot" diseases* – torhənnawen ti n- tākusse

Earlier, when the herds were still large and sufficient milk was available throughout the pastoral cycle, the Kel Alhafra say they rarely suffered from disease and especially not from so many diseases classified as "hot". Today, only during the rainy season, *s-akāsa*, are they fit and have less complaints than in the other months of the year. However, a new fever, *tenāde tāšrayāt*, now appears even during *akāsa*, along with *tenāde tamāssāyarāt*, "the fever at the end of the rainy season" (malaria), both of which have increased in prevalence and severity during the past decade. "The time of the fever", *azzāman wa n-tenāde*, now sets in in mid-September, when the star *γuššāt* (Canopus) appears in the eastern sky. *tenāde tamāssāyarāt*, malaria, ravages entire encampments that are staying near the river, and the change in seasons and the general supplementation of the diet with *allon*, cereals, brings in addition *tenāde ta n-āmāγrəs*, the fever that accompanies dietary change, debilitates the human organism, *tarəkkəm n-tayəssa*, and promotes the appearance of other disorders. In the cold months of *tajrəst*, when the temperatures fall to 0 °C, and humans and animals suffer from the frosty atmospheric conditions, respiratory diseases in particular emerge, such as *iḍmārān*, bronchitis, *ǝjjǝburu*, colds and coughing, *tāsut*, but also *tākmo n-iγāssān*, bone and joint pains. Because people do not wash very often during the cold months of *tajrǝst*, the Kel Alhafra observe that the lack of hygiene encourages the dissemination of parasites like lice, *tilken*, and also favors diseases such as *ahǝnnǝj*, eye inflammations, or *ašyoḍ*, scabies. When the days become warmer and the last goat milk has run out, malnutrition sets in, *azzāman wa n-iba n-imǝnsiwān*. Once again the human organism is debilitated by *āmāγrǝs*, the lack of the customary foods, and *āmāγras* (dark lesions) as well as *isibān wi ihee ukmāš*, itchy blisters, appear on the skin. The Kel Alhafra say the monotonous diet of *ewelān* also causes *ermās*, stomach problems and bone pains, *tākmo n-iγāssān*. In addition, the strong sunlight provokes *āhunšar,* nose bleeds, headaches, *tezẓort n-eγāf* and *tenāde ta n-afālla,* the fever of the head, which can suddenly afflict entire families, even if on the previous day, everyone had been vigorous in their normal activity with no indication of impending trouble.

The Kel Alhafra agree that disease incidence has increased and that individual diseases are no longer restricted to certain seasons but occur throughout the year. *tākmo n-iγāssān*, bone pains, for example, and *tilāwayen*, joint pains (rheumatism), used to be associated with the cold months of *tajrǝst* or the dry season of *ewelān*, afflicting predominantly older people. Now, however, everyone, children included, suffers from bone, joint and limb pains all year round. Contagious diseases like *tassididet*, measles, and *tenāde ta n-afālla*, meningitis, were also largely restricted to the cold months of *tajrǝst* or the dry season of *ewelān*, with epidemics giving rise to such epithets as *"awātay wa n-tassididet"* – "the year of the measles" or *"awātay wa n-tenāde ta n-afālla"* – "the year of meningitis". Today, however, these diseases are no longer sporadic and co-occur unpredictably throughout the year: "they no longer stop" – *"torhǝnnāwen aba-s badādnāt",* was the lament of 74-year-old Zainabu under the leather roof of her tent in an encampment at Inkomen.[244]

Characteristic diseases of the female life cycle
The table above summarizes those diseases that the Kel Alhafra women identify as characteristic for the various stages of their life cycle. According to their mothers, infants, *imānkāsān*, and small children, *imārkāsān*, suffer most from stomach and digestive complaints, as well as *ākorkor*, a mycosis of the scalp, eruptive skin rashes, *isibān fāll tayǝssa*, and fever, *tenāde*. When they are slightly older, the girls predominantly suffer from infectious diseases like

244 Conversation at Inkomen with with Zainabu Wālāt Muḥammad, November 2005.

Table 4.3. *Characteristic diseases of the female life cycle*

Life cycle		Characteristic diseases
āmankas *tamārkəst*	Infant (7 days to 2 years) Small child (0–5 years)	*tezzort n-tāsa* – adbominal pains *tufit* – diarrhea *tenāde* – fever *ubšej* – chickenpox *ahənnəj* – eye inflammation *ākorkor* – dermatophytosis (fungi on the scalp) *əjjəburu* – common cold *isibān fāll tayəssa* – spot on the body *tezzort n-eyāf* – headaches *sāqqārnen* – whooping cough
talyāḍt *tābārmawāḍt*	Child, girl (5–12 years) Adolescent (12–20 years)	*tenāde* – fever *iḍmārān* – bronchitis *sāqqārnen* – whooping cough *tassididet* – measles *ubšej* – chickenpox *šāggāy* – German measles (rubella) *eyāf wa lābasān* – "the bad head" (meningitis)
tamawāḍ *tamaḍt*	Young adult (18–30 years) Woman (30–50 years)	*tākmo n- ārori* – "back pains", dysmenorrhea *təlleyāf* – vertigo *ibsan* – vomiting *tākmo n-ulh* – heart problems, nausea *tākmo n-iḍarān* – pains in the legs *ābiwəs* – birth wounds *tedeje ta n-aḍu* – "the stab of the air" *tenāde* – fever *tassididet* – measles *ubšej* – chickenpox *sāqqārnen* – whooping cough *timāzzujen* – ear inflammations *azəlmaz* – throat inflammations *əjjəburu* – common cold *tākmo n-iyāssān* – bone pains *āmāyras* – "that which kills" (syphilis) *iba n-imənsiwān* – malnutrition *tāhafnent* *tākmo n-ermās* – stomach problems *tawārāywārāy* – "that which colors the skin yellow"
tamyārt	Old woman (≥50)	*tākmo n-iyāssān* – bone pains *tilāwayen* – rheumatism *āmazla* – common cold (sinusitis) *tākmo n-arori* – back pains *tezzort n-ermās* – stomach problems *tezzort n-isenan* – toothache

sāqqārnen, whooping cough (pertussis), *tassididet,* measles, *ubšej,* chickenpox (varicella), and *šāggāy,* German measles (rubella): these growing young
girls are physically active, frequently visiting their friends in neighboring encampments where they pick up the diseases and bring them into their home
tent. When a young woman finally enters the phase of the monthly "loss
of prayer", *iba n-amud,* i.e. she begins menstruating, ailments specific to
women, *torhənnawen n-tiḍeḍen,* begin to dominate. However, at this stage,
the women list not only the troubles that accompany menstruation, pregnancy

and birth, but also infectious diseases such as measles, *tassididet*, chickenpox, *ubešj,* and whooping cough, *sāqqārnen.* It is interesting that malnutrition, *iba n-imənsiwān*, is only cited during this stage of life, and also that the number of named problems is greatest among young and adult women. Diseases associated with old age include bone pains, *tākmo n-iɣāssān*, joint pains (rheumatism), *tilāwayen*, as well as dental problems, *tezzort n-isenan*, and stomach complaints, *tezzort n-ermās.*

The Kel Alhafra women associate the reproductive phase of their life with the most risks and diseases. During this phase, the female cycle, pregnancy and birth tie the woman irreversibly to natural powers, such that in the desert she is continually walking a fine line between life and death. This condition between creation and destruction, between hot and cold, endows her not only with a special status but also attracts the noxious, demonic powers of the *kel tenere*, an additional danger to which the woman during this period is particularly susceptible.

However, the mothers also view their infants and small children as being particularly vulnerable to diseases, and the number of listed diseases only declines when the child is past five years of age.

New diseases – *torhənnawen tišraynen*
Western medical terms such as polio, meningitis, tuberculosis, pneumonia, diphtheria and malaria have no single equivalents in the Tamasheq spoken by the Kel Alhafra. Unlike diseases such as measles, *tassididet,* nightblindness, *dāmbāraku,* chickenpox, *ubšej,* German measles, *šāggāɣ*, and whooping cough, *sāqqārnen*, with which the Kel Alhafra have been familiar for a long

Figure 4.9. *Perceived frequency of disease categories at different stages of the female life cycle*

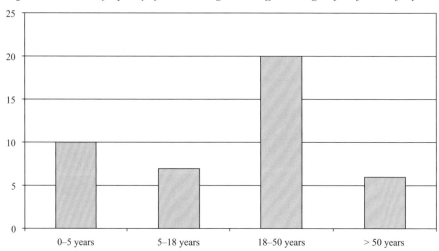

time and which have unique, specific names, "newer" diseases which the Kel Alhafra have known about for a much shorter period (which does not necessarily mean, however, that they did not exist previously) are described in their language with auxiliary constructions that evoke certain associations. These constructions, however, sometimes convey a very imprecise word-image, which can lead to confusion and errors not only in translation but also in the understanding of the Kel Alhafra themselves. In an educational campaign in 1989, UNICEF and the Ministère de l'Education de Base de la République du Mali (DNAFLA) issued a health brochure,[245] in which *tāhafnent* was identified as malaria and *āmāγras* as leprosy. These new definitions are totally at odds with the original associations of these disease terms. For the Kel Alhafra, *tāhafnent* is a condition that can indeed accompany malaria, *tenāde tamāssāγarāt*, but is also associated with other diseases. Likewise, in the Kel Alhafra understanding, depending on further specification, *āmāγras* covers a range of diseases that are visible on the body's surface, from syphilis to leprosy or vitiligo, and only with the more precise terminology, *"āmāγras wa āfnoozān"* – *"āmāγras* that reduces" is the condition specifically recognized as "leprosy".

To describe "new" diseases, the Kel Alhafra often modify the term for an existing, similar disease with the adjective, *talābasāt*, "bad", leading to such constructions as *"tāsut talābasāt"*, "the bad cough" for tuberculosis, *"iḍmārān wi lābasnen"*, "the bad bronchitis" for pneumonia *"aẓəlmaẓ wa lābasān"*, "the bad throat inflammation" for diphtheria and *"eγāf wa lābasān"*, "the bad headache" for meningitis. For diseases whose primary symptom is a fever, word constructions containing *tenāde* (fever) are common: *tenāde ta bəddən* describes a fever "that cripples", i.e. that leaves permanent damage, and can thus refer to either polio or meningitis; *tenāde ta n-afālla* means "the fever from above", which leads to a stiff neck and is most often used in cases of meningitis; *tenāde talābasāt* or *tenāde ta māqoorāt,* the "bad fever" or "the big fever" may designate meningitis, polio or any other disease accompanied by a high fever; *tenāde tamāssāγarāt*, "the fever at the end of the rainy season" signifies malaria, while *tenāde tāšrayāt*, the "new fever" may be used for meningitis or malaria but also as an alternative for *tenāde ta n-Abidjan*, a fever from Abidjan brought back by returning migrant workers from the Ivory Coast and that may refer to malaria but also to another "new fever", i.e. AIDS.

The Kel Alhafra are, in general, not informed about the HIV virus, even though migration, high male mobility, unprotected sexual intercourse and the smuggler routes that cross Azawad from Algeria provide a setting in which

---

245 *Musnāt i-efes. āssexāt 1+2*, Bamako: Ministère de l'Education de Base de la République du Mali (DNAFLA), UNICEF, 1989.

AIDS could spread. A traditional healer in Ber told me he believed that in general people would misrecognize AIDS as an end stage of tuberculosis or other fatal diseases. When questioned, individual Kel Alhafra who have heard about HIV through the radio or television maintain that AIDS does not exist in their society, that it is a disease of homosexuals of whom there are none among them: *"meddān wi əmārhānin germa-nāsān, a-wa wāddey imukān dāy tamətte ta-nanāy"* – "men who love one another, that is impossible in our society".

The Kel Alhfra comprehension of the "new" diseases is as imprecise as the Tamasheq descriptions they use for these ailments. They do not know, for example, how *tenāde tamāssāyarāt*, "the fever at the end of the rainy season", is transmitted, nor in what forms it can manifest itself. They assign the inexplicable to the realm of the *ğinn* and the *kel tenere*: if a child is suffering from fever and shivering, they are more likely to attribute this to evil spirits than to malaria. Although previous authors have allocated illnesses whose cause can be traced back to the *kel tenere, torhənnawen n-kel tenere*, to the domain of mental diseases, like Hureiki I believe that such a classification should be treated with caution.[246] If the Kel Alhafra ascribe the cause of a "new" disease to the *kel tenere*, this disease need have no psychopathological features, merely characteristics that for the Kel Alhafra are obscure or inexplicable.[247]

The Kel Alhafra also use the designation "new" disease for those ailments whose prevalence has increased and that in the past had a less significant impact on the population's health. Such diseases include *ākorkor*, mycoses (dermatophytosis), *tākmo n-iyāssān*, bone pains, *isibān,* skin rashes of all types that are unfamiliar to the Kel Alhafra, and *taqāst,* dental problems. Aïcha, a woman of nearly seventy from In Astilan, attributed the increase in these diseases to new foods that have entered the Kel Alhafra diet from outside and are connotated as "hot", including tea and sugar, *ātay d-əssukar.*[248]

---

246 Although Hureiki writes that "spirits primarily cause mental diseases", a few lines later he states that, "it would be too simple to presume that the Tuareg view all mental diseases as the work of spirits and all physical disorders as having a natural cause". Further on he writes that, "spirits are responsible for both mental diseases as well as the majority of somatic diseases that are classified as cold". Jacques Hureiki, *Tuareg. Heilkunst und spirituelles Gleichgewicht* (Schwülper: Cargo, 2004) 97–98.

247 Bernus writes that "Mental diseases are fairly widespread among the Tuaregs. They are attributed to the evil spells of supernatural beings, the ginns. That is why *tuwurna tan kel əsuf* or *tuwurna tan el jeniən* designates mental illness in general – as distinct from madness or congenital idiocy – and meaning 'the disease of the bush' (*kel əsuf*, those of the solitude, those of the bush, is the synonym for 'ginns' or 'devils')." Among the Kel Alhafra, however, the term *torhənna ta n-kel tenere* need not explicitly refer to a mental illness. See Edmond Bernus, "Maladies humaines et animales chez les Touaregs sahéliens", *Journal de la Société des Africanistes* 39.1 (1969):122.

248 Interview in an encampment at In Astilan with Aïcha Wālāt Muḥammadou, February 2006.

4.3. Disease causation – āssəbabān n-torhənnawen

To come closer to appreciating how the Kel Alhafra understand disease, acquaintance with their belief system and their perception of the relationship between this, the existential, world and the next world is absolutely essential. Although research to date on the etiology of diseases among the Tamasheq has made a subdivision into "natural" and "supernatural" causes, this does not correspond with the categorization employed by the Kel Alhafra.[249] During an illness, every member of the Kel Alhafra acknowledges a connection between God and the suffering placed on them.

For the Kel Alhafra, all of creation, *āddunya,* but also *ākall,* this lifeworld in the sense of nature, are essentially teleologically determined. In nature nothing is driven by its own forces, there is no causal nexus or natural law in the form of a physical connection between cause and effect. God alone is reality and responsible for every single event and being. In this theistic understanding, the creator alone is responsible for all diseases.[250] There may indeed be bacteria, *mikrobtān,* poisons, *āssāmān,* the cold, *təssəmḍe,* the heat, *tākusse,* and other things that elicit diseases, but nothing happens independently of the will of God, *derhan n-Māssināɣ.* He both endows these causal factors with their disease potential and characteristics, and grants to a therapeutic method its healing powers. For the Kel Alhafra, disease represents a manifest form of the supernatural power of God, *temātert n-Māssināɣ,* and thus cannot be simply perceived as bad or evil, because God is merciful and does not meaninglessly impose a burden on humans. Disease, rather, reflects *tāmusne ta wār ti tənhəy,* "the knowledge of the invisible", which encompasses a hidden divine wisdom that it not always comprehensible or obvious to humans.[251] Through suffering, *aɣāna,* the individual comes closer to God, must submit him– or herself to God's will and recognizes in his or her weakness the boundlessness of divine power.

A human can have no influence on the appearance and causes of diseases, except in so much as he or she sins, earning as a result God's punishment,

---

249 See among others Barbara Fiore: "La Maladie 'naturelle' et soins chez les Touaregs", in Walett Faqqi, *Isefran,* 53–62; Le Jean, *Médecine traditionnelle;* Hureiki, *Tuareg;* Bernus, *Maladies humaines et animales.* etc.

250 See also here the Koranic understanding 6:17: *"wa 'in yasaska –llahu bi-ḍurrin fa-la kāšifa lahu 'illa huwa wa 'in yasaska bi-ḫairin fa-huwa 'alā kulli šay'in qadīrun",* – "and if He visits thee with good, He is powerful over everything, He is Omnipotent over His servants".

251 *"'innama-l-ġaybu li-llāhi"* Surah 10:20. but also surah 6:59: "With him are the keys of the Unseen; none knows them but He. He knows what is in land and sea; not a leaf falls, but He knows it. Not a grain in the earth's shadows, not a thing, fresh or withered, but it is in a Book Manifest."

ālγazzāb, in the form of an illness for which the individual is then responsible. The Kel Alhafra believe that everyone must look after and preserve their health as a part of God's creation and that a sick person must do everything in her or his power to achieve a cure. At the same time, however, everyone has a day predetermined by God on which he or she will die, *ašāl wa n-tāγrəst təmda*. Like disease, the event of death is never arbitrary but is rooted in divine providence and cannot be influenced by human beings. Nevertheless, every sick person contemplating the divine power is expected to appeal to God for a cure. Since, though, God alone is responsible for life and death, the Kel Alhafra are deeply suspicious about the effectiveness of both traditional and modern medication. God's knowledge encompasses everything, and when a life has reached its appointed end, nothing can delay the predestined death.[252] A therapy can never counteract divine providence and may only be effective if the disease has been sent as a test and purification or as a punishment[253] intended to bring the suffering individual closer to God and to lead him or her back to the righteous path. Only God's mercy in the form of a cure for the disease can release one from one's torments.

4.3.1. Disease as test and purification

For the diseases in the discussion that follows, which are elicited by natural elements and the stars, by natural catastrophes, poisonous animals, infection, accidents and hereditary factors, humans beings, according to the Kel Alhafra, bear no responsibility; such causal events have been scheduled by the divine power long before their appearance in this lifeworld, *fāll tesāyt n-ākall fuk*,[254] and are sent to believers as a trial and purification, to test their patience, *tāẓidert*, and piety, *āliman*.

Influence of elements and stars

A cold wind, *aḍu sammeḍān*, sent by God to sweep across plains and dune valleys, especially during the cold months of *tajrəst*, can, according to the Kel Alhafra, precipitate bronchitis, *iḍmārān*, the common cold, *əjjəburu*, sinusitis,

---

252 See surah 63:11: *"wa lan yu'aḫḫira-llahu nafsan 'iḏan ğā'a 'ağaluhā wa-llahu ḫabīru bi-mā ta'malūna"* – "But God will never defer any soul when its term comes, And God is aware of the things you do".

253 In this context, certain Kel Alhafra sometimes cite the following saying of the Prophet from *Ṣaḥīḥ al-Buḫārī:* "Neither tiredness nor sickness, neither care nor grief, neither pain nor sorrow afflicts a Muslim, not even a single miniscule thorn can prick him that is not God's punishment for his errors."

254 See surah 57:22: *"mā 'aṣāba min muṣībatin fi-l-'arḍi wa la fī 'anfusikum 'illa fī kitābin min qabli 'an nabra'ahā 'inna ḏālika 'alā-llahi yasīrun"* – "No affliction befalls in the earth or in yourselves, but it is in a Book, before We create; that is easy for God."

amāẓla, and other diseases of the cold, *torhənnawen n-təssəmḍe.* In contrast, a hot wind, *aḍu wa ikussān,* whipping the face during the dry season of *ewelān* provokes *tibyay,* earache, *teẓẓort n-timāẓẓujen,* and asthma, *təssāh.* Anyone traveling or working while a hot wind is blowing may suffer from headaches, *teẓẓort n-eyāf,* and bone pains, *tākmo n-iyāssān.*

Anyone exposing him- or herself to the burning hot sun, *tāfukk təssāry,* risks not only sunburn, *isəryitān n-elām* (sing. *asāry n-elām*), but also nose-bleeds, *āhunšar,* due to overheating of the blood, as well as *tilāwayen n-tākusse,* "rheumatism of the heat" and *tenāde ta n-eyāf,* "the fever of the head" (meningitis).

The thermal nature of the element earth conforms with that of the seasons, *ākall idaw āẓẓāmān.* Anyone sitting on the earth or more specifically sand, *ešəš,* heated by the sun may suffer from *tijdil āwas,* bladder complaints, or *aẓāndi,* hemorrhoids. Sitting on cold earth, *ākall wa sammeḍān,* on the other hand, might provoke *tijdil āwas, tākmo n-iyāssān,* bone pains, *tākmo n-ārori,* backache and *tākmo n-asəjbas,* pains in the small of the back.

Sometimes the Kel Alhafra must protect themselves from the moon. The beams, *ešelal,* of the full moon, *tamāllān n-iyor,* can trigger headaches, *teẓẓort n-eyāf,* and *temāslāyt,* an allergic cough.

Rain, *ajənna,* in the desert can be followed by a period of bitter cold that the Kel Alhafra call *talāfa,* which also means "to shiver with cold". In such cold conditions, humans or animals soaked by rain risk being smitten by *tābbašār,* an "inner fever", which can cause irreversible paralysis within 24 hours. Rain is in general held responsible for provoking "cold" diseases, *torhənnawen n-təssəmḍe,* although the Kel Alhafra are of the opinion that rain can only elicit disease in weak humans or animals.

Natural catastrophes

The Kel Alhafra believe that all events taking place on the *tesāyt n-ākall,* as their lifeworld, have been decided far in advance by God, long before human beings encounter them. Natural catastrophes, *muṣibātān,* such as drought, *mānna,* bad harvests, *ixšad n-adomm,* pests in the form of locusts, *tašwālen,* or the gypsy moth caterpillar, *tiẓəlfen,* as well as the consequences of these catas-trophies such as malnutrition, *iba n-imənsiwān,* hunger, *jələk,* and an abrupt dietary change, *āmāyrəs,* can all be the harbingers of disease.

Large-scale destruction and upheaval contain the core of change, which is particularly difficult for the older Kel Alhafra. Since Azawad has been inflicted by more droughts, since sorely needed rainfall has become sparse, and since the people have had to endure famine, war, flight, disease, and are forced into a perpetual battle to survive, an apocalyptic attitude has spread among older members of the society. Idealizing the past, they describe the accumulation of catastrophes in the past 35 years as *xārāuxārāu*, "terrible things", and see them as heralding the approaching end of the world, *taməddāwt n-āddunya*. Young people, however, want to live. They want to come to terms with the modifications to their environment, to confront the social changes and seek ways into a better future. They view catastrophes and the concomitant suffering as divine warnings, to which they should respond not only by adaptation and reflection, but more importantly by turning their minds back to religious values through a reinterpretation of their Islamic identity.

Poisonous animals and accidents

If a Kel Alhafra is bitten by a snake or stung by a scorpion, if a spider deposits its noxious poison in food, if someone comes into contact with a poisonous plant, injures him- or herself accidentally or suffers from the aftereffects of strenuous physical activity – in none of these cases does the individual bear guilt for his or her sick condition. The creator wishes to test their faith in God, *tāwākkul*. This creator, however, is a God of mercy, *Māssināy n-ārrāxmāt*, and a God of justice, *Māssināy n-ālhāqq*, who only inflicts on humans as much as they can bear and what they deserve.

Infections and hereditary transmission

First and foremost, the Kel Alhafra view infection as the creation of a condition of sickness in a formerly healthy person. Since God alone can create, once again he alone is the origin of the illness. While the Kel Alhafra have empirical experience of the mechanical transmission of a disease, they can provide no concrete explanations for such transmission and cannot construct a theoretical picture for the process of an infection. In the absence of such conceptions, infectious diseases are often misrecognized as hereditary diseases, as is the case for tuberculosis, *tenāde talābasāt*, and skin mycosis, *ākorkor*. Because entire families may be afflicted by these diseases, the Kel Alhafra conclude that God has marked the family with the disease and that it is passed on from generation to generation, although such a "hereditary line", *etāri dāy imārawān*, may be broken or modified by the creator's will. The wind, *aḍu*, can also spread diseases, against which the infected individual is defenseless, just as he or she carries no guilt for afflictions and suffering passed on by the parents.

4.3.2. Disease as divine punishment

If diseases are sent as divine punishment, the individual concerned shares the responsibility for his or her condition. A debt, *ābākkaḍ*, has been imposed, such that through suffering one may reflect on and recognize one's weakness, helplessness and subjection to the all-encompassing divine power.[255] *"a-fal osās āwadəm har iksuḍ Māssināy"* – "if a human has difficulties, he is re-minded of God", the Kel Alhafra say. Through suffering the sick person comes closer to God and appeals to Him for forgiveness for all sinful behavior and in-attention to the divine creation.

Unhealthy conduct and bad habits

The Kel Alhafra argue that it is the duty of every believer to take care of his or her health, this being a gift of God. Because the body is conditioned by oppo-sitional qualities, everyone should strive continuously to equilibrate these in-ternal forces. Particular attention must be paid to the food one eats, and certain food combinations, inedible and potentially harmful foods must be avoided. Anyone indulging without restraint – be this, for example, excessive tea con-sumption or simple greed – should not be surprised if this results in indisposi-tion. The Kel Alhafra also view lack of hygiene, *iba n-ašəšədaj*, as a self-im-posed cause of various diseases such as eye inflammations, *ahənnəj,* worms, *imijlān,* syphilis, *āmāyras*, and scabies, *ašyoḍ*. A lack of cleanliness can also lead to the consumption of spoilt food and the concomitant health problems, to the spread of vermin, and, in humans, to psychic disturbances. The Kel Al-hafra view those who neglect themselves and their bodily hygiene as having a "disturbed spirit", *ənniyāt wār-hin osja*, and as no longer being in a state of psychic or physical purity. Such a condition attracts the *kel tenere*, who, hav-ing settled inside such individuals, provoke abnormal behavior or disease. A sedentary lifestyle, *azuzəy*, and a lack of exercise, *iba n-amrumər*, can also, the Kel Alhafra say, elicit certain diseases such as *tāhafnent*, constipation, *tayārt n-tāsa*, and hemorrhoids, *aẓāndi*, for which, once again, the person concerned bears resposibility.

Transgression of proscriptions and taboos

Certain norm-breaking and forbidden actions can also transform the actor into a condition of impurity in which he or she becomes susceptible to dis-ease. Transgressions, *teḍləmen* (sing. *taḍləmt*), that are considered dangerous, sources of misfortune and that lay one open to disease include rape, *ejāḍāl fāll tamāḍt*, homicide, *tenāye*, incest, *ādobān dāy əddināt n-ehān wār immukān,* adultery, *āhalis itikar hənni-ənnes* or *tamāḍt tikarāt āhalis-ənnes,* corporal punishment of children, *təwwat n-aratān*, defilement of the holy-connotated

---

255 See here surah 4:123: *"... man ya'mal su'an yuğzabihi wa la yağid lahu min dūn-i-llahi walīyan wa la naṣīran."* - "Whosoever does evil shall be recompensed for it, and will not find for him, apart from God, a friend or helper."

direction of prayer, *asəssikəd edāgg wa n-ālqiblāt*, sleeping with one's head to the north, *tenāse tijəd eɣāf s-afālla*, disrespect toward one's parents-in-law, *wār isəmɣar iḍulān-ənnes*, totally undressing the body, *ukəs n-iməlsan*, and having sexual intercourse with a woman during her menses, *tenāse s-tamāḍt ta tənhay tāɣimit*. If such offenses are perpetrated, God allows the *kel tenere* to become active. Attracted by *təšoṭṭ*, the evil eye of the sinner, *anāsbākkaḍ*, the *kel tenere* afflict him or her with all sorts of diseases. Through the suffering, though, he or she must reflect on the divine truth, *ālhāqq*, and, in a repentant state, *tātubt*, petition the creator for forgiveness, *tenāšše*.

The *kel tenere*, however, wait everywhere for any opportunity to tamper with humans. A Kel Alhafra should therefore avoid those places favored by the *kel tenere*, such as lonely regions in the desert without vegetation, *təfārre n-tināriwen,* sites where people have died, *idāggān wi n-nānāmetān*, or nocturnal walks, *tikle n-ehāḍ,* in order to evade the risk of encountering the temptations of a *ǧinn*, who may lead one onto the wrong spiritual track, *anāfraɣ n-tayətte*, such that, in the worse case, one will lose sight of the holy center of Mecca and become an apostate, *ažāhal*.

5. Therapeutic Networks

In his book, *Patients and Healers in the Context of Culture*, Kleinman describes how three overlapping and interdependent health domains can be identified in all complex cultures.[256] Before applying his scheme to the Kel Alhafra, I will begin with a brief summary of its essential features. Kleinman first defines an informal sector, the "popular sector of health care",[257] which has the broadest scope and covers health care performed by the individual, families and social networks on a daily basis according to a community's general codes and norms. It covers nonprofessional lay activities, in which illness and disease are first defined culturally before curative actions are undertaken. The second of the sectors defined by Kleinman, the "folk sector of health care",[258] is the realm of nonprofessional specialists who are not part of the official medical system but who can work close to members of the professional sector and take up an intermediate and intermediary position between the informal and professional sectors. These "folk healers" represent a heterogeneous group and often offer their clients a blend of spiritual and secular forms of therapy. The third, "professional sector of health care"[259] comprises the organized groups of state-recognized practitioners of modern, scientifically based medical care (biomedicine). Kleinman, however, emphasizes that it is not only the various types of doctor, nurses and midwives that should be ascribed to this sector but also traditional medical systems such as Ayurveda, Chinese or Galenic-Arabic medicine which have become professionalized to varying degrees in many countries.

As I will show, the Kel Alhafra use a plural medical system in which the health-seeking behavior of its members tests the effectiveness, the possibilities and the healing options of the various sectors. In each of the levels defined by Kleinman, different roles and rules are applied, and these determine their accessibility. Certain groups, such as women, children, old people or the socially disadvantaged, can, for various reasons, be denied access to parts of or entire sectors.

The help seeking behavior networks of each group are different, but it would be beyond the scope of this work to analyze them all. Therefore I focus particularly on Kel Alhafra women and children, whose networks usually extend only as far as the folk sector.

---

256 Arthur Kleinman, *Patients and Healers in the Context of Culture* (Berkley: University of California Press, 1980) chapters 2 and 3.
257 Kleinman, *Patients and Healers*, 50–53.
258 Kleinman, *Patients and Healers*, 59–60.
259 Kleinman, *Patients and Healers*, 53–59.

5.1. Informal sector: Women as primary health resources

The enormous distances that usually separate a sick Kel Alhafra woman or her children from neighboring encampments, from the Saturday market in the nearest settlement or from state-run health centers mean that she must primarily rely on her own healing skills.

When a child falls sick, the mother will first apply the knowledge she has learned from her own mother about the "traditional household remedies" based on plants, minerals, animal products or foodstuffs. Older women among the Kel Alhafra are especially knowledgeable about the efficacy of certain plants and other natural products, and younger members of the community readily turn to them for advice. These older women, however, are not healers in the sense of a *tenāsāfārt*, a traditional healing practitioner from a family of healers, but female members of the encampment who have gained their knowledge through practice and experience. These are the women who assist mothers to give birth, who are usually past child-bearing age, have overcome their cyclical bondage to the natural powers and who, through their dialog with the fate-determining divine power, have moved into closer communion with the creator and can petition for a cure in unrestrained prayer.

When a woman or one of her children falls sick, she, assisted by other female members of the family and encampment, will attempt to alleviate the

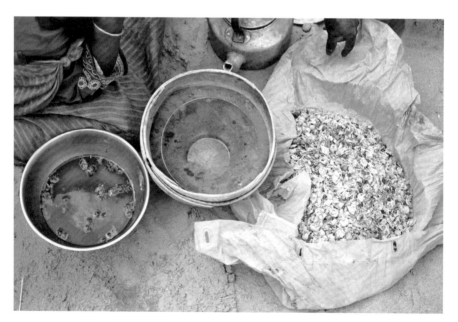

Figure 5.1. *Women prepare a traditional medicine with* ahəjjār *(Acacia nilotica seed capsules). (In Astilan, February 2005).*

suffering herself. The ingredients she needs for the traditional medicines are either to be found in her immediate environment or can be procured in a neighboring encampment. A Kel Alhafra woman who has fallen sick will demonstrate a high degree of self control and will hide her problem for as long as possible, confiding, if at all, only in other women. She will only turn to her husband for help when, for example, she is no longer capable of fulfilling her usual daily tasks or when the pain becomes so intense she can no longer sleep. A woman will only break out of her internal networks when an illness or disease is well advanced. The family head will then acquire from the market in Ber additional traditional medicines or even modern drugs offered by traders, the *kel mamāla* (who often lack any extensive medical knowledge), or recommended by tradional healers, the *ināsāfārān*.

The pharmaceuticals either come from wholesalers located in southern Mali, or from Algeria. The latter are particularly popular because they are cheap. The most common modern drugs used by the Kel Alhafra are paracetamol, aspirin and chloroquine. Others are selected depending on the illustration on the packaging, with preference given to those that show what they are good for. The women emphasize, however, that they always try traditional medications first, and only when these prove ineffective do they turn to other remedies. *"isəfrān wi n-lāytor safārān ašāmol n-torhənna šik"* – "modern compounds cure symptoms rapidly", said Tahurut, a Kel Alhafra in her fifties in an encampment at Inkomen, "but modern medications do not cure the sickness, and sometimes it reappears in another part of the body" – *"mušān isəfrān wi n-lāytor wār safārān torhənna iman-ənnes d-torhənna taqqālid ālwāqq tənniyād dāy tayəssa"*. "For example, if someone is suffering from stomach ache", she continued, "and it is treated with modern drugs, the sick person will then perhaps suffer from headaches".[260]

Only when self-medication does not work and the sick woman's energies are exhausted does she turn for help to the next, and more costly, level of medical care.

5.2. Folk sector: Treatment between the sacred and the secular

Only when the female and family networks have failed will a sick woman or the mother of sick children seek out someone outside these circles known to possess healing powers. These individuals are also members of the woman's community, share her cultural background and worldview and can thus

---

260 Conversation in an encampment at Inkomen with Khadījatu Wālāt Muḥammad, Asiātu Wālāt Ḥāmmadu, Faḍimāta Wālāt Amnuḥen, Faḍimāta Wālāt Almunser, November 2005.

be trusted. Such healers will either be religiously inspired, like the marabouts who can mobilize divine powers through the words of the holy text, or who, like the *ināsāfārān*, can equilibrate the body's imbalances using therapies based on their particular medical knowledge. Both types of healers are endowed with *ālbarāka*, the divine power of blessing, and in the healing process play the role of intermediary between the divine power and the sick person.

The Kel Alhafra rarely seek out the assistance of the *kel toxni, imāssāḥārān* (sing. *emāssāḥār*) or *ināmenšāyān* (sing. *enāmenšāy*), i.e. those who are specialized in sorcery, *ešāyāw,* or black magic, *asəmmajru*.[261] These groups are not simply feared but also deeply despised, their powers unable to compete with God's omnipotence. A demon, *ǧinn*, can only be driven out of a possessed person's body by the purifying, holy words of the Koran. Illness tests the individual's piety. It is a reminder of divine power and should lead the sick person back onto the righteous path, *tābarāt ta tāhuskāt*. Healing, *tamazzuyt*, can only be achieved through God's mercy and grace, *ārrāxmāt d-ānnoymāt n-Māssināy*.

The healing approach of both the marabout and the *enāsāfār* is a holistic one that takes into consideration all aspects of the patient's life. According to the Kel Alhafra, a human's thermal balance can be thrown into disorder not only by the natural surroundings but also by physical impairments and emotional pain arising from disturbed interpersonal relationships. The role of the marabout or traditional healer, *enāsāfār*, is to use his or her supernatural knowledge to restore the patient's psychic and physical balance. Reflection by the sick person on God's allmightiness is a crucial aspect of the healing process. It is through these cultural connections that a Kel Alhafra feels much greater affinity to a divinely inspired marabout or a traditional healer with *ālbarāka* than to a biomedically trained doctor.

5.2.1. From *ālfāqqi* to marabout

An *ālfāqqi*[262] has mastered both spoken and written Arabic, *issan teyāre n-tārābt*, can recite the Koran by heart, *issan āššāreya n-islam*, and functions in the Kel Alhafra society as a religious expert, *issan āddīn*, and as a performer of religious rites such as marriage, baptism, circumcision, and burial. He additionally plays the role of witness, *ijīha*, arbitrator and judge in cases of liti-

---

261 On the significance of the *kel toxni*, the *imāssāḥārān* and the *ināmenšāyān*, see chapter 4.1.4.
262 The Tamasheq word *ālfāqqi* is derived from the Arabic *faqīh,* which itself draws on the Arabic root *faqiha* "understand", "grasp" (in second radical, "to teach" or "instruct") and designates Islamic jurists, experts in *fiqh* (Islamic legal science), and theologians.
Foucauld defines the *"elfaqqi* (pl. *elfaqqīten)"* as *"a well-read Muslim"* (a man who knows the Koran by heart). See Foucauld, *Dictionnaire Touareg-Français*, vol. III, 999.

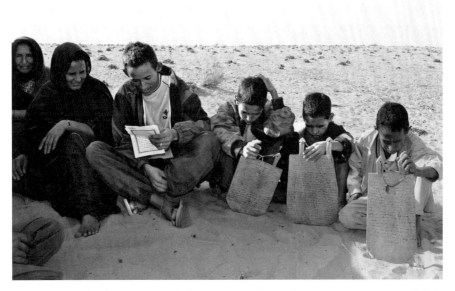

Figure 5.2. *A* tālfāqqit, *a Koranic scholar instructing her students in an encampment at Inkilla (November 2005).*

gation, *iqqal ālqaḍi*, and teaches young children at elementary level in a small Koranic school for a group of encampments, *isaɣrā dāɣ mādrāsā*. The special scholarship and erudition of the *ālfāqqi* is not restricted to men, and Kel Alhafra women can acquire Koranic learning and as *tālfāqqit* pass this on to young students.

In cases of sickness, a Koranic scholar, *ālfāqqi*, will prepare a curative amulet, *tikarḍiwen*, in which auspicious Koranic surahs are sewn into the leather. He also reads from the holy book to sick and dying people to palliate their suffering through the healing magic of the divinely revealed words. Among the Kel Alhafra, an *ālfāqqi* need not be a marabout. He will only receive this designation when he knows fully how to apply his special knowledge of the holy book and the healing practices derived from it, when he has achieved religious steadfastness and strength, when he can enter into direct contact with the supernatural powers and when he can encounter the dark powers with as much fearlessness as he can negotiate with the luminous energies. A marabout is a Koranic scholar endowed with *ālbarāka*, the divine power of blessing and healing.[263] Female Koranic scholars, *tālfāqqiten*, point out that although they

---

263 The Kel Alhafra are a subgroup of the tribal association of the Kel Ānṣar who as *inǝslǝmān* (sing. *anǝslǝm*), a mostly pacifist Tamasheq class, have devoted themselves since the 11/12th century to the study of the Koran and Arabic science. Among the Kel Alhafra there

know the magic practices of *"maraboutage"*, they do not wish to practice it, in part because they do not want to interfere in a domain considered male, in part to avoid exposing themselves to the pernicious powers of the *kel tenere*. Faḍimata, a *tālfāqqit* in an encampment at Inkomen, who teaches students and recites the Koran for the sick, stressed the Kel Alhafra understanding that a woman's female nature renders her much more susceptible than a man to the malign powers of the *kel tenere, tamāḍt tināmeḍḍāt n-kel tenere i-āhalis*. There are therefore many diseases that she as *tālfāqqit* can recognize but which, due to her innate feminine inferiority, she is not able to heal, *əllanāt torhənnawen ajootnen wi əzzayāɣ mušān a-ɣās nākku tamāḍt, wār ādoobey a-has nəttajāɣ asāfar*.[264]

The marabout's significance as a healer among the Kel Alhafra resembles that of the old Arabic seer-doctor, the *kāhin*, whose task it was to negotiate with the fateful powers to expel the sickness – understood by the pre-Islamic Arabs to be caused by a *ǧinn* – out of the patient's body.[265] Although the Arabic-derived Tamasheq term *ālšin* is today used by the Kel Alhafra as the equivalent to the Arabic *maǧnūn*, "possessed by a *ǧinn*", or "insanity", in the Kel Alhafra understanding, someone possessed by a *ǧinn* is not necessarily insane (and likewise, the ancient Arabs obviously did not suffer from mental diseases alone). A sickness is ascribed by the Kel Alhafra to the pernicious powers of the *kel tenere* or *ǧunūn* when it displays characteristics that are obscure and unpredictable. The Kel Alhafra do not recognize psychic disorders in the western sense, merely the deformation of the natural human spirit when it is in a state of possession. Like all illnesses, emotional disturbances are perceived as disruptions in the relationship between human beings and the creator, who mobilizes the tempting powers of the *kel tenere* as a punishment or trial.

Although authors who have studied the function of marabouts among the Tamasheq have assigned to them a role as healers of psychic disorders, for the Kel Alhafra this is true only up to a point. A marabout will certainly be consulted in cases where the illness is poorly defined or chronic, cannot be interpreted or cured by a traditional healer, *enāsāfar*, and shows psychic symptoms, for example when the heart as the seat of the soul is afflicted (a connection is

---

are, therefore, well-established families of marabouts, in which *ālbarāka*, the divine power of blessing, is passed down patrilineally from generation to generation. The Kel Alhafra say, though, that certain marabouts have received their knowledge and the divine blessing through revelation or in making a pilgrimage to Mecca and need not necessarily belong to a family of marabouts.

264 Interview in an encampment at Inkilla with Faḍimata Wālāt Alyāḍ, November 2005.

265 For the significance of the old Arabic *kāhin* see Felix Klein-Franke, *Vorlesungen über die Medizin im Islam* (Wiesbaden: Franz Steiner, 1982) 15.

never made between psychic problems and the brain). However, as already mentioned in chapter 4.1.2., illnesses that bring a Kel Alhafra to a marabout include those that are unknown or new to the population and which do not respond to the traditional therapeutic methods of the *ināsāfārān*. The Kel Alhafra turn to a marabout when the believer can no longer draw on his or her own physical and psychic resources to fight the disease or when, for examples, these resources have been appropriated by a *ǧinn*, and the sick individual needs an intermediary to restore the connection between him or her and the divine powers.

The Kel Alhafra say that marabouts are consulted more today than in the past, even though their services often cost more than those of an *enāsāfār*. Nevertheless, the marabouts are a daily presence in Kel Alhafra society: they live among them. Their practices have general societal validity, are available to anyone who is Muslim and can be applied anywhere through the faithfully recited holy words of the Koran. Within the current upheaval between traditional and modern medical practices, between nomadic and sedentary lifestyle, between rebellion and capitulation, there has been a return to religious values and a reinterpretation of their religious identity. In this reevaluation, the position of the marabouts has also been reassessed, and they are now perceived as both upholders of social stability as well as playing an influential role as mediators between the divine powers and humans in all aspects of the healing process.

5.2.2. From *enāsāfār* to "Agent de Santé"

For the Kel Alhafra, an *enāsāfār* (male) or a *tenāsāfārt* (female) is a traditional healer from a family of healers, *ehān n-ināsāfārān*, whose specialized knowledge is passed on from father to son or from mother to daughter.[266] A healer family is endowed with *ālbarāka*, the divine power of blessing, which enables the practitioners to apply their therapies to sick individuals to restore the body's lost equilibrium.

Through his questions, an *enāsāfār* first establishes the specific thermal temperament of his patient. The sick person is then asked to describe his or her symptoms, *ašāmol n-torhənna*, so that together with his own observations, the healer can create a picture of the sufferer and their situation. The *enāsāfār* en-

---

266 Although Touré in her article "Une innovation sanitaire: l'appropriation des médicaments par les populations touaregs du Mali" writes that "traditional medicine is essentially an affair of women, who practice their skills only among their family or friends", this statement does not apply to the Kel Alhafra region north of Ber. There the majority of the traditional healers, that is *ināsāfārān*, are men, who also offer their services on the weekly Saturday market in Ber. See Laurence Touré, "Une innovation sanitaire: l'appropriation des médicaments par les populations touaregs du Mali", in *Panser le monde, penser les médecines: Traditions médicales et développement sanitaire*, ed. Laurent Prodié (Paris: Karthala, 2005) 270.

quires about signs such as fever, *ašāmol sund tenāde*, visible manifestations on the surface of the body, *ašāmol n-torhənna tāhanāyād fāll elām*, about urination and stools, *tulāt n-isbəkkitān d-āwas*, and about the places where the sick person has spent time in the previous few months, *edāgg d-āttāyān wi iskālāt n-iha āmarhin dāy oran wi išraynen*. He also gathers information about what the patient has been doing recently, *edāgg d-āttāyān wi iskālāt n-iha āmarhin dāy oran wi išraynen*, what he or she has eaten, *ma ija āmarhin dāy əssəbuy wi išrāynen d-ma ikša*, about the patient's appetite, *əndek a-wa itajj dāy tetāte*, what changes or particular incidents have occurred, *ma dar olāh ehān d-irəzzej d-aməzzoy*, and also about the general condition of the family, their animals and their encampment, *dar olāh ehān d-irəzzej d-aməzzoy*. With this information, the *enāsāfār* can determine what factors have acted on the patient, what has brought about the internal disequilibrium, the nature of the prevalent condition, and what therapies will be adequate to heal it.

Earlier, according to the Kel Alhafra, the *ināsāfārān* of certain fractions had moved with and among the nomads as their encampments pursued the seasonal cycle. However, since the years of drought and war much has changed. Following their return from exile and refugee camps, most families of healers became sedentary to compensate for the loss of their herds and earn a livelihood by practicing their healing craft among the villagers and townspeople, while also treating nomads visiting the weekly market. But not only has their clientele changed, in competition with other healers in the village or city, they have forfeited their formerly special position within their nomadic group. Furthermore, not only must the *ināsāfārān* compete with healers from other fractions and ethnic groups, they have also been obliged to adapt their healing knowledge to the new circumstances in which the nomads find themselves. To maintain their position, not only must the traditional healing repertoire of the *ināsāfārān* integrate new diseases, their therapies have to be fundamentally revised to take into account the general changes in nutritional habits, the preponderance of diseases classified as "hot", the disappearance of certain medicinal plants from the area and the appearance of modern drugs on the local markets.

Although the *ināsāfārān* previously administered solely traditional medicines of plant, mineral or animal origin, today they also prescribe modern drugs. Because the Tamasheq now have access to both traditional medications but can also self-administer chemical drugs purchased at the weekly markets, the *ināsāfārān* subdivide their patients into two groups: those accustomed to traditional medicine and those who use modern medicines. When they fall sick, the first group use only traditional remedies and therefore respond better to the traditional, natural therapies. If, however, they become seriously ill, they respond rapidly to modern medications and can be effectively cured. The second group,

in contrast, who regularly use modern drugs, are considered particularly difficult to cure. The *ināsāfārān* concede that pharmaceuticals have almost immediate effects, but they combat only the symptoms of a disease and do not eliminate
the real sickness from the body. A sick person in this group has internalized an
"undigested" disease history, and every time he or she falls ill again, the modern drugs alleviate the external signs but leave the core of the disease untouched.
Because such a person's body has become accustomed to the modern compounds, traditional therapies either have little effect or take an especially long
time to elicit a response. A patient habituated to pharmaceuticals can only be
treated with such chemical drugs, otherwise he or she will die. According to the
ināsāfārān, only when the acute symptoms have vanished, can the patient try to
restore his or her internal equilibrium using traditional healing methods.

The *ināsāfārān* themselves state that they will treat everything that is not
strongly infectious – including diseases in the "hot", *wa n-tākusse*, and "cold",
wa n-təssəmḍe, categories as well as psychic problems – with traditional, natural remedies. The patient will be familiar with the medical discourse that an
enāsāfār uses, will recognize most of the natural products used in the therapy,
and if a modern drug is prescribed, it will usually be one known from the drug
stalls at the weekly market. When this is not the case, the patient will not feel
inhibited questioning the *enāsāfār* about the unfamiliar product. An *enāsāfār*
will usually have acquired his knowledge about modern drugs through his
own personal experience, although a few have received additional training as
an "Agent de Santé" or an "Agent de Santé Itinérant" within the framework
of a health project. The healers who deal simultaneously with both traditional
as well as modern medications are almost exclusively male. The vast majority of female healers, *tināsāfāren*, apply only traditional therapeutic methods.
Female healers do not offer their services within the male domain of the markets, they have limited access to modern drugs and, by and large, they deploy
their medical knowledge solely within the female and family sphere enclosed
by house and tent walls.

It needs to be emphasized though that among the Kel Alhafra there is no
tradition of healer families. There are well-established families of *ālfāqqitān*
and marabouts, but no *ināsāfārān*. I was told by the women that there was a
woman with "special healing knowledge" in an encampment near the well
at Inkomen, but she did not belong to a family with an explicit tradition of
healers. None of the questioned Kel Alhafra women reported having visited
a *tenāsāfārt*. If the internal networks for self-treatment fail, a Kel Alhafra
woman, accompanied by a male member of her family, will seek out a practicing, sedentary *enāsāfār*, from a neighboring fraction such as the Kel Inagozmi,
at the weekly market in Ber.

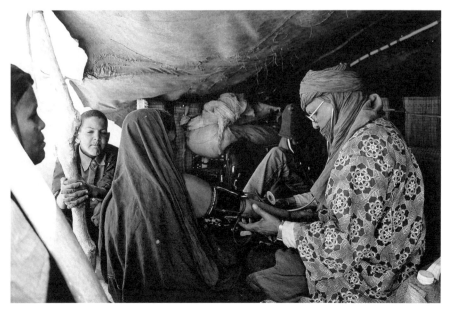

Figure 5.3. *A "modern* enāsāfār*" or "Agent de Santé" at work in an encampment
(Inkilla, November 2005).*

5.3. Professional sector

5.3.1. Between *lāytor* and "modern *enāsāfār*"

When I asked the Kel Alhafra women for their opinion of western-trained doctors, after some consideration they hesitantly replied: *"lāytortān? infa hārāt"* – "Doctors? Well, they do serve some purpose".[267] And indeed, when neither the traditional healer nor a marabout can cure a sickness, and the condition has become acute, then, and as a last resort, the Kel Alhafra finally turn to doctors in a health care center or hospital. However, as I will discuss in more detail in the next section, before they can do so they must overcome several hurdles.

Not only do the majority of the doctors working in the hospital in Timbuktu come from other ethnic groups, they are also members of a different social and economic stratum than most of the Kel Alhafra, have developed a different worldview through their education and their sociocultural context and usually speak a different language. For the Kel Alhafra, doctors represent something foreign, whose work and discourse they do not understand. At the same time the *lāytortān* working in the state-run health centers personify an institutionalized relationship to the Malian regime, creating additional grounds for mistrust.

---

267 Conversation in an encampment at Inkomen with Khadījatu Wālāt Muḥammad, Asiātu Wālāt Ḥāmmadu, Faḍimāta Wālāt Amnuḥen, Faḍimāta Wālāt Almunser, November 2005.

"nəksuḍ lāɣtortān" – "we are afraid of the doctors", some of the women declared. They feel insecure in the consultations in which they encounter primarily male doctors: *"nahiyas s-a-fāl nosa lāɣtor a-han ājjāj a-wa irha, wār ədoobād a-hānāɣ ijrah"* – "we feel helpless, and they cannot really understand us".

If a Kel Alhafra describes her perceptions of her illness to a doctor, not only do language barriers make it difficult to build up a relationship of trust, in translation, the metaphoric meaning of symptoms and organs, figures of speech and the localization of the problem risk being misunderstood or distorted. In turn, the nomads do not understand the doctors' medical discourse and experience a sense of inferiority vis-à-vis the more literate and better educated "experts". Conviction in the doctor's reliability is, for the Kel Alhafra as for others, a basic prerequisite for building up a relationship of trust between doctor and patient: if the Kel Alhafra do not understand exactly what the doctor is doing during a medical examination, or why they receive certain injections or are prescribed certain drugs, if they are treated condescendingly or their sense of modesty is transgressed, the already substantial barriers between the nomads and the doctors are simply magnified.

The Kel Alhafra regard western-trained doctors neither as trustworthy partners nor as advisors. A *lāɣtor* is an official of an medical organization who fights disease symptoms with theoretical knowledge and modern chemical drugs. He is neither religiously inspired nor does he possess *ālbarāka*, the divine power of blessing. He is an instrument who can provide rapid, but superficial, relief from suffering by using particularly efficient medications. Nevertheless, the Kel Alhafra do not see the *lāɣtor* as competing with the marabout: the former cannot fully rid the body of its illness because his treatments do not incorporate the component of religious purification. Furthermore, the two types of healer operate on different planes, the religious and the secular, which do not interfere with one another.

If, however, like several healers in Ber, an *enāsāfār* endowed with *ālbarāka* acquires supplementary knowledge from modern medical practice so that he can undertake small operations and provide immediate assistance in emergences, he unites in one person the ability to apply these modern techniques as well as the traditional therapies that restore the body's natural equilibrium; he functions in the secular and the sacred realms. Such a "modern" *enāsāfār*, sometimes known as an "Agent de Santé",[268] today competes with the doctors. He stands

268 "Agents de Santé" or "Agents de Santé Itinérants" is the designation used in Mali for persons active in the area of health care who have received some medical training. They are all men, who have acquired a certain degree of basic medical knowledge either in the army, in the refugee camps, or through an organization. There is large individual variation in the degree and type of this knowledge. Some of these "Agents de Santé" are traditional heal-

closer to the nomadic population and, in the future, his importance in the therapeutic networks of the Kel Alhafra is likely to increase, so long as the fee for his consultations and medications remains negotiable and cheaper than those of the health care centers and doctors. The *ināsāfārān* today behave like businessmen, they practice on the markets and they sell their medical knowledge and therapies. If an epidemic breaks out outside the village, they will often collaborate with the local health care center, stock up with drugs and then go out to the stricken encampment(s) and sell the drugs to the nomads. The Kel Alhafra will often summon an *enāsāfar* to visit a seriously ill person in a distant encampment rather than taking him or her to the state-run health services, first because of the greater degree of trust, and second, because this is cheaper and quicker than hiring a vehicle for transport or organizing an ambulance from Timbuktu.[269]

5.3.2. Access to state health care institutions

For the Kel Alhafra, the nearest state health care center (CSCOM – Centre de Santé Communautaire)[270] is at Ber on the banks of the Niger, which lies 120 km from the center of the nomadic region (In Agozmi) and 250 km from its

ers, *ināsāfārān*, who now combine and offer experience in western medical practice alongside their traditional therapies. The "Agents de Santé" occasionally cooperate with a local CSCOM, and such healers from among the nomadic population often make visits to neighboring encampments. They acquire their drugs and other medical materials either in the CSCOM or, increasingly, at the local weekly markets.

269 In his study on the use of the health care centers in Ber and Tehārje, Elmouctar found that 46.3% of the patients had first consulted a marabout and 31.7% a traditional healer before going to the CSCOM. See Mohamed Elmouctar, "Logiques de production et utilisation des services de santé en milieu nomade au Mali: Cas de la commune de Ber (Tombouctou)", (Thèse de doctorat, Université de Bamako, 2007) 97.

270 In Mali, a CSCOM (Centre de Santé Communautaire) is a health care center administered by a village's inhabitants. The Mali health care law defines a CSCOM as follows: "A basic health care facility constructed in a health district by a community health association; the CSCOM comprises at least a dispensary, a maternity ward and a store of essential drugs." (See République du Mali: Loi N° 02-049 du 22 Juillet 2002, Définitions).

CSCOM status is accorded an institution when it is administered by an ASACO (Association de Santé Communautaire). The ASACO is a nonprofit organization, under contract to the state's public services. In the Malian health care law, an ASACO is described as follows: "A group of public health care service users who can be authorized to create and run a health care establishment called a 'Centre de santé communautaire'." (See République du Mali: Loi N° 02-049 du 22 Juillet 2002, Définitions).

Under ideal circumstances, the CSCOM team comprises a doctor, a nurse and/or a midwife and should provide for the basic health care needs of the population in the areas of curative, preventive and proactive medicine, such as general medical services, maternal care, vaccinations and preventive medical check-ups.

According to the health care policies of Mali, the country is subdivided into "health zones", the aim being that every member of the population lives within 15 km of a local CSCOM. According to a study undertaken by the "Systèmes Local d'Information Sanitaire (SLIS)", the 15-km accessibility of a CSCOM should have risen from 66% in 2001 to 68% in 2002, with Bamako

most northern well at Arūj. "When they fall sick, the people don't even think about the health care center" – *"kunta āwadəm irhiin, wār nəzinəzjumut edāgg n-lāɣtor",* said Faḍimata in an encampment at Inkomen, "it is too far away and, in any case, we cannot afford it" – *"edāgg wa n-lāɣtor ujəj d-wār nəla aẓrəf inuflāyān".*[271]

The health care center in Ber lies 60 km from its "Centre de Santé de Ré-férence" (CSREF)[272] in Timbuktu. The building has a consultation room, a sick room, an office for the state nurse and a pharmacy. A shed is used to accommodate outpatients requiring an infusion; the patient reception is located on a roofed terrace. The health care team in Ber comprises a state nurse, his assistant, the manager of the pharmacy and a midwife (although during my stay in 2005, this post was vacant), all of whom are Tamasheq. The Ber CSCOM together with those in Tehārje (a state nurse, a nursing assistant) and Zārho (a state nurse, a midwife, a pharmacy manager) serves the 25,000 inhabitants of the commune of Ber spread out over an area of 72,000 km^2.[273]

For members of the state communal health care association (ASACO),[274] a consultation costs CFA 300; nonmembers pay twice as much, i.e. CFA 600. None of the Kel Alhafra I talked to were members of the Ber ASACO, and a simple consultation (i.e. medical examination by the nurse and a prescription for medication) costs between CFA 1,500 and 3,000,[275] to which have to be added the costs of transport. For a patient who travels to the health care center by camel or donkey, the price of an outpatient consultation is about equivalent to the value of a well-fed goat, around CFA 4,000–5,000. "Many of us cannot afford to go to the CSCOM", said Faḍimata, a statement supported by other Kel Alhafra women. For them, article 46 of the Malian health care law is more

---

having the highest accessibility (95%) and the region of Timbuktu the lowest (27%). (SLIS: Annuaire statistique sanitaire du système locale d'informations sanitaires, Bamako: 2002).

271 Interview in an encampment at Inkomen, November 2005.

272 In Mali, the CSREF (Centre de Santé de Référence) is administered by the regional health care authority (Diréction Régional de la Santé) and serves a district as the medical reference center for the surrounding CSCOMs. It is also responsible for transferring patients to the regional hospital. The CSREF director oversees the running of all the CSCOMs in his district. A CS-REF is defined as follows in the Malian health care law: "The Centres de Santé de Référence are the health care centers in the towns of the health care district functioning as primary technical reference centers and providing those public health functions defined in the sector-based health care policies." (See République du Mali: Loi N° 02-049 du 22 Juillet 2002, Article 26).

273 In Mali the state health care infrastructure is concentrated in the south and in urban centers. According to an ECHO (European Community Humanitarian Office) study in 1998–1999, in Mali 57% of the state-employed doctors, 47% of the nurses and 64% of the midwives are located in the capital of Bamako. See ECHO, Rapport d'évaluation des actions humanitaires financées par ECHO dans le Nord-Mali et le Nord-Niger, 1998–1999. April 2000.

274 See footnote 270.

275 See also the data in Elmouctar, *Logiques de production et utilisations des services de santé.*

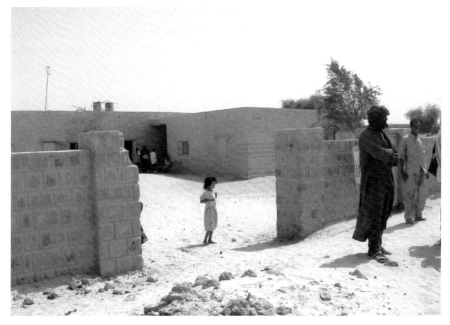

Figure 5.4. *The CSCOM (Centre de Santé Communautaire) in Ber.*

a political ambition than a reality: "The financial costs for participating in the health care system should not hamper the access of the population to health care services".[276]

The Kel Alhafra only take a sick person to the state health care center when their own curative resources are exhausted and the patient's life is in danger: *"edāgg wa n-lāγtor nətakkās-t dāγ ālwāqqātān wi išraynān"* – "we only go to the CSCOM at the last minute", confirmed the 40-year-old Salma in an encampment at In Astilan.[277] At this stage, though, a sick person can no longer be transported on the back of a donkey or camel, and organizing motorized transport to the health care center requires time (up to five days to go by camel from the northern part of the nomadic range to Ber to fetch help) and cash that the Kel Alhafra often do not have: a rented vehicle costs between CFA 45,000–60,000, and their financial resources are tied up in animals that would first have to be sold on the marked to pay for such means of transport. This is not a realizable option for many Kel Alhafra families. Furthermore, ambulances from Timbuktu will not go out to the remote areas of northern Azawad because the state health care budget does not cover the fuel costs. *"wār nəla RAC i-sənāγra torāft ta n-lāγtor"* – "We also have no RAC [Race

---

276 See République du Mali: Loi N° 02-049 du 22 Juillet 2002, Article 47.
277 Interview in an encampment at In Astilan with Salma Wālāt Akola, February 2006.

Communication System],[278] to call for an ambulance from Timbuktu", said Faḍimāta, a mother of two children in Buneyrub, *"mušan wār-ti tǝkkǝd γās edāgg wa nānāγ"* – "but even if we did, they probably still wouldn't come out to us".[279] If an attempt is made to transport a seriously ill person to Ber, the Kel Alhafra say that very often he or she will die during the journey. As Tiyāyya put it, "How can you bring a sick person alive to Ber if you must tie him to a camel and throughout the journey he sways from left to right and is always on the verge of falling off?" – *"ǝndek ǝmmukās ǝmmǝk wa s-han nǝkkel āmarhin har Ber, kunta tǝjīt fāll amǝnis d-dāγ āsikǝl iha miši najāḍāl fāll išrut-ǝnnes wa n-ayǝll meγ wa n-tašālje?"*[280]

The Kel Alhafra women and children feel themselves to be excluded from the health care center not only by enormous distances, but also by sociocultural barriers. The women cannot undertake the journey to the CSCOM without the permission of a husband or male relative, and they must be accompanied by a man. *"meddān ǝsikālān ālwāqq fuk fāll imnas-nāsān, ādoobān tikāwt n-edāgg wa n-lāγtor a-fāl illan γor edāgg n-ewet"* – "the men are constantly traveling with their camels and can visit the health care center when they are at the market", said Faḍimāta, "they know the region and don't get lost" – *"meddān issanān ākall ǝmma-tān iba"*. "But we women, who remain in the tents and encampment, how can we go to the health care center without male assistance?" – *"mušan nākkāneḍ tiḍeḍen, ālwāqq fuk nākkānāḍeḍ ihānān dāγ amǝzzoγ, ǝndek ǝmmǝk wa s-iman-naj edāgg wa n-lāγtor?"* "Alone we would lose our way and die" – *"iman-nānāγ a-hanāγ iba meγ nǝmmut"*. "Furthermore we often don't have the cash", Aïcha added, *"ālwāqq wār nǝha aẓrǝf iman-nānāγ"*, "the men have to wait until market day to sell an animal so that we can pay for a consultation" – *"meddān aqqālān ašāl wa n-ewet a-hin šinšinān hārāt dāγ irǝzzejān a iha aẓrǝf n-edāgg wi n-asāfar"*.[281] A father can take a child to the CSCOM on a market day, so long as it is older than two years and is already weaned, otherwise the mother must come too, rendering the situation much more complicated. In general, an acutely sick child is treated by the Kel Alhafra themselves and resort is only made to the CSCOM when the illness has become chronic, when neither a marabout nor an *enāsāfar* can help, when the parents are at a loss what to do next and when

---

278 RAC (Race Communication System) – an automatic, high-frequency radio and telephone system for communication in remote areas. Some fractions in Azawad are connected to the RAC network and in an emergency can call for help from Ber or Timbuktu.

279 Conversation in an encampment at Buneyrub with Faḍimāta Wālāt Muḥammad, Tiyāyya Wālāt Muttalāmīn, Aïcha Wālāt Muḥāmmadou, February 2006.

280 Conversation at Buneyrub, February 2006.

281 Conversation at Buneyrub, February 2006.

they are camped relatively near to a health care center. [282] However, the Kel Alhafra point out, in the far north of Azawad, everything cannot be abandoned just for the sake of a sick child: "The animals need to be watered" – *"āhuššāl i-āwadəm a isass irəzzejān",* "someone must fetch water from the well" – *"āhuššāl i-āwadəm har ikka əwwi-dd aman γor anu",* "someone must take the herds out to the pastures" – *"āhuššāl i-āwadəm har āwwāḍ edāgg wa iha akāsa",* "protect the family and property" – *"āhuššāl i-āwadəm har ijənniyāt əddināt-ənnes d-ehāre-nāsān".*[283] Among the Kel Alhafra, male labor is essential for the daily activities with the animals and wells. When pastureland is sparse and the nomad tents are scattered far from one another, a father cannot abandon his wife, children and animals to care for themselves in order to travel for four days by camel to Ber with the animals he wants to sell in order to raise the money needed to take a sick child to the CSCOM.[284]

Even if the Kel Alhafra have pitched their tents near the river and are temporarily living nearer the health care center, they do not necessarily visit it more often than when they are living in the far north. The women believe that they are put down by the CSCOM staff as "women of the bush", as *"tiḍeḍen n-ajāma"* or "broussardes", while also admitting that they do not know how they should behave themselves, *"wār nəjjəš lākkol, wār nəssan a-wa itajjān γor edāgg wa n-lāγtor"* – "we have not attended a state school and we feel out of place there", said Tin Albarāka in an encampment at Intikewen.[285] On the other hand, women who have already been to the CSCOM report that they have no trust in the staff: "they are like traders on the market" – *"əddināt wi iššāγālān γor edāgg wa n-lāγtor wālan sund kel mamāla",* "they sell drugs at high prices and then pocket the money for themselves" – *"išanšān-hin timāγwānen izzəwātnen, ḍarāt a-wen itajjān āẓrəf dāγ əlšitān-nāsān",* said

---

282   In response to the questionnaire conducted by Elmouctar in the nomad encampments within 35 km of the health care center in Ber, 56% of the mothers stated that it was not possible for them to get to the CSCOM in Ber. See Elmouctar, *Logiques de production et utilisations des services de santé,* 86.

283   Conversation at Buneyrub, February 2006.

284   In his study on the use of the health care centers in Ber and Tehārje, M. Elmouctar also shows that during the study period from August to September, the majority of the patients attending the CSCOM in Ber were men (47.31%), 30.65% were women and 22% children; 94.69% of the patients were inhabitants of the village itself. See Elmouctar, *Logiques de production et utilisations des services de santé,* 89.

285   Conversation with Tahurut Wālāt Ibrahim and Tin Albarāka Wālāt Muḥammad Ousmane at Intikewen, November 2005.
      For his study on the use of the health care centers in Ber and Tehārje, Elmouctar made a qualitative assessment of the attitude of nomads living within 35 km of Ber to the CSCOM. Of the 237 interviewed nomads, 81.4% had never attended a school. See Elmouctar, *Logiques de production et utilisations des services de santé,* 92.

Tāhurut, "and, moreover, they never have time and don't listen properly to what you are telling them" – *"əlan əššāɣāl ālwāqq fuk d-wār hanāɣ-əsījidān"*. "You are simply prescribed any old drug, and once I'm outside I no longer know what it is good for and when I should take it", another woman added, *"isəfrān wi n-lāɣtor safārān ašāmol n-torhənna, mušān torhənna iman-ənnes taqqālid dāɣ taɣəsssa".*[286]

Apart from the barriers posed by distance, economic conditions, their dependence on male family members, lack of education and a lack of trust in the CSCOM staff, the Kel Alhafra women also have to contend with the effectiveness (or, rather, lack thereof) of the modern medicines that they are offered. Faḍimatu from Intikewen described how she had gone to the CSCOM in Ber for treatment of *āmāɣras* (syphilis). There she was told that she would require three injections over the course of three months to treat the disease. Although the first injection was free, she could neither remain in Ber for three months nor return every month: "how can I do that when my family is at the Tin Timāɣayān well [about 140 km north of Ber]?" – *"əndek a-wa mārājāɣ əkka lāɣtor, ehān-in ɣor anu n-tin timāɣayān?"* Because she felt even sicker after the first injection, she retreated into the desert and broke off the course of treatment.[287] One of Faḍimatu's neighbors told me how she too had gone to the health care center in Ber to be treated for *āmāɣras*. She received all three injections and felt better afterwards, but the disease was still there. "Modern drugs dispel the symptoms", she said, "but the disease itself cannot be eliminated, it remains in the body" – *"isəfrān wi n-lāɣtor safārān ašāmol n-torhənna, mušān torhənna iman-ənnes taqqālid dāɣ taɣəsssa".*[288]

The Kel Alhafra women do not understand why a pregnant woman should go to the CSCOM for a preventive medical checkup. "Pregnancy and birth are not the concern of doctors and certainly not male ones" – *"abārkot d-tiwit waddeɣ dāɣ hārātān n-lāɣtortān kāla n-meddān lab"*, said Tin Albarāka at Intikewen. A pregnant woman will only be taken to the CSCOM in Ber if she is having problems giving birth and her life is in danger. Tin Albarāka pointed out, however, that she did not know a single woman who had given birth in a CSCOM.[289]

---

286 In his study, Elmouctar mentions that of 66% interviewed women, 43.9% stated that they were afraid of the CSCOM health care personnel. See Elmouctar, *Logiques de production et utilisations des services de santé*, 80.

287 Faḍimatu Wālāt Muḥammad Attaher at Intikewen, November 2005.

288 Aminatu Wālāt Ayya in an encampment at Intikewen, November 2005.

289 Tin Albarāka Wālāt Muḥammad Ousmane, Intikewen, November 2005.

When I asked the Kel Alhafra women for their opinion of the regional hospital[290] and the other health care institutions in Timbuktu, Faḍimatu's response echoed that of the women when asked about their attitude to western-trained doctors, *"infa hārāt"* – "they serve some purpose". However, the nomads only go to the hospital in Timbuktu if they are transferred there from the CSCOM in Ber, when they require an examination that needs instruments, machines or specialists that are not available at the CSCOM, when they need drugs or vaccinations that are only available in Timbuktu or when they happen to be camped near the city. One woman, however, said that "one only goes to hospital in Timbuktu to die" – *"əddināt əkkan edāgg n-lāᵧtortān ᵧor tinbətku i-əmmutān"*. The Kel Alhafra are intimidated by the size of the hospital, and once again, language and cultural barriers are an impediment to building up relationships of trust with the medical personnel who are usually from other ethnic groups. For special investigations, surgical interventions and hospital stays, many Kel Alhafra, therefore, prefer to go to Algeria. The Algerian health care institutions are not much further from Azawad than those of Timbuktu, the Kel Alhafra are familiar with the Arabic spoken by the Algerian medical personnel and, since 1974, the services of the relatively well-functioning health care system in Algerian are in general free of charge (in contrast to a inpatient stay in an 84-bed regional hospital in Timbuktu which costs about CFA 10,000 per day).

While the women were discussing state-run heath care at the CSCOM, a man who was passing by joined in: "whoever goes to the health care center is a coward and does not endure what God has inflicted on him".[291] This statement reflects a view widely held among the Kel Alhafra. As God-fearing Muslims, the more devout among them in particular reject modern medicine, perceiving in it a danger to belief. As a divinely sent trial and catharsis, sickness must, in their opinion, be borne with patience and piety. Medical intervention cannot postpone the divinely predetermined end of an individual's life and, when sick, many Kel Alhafra demonstrate either a certain degree of fatalism or seek out only a divinely inspired marabout or *enāsāfār*. In his study, Elmouctar confirms this behavior: 57.4% of those he interviewed living relatively close

---

290 The "Hôpital Régional" in Timbuktu serves as a reference center for the other health care structures in the region. In 2006, the hospital comprised nine departments: pediatrics, odontostomatology, radiology, laboratory and pharmacy, gynecology and obstetrics, orthopedics, physiotherapy and surgery. See Elmouctar, *Logiques de production et utilisations des services de santé*, 2007, 41–42.

291 In his study on the use of the health care centers in Ber and Tehārje, Elmouctar states that between August and November 2005, only 5.3% of the CSCOM patients in Ber came from nomad encampments. See Elmouctar, *Logiques de production et utilisations des services de santé*, 96.

to Ber and Tehārje first sought out a marabout or another kind of healer before
turning to the health care center.[292]

5.3.3. *"tiksənna infa hārāt"* – "vaccination is of some benefit": Attitudes toward immunization

The Kel Alhafra women perceive vaccination as the equivalent to receiving an
injection *inaẓmayān* (sing. *ānaẓmay*). Along with infusions, *perfəsion*, injections are considered to the most effective form of modern medication. During
a discussion in an encampment at Buneyrub, the women told the wildest stories about injections. "If an injection is done badly, it can make you lame" –
"kunta ānaẓmay wār təkna tijālt-ənnes ad təyšed aḏār-ənnes", said Aichata.
She had heard of a man who was suffering from *tenāde tamāssāyarāt* (malaria)
at the end of the rainy season who went to a health care center. There he received an injection in his thigh, after which his leg became stiff. "Yes, injections can cause paralysis" – *"iya, ānaẓmay iyšadān iḏārān n-āwadəm"*, Mariamma agreed, "they are dangerous, but also very effective" – *"inaẓmayān wi
lābasnen, mušan wi yāhuskātnen day"*. Some women have had experience of
injections at health care centers, in particular for *amāyras* (syphilis), and most
of them declared that they had helped. Tin Albarāka, an 18-year-old mother
of twins, told us about a neighboring Arab whose son was suffering from a
bloated stomach and parasites. The father himself had given the child an injection using the same compound (ivermectin) that he used for his animals: "He
gave him the injection in the upper arm, and afterwards the boy recovered" –
"itaj ānaẓmay dāy āfus-ənnes, ḍarāt a-wa izzay". Among the pharmaceutical products they are prescribed, the Kel Alhafra view injections as being far
more effective than medicines that are administered orally. If someone is seriously ill and consults a western-trained doctor, upon his or her return the relatives will immediately ask: *"a-t ajen tijar ānaẓmay?"* – "Did you get an injection?" In the opinion of the Kel Alhafra, only those who receive an injection
or *perfəsion*, an infusion, have been taken seriously and treated with an effective therapy.

Often, however, no differentiation is made between an injection as a form
of therapy and an injection as preventive medicine. The women do not understand precisely what the effect of a vaccination, *tāksənnet* (pl. *tiksənna*),
is. *"wār nəssan a-wa infa tiksənna"* – "we don't know what vaccinations
are good for", said Aichata, and Tahurut added, "they are certainly useful for
something, but we don't understand their purpose" – *"ānaẓmay infa hārāt,
mušan wār nəjrah a-wa infa"*. A mother of six sons, however, joined in and re-

---

292 See Elmouctar, *Logiques de production et utilisations des services de santé*, 121.

buked Tahurut: "But we've heard that vaccinations can prevent diseases, and if that is really so, then we need a vaccination against *āmāɣras* (syphilis)" – *"nǝsla ānaẓmay inǝtākkās torhǝnna; a-fal a-wen-dāɣ a-najj infān n-āmāɣras"*. "And against *sāqqārnen* (whooping cough)" – *"d-ānaẓmay infa sāqqārnen"*, Aichata added, "but the health care teams don't come out to us" – *"mušan ǝddināt wi n-isǝfrān wār ǝjjǝšān imǝzzāɣān-nanāɣ"*. "Sometimes they stop over at the well" – *"ālwāqqātān ǝddinat wi n-isǝfrān ǝqqǝlān ɣor anu"*, said Faḍimata, "but there are only men and a few children at the well" – *"mušān ɣor anu wār illa dihen meddān d-aratān bās"*, "and the children take to their heels at just the mention of the word health care team" – *"a-fāl aratān išilān šik kunta sallān hārāt n-ǝddināt wi n-isǝfrān"*, said Aichata, laughing. The women complained that the few health care teams that did penetrate Azawad nevertheless did not come out to their encampment. Furthermore, the women were not informed in advance of their rare appearances: "If we knew that they were coming into our area, we would go to the well" – *"kunta nǝssan ǝddināt wi n-isǝfrān osān ma lǝmmiḍ anu nākkānen"*, said Mariamma. She continued, "and we would also have our children vaccinated, if we had the opportunity" – *"nǝksǝnnāt ilyāḍān-nanāɣ kunta immukān"*.

The few women whose children have been vaccinated by a mobile health care team said, however, that they did not know for what diseases their children had been immunized. Faḍimata related how, once, a doctor in a mobile team had said to her that her children would receive an injection but a second one would be necessary later for the treatment to be effective. "But they never returned" – *"mušan wār iqqǝlān-dd ḍarāt a-wen"*, she said, "and I have no idea now whether or not my children have been immunized" – *"wār ǝssenāɣ a-fāl aratān-in iksǝnnān fāw"*.

To reach the remote areas of Azawad, a mobile health care team requires not only precise information about the region, but also adequate equipment and materials to protect the vaccines from heat and breakage during the long drives over bumpy and difficult terrain. Even in a refrigerated box, in temperatures that might reach 50 °C in the shade, the vaccines have a limited shelf-life. In addition, the Malian public health system simply cannot afford to pay for transportable refrigerators and the high fuel costs required for a vaccination campaign, and if an international organization launches an initiative, it is always geographically selective and does not cover the far north. Some children have benefited from such initiatives when the Kel Alhafra lived in the southern parts of their nomadic range. However, it appears that the manner and form of information and explanation given to the parents about the vaccinations have been insufficient for the adults to get an intelligible picture of the mode of action and the benefits of immunization.

6. Clinical Status of Women and Children: A medical study among the Kel Alhafra

Anna Münch[1], Birama Diallo[2], Jakob Zinsstag[3], Jan Hattendorf[3], Bassirou Bonfoh[3-4]

1 Institute for Islamic and Middle Eastern Studies, University of Bern, Switzerland / Center for Health and Wellbeing, Princeton University, USA

2 Institut du Sahel, Bamako, Mali

3 Swiss Tropical and Public Health Institute, Basel, Switzerland

4 Centre Suisse de Recherche Scientifique CSRS, Abidjan, Côte d'Ivoire

6.1. Approach and methods

During the time I was undertaking research among the Kel Alhafra, two medical investigations were carried out, both approved by the Ethical Commission of the University of Bamako. In the first, a Malian doctor studied the use of the health care centers in Ber and Tehārje by the Tamasheq living in the province of Ber [Mohamed El Moctar: *Logiques de production et utilisation des services de santé en milieu nomade au Mali: Cas de la commune de Ber (Tombouctou)*. Thèse de doctorat à la Faculté de Médecine, de Pharmacie et d'Odonto-Stomatologie, Université du Mali. Bamako: 2006. 105 p.]. A second, clinical investigation was undertaken by another Malian doctor among the Kel Alhafra in the research area.

Between 10 October 2005 and 10 February 2006, seven field missions were conducted, in which, using a standardized questionnaire (source: Swiss Tropical Institute, Basel, Switzerland; see Appendix), Kel Alhafra women and children were asked about topics such as the performance of their daily tasks, nutrition, number of children, immunization and their use of health care institutions. The purpose of the study was explained to the women, and they were only examined clinically if they gave oral consent. The questionnaire was in French. None of the participating Kel Alhafra women could speak, read or write French. They spoke Tamasheq and Ḥassanīa Arabic; a few could read and write Arabic. An interpreter was therefore necessary for this part of the study. During these field missions, I undertook 53 unstructured interviews in Tamasheq with the women participating in the clinical study. The women were asked, for example, about their pregnancies, number of children, miscarriages, the histories of children who had died, eating habits, diseases, therapies that they used and about their opinions of health care centers.

The women who were examined clinically by the doctor are referred to here as the "clinical group"; the interviewed women as the "interview group".

Table 6.1. *General information*

Field mission	Date	Date	Location	Number of encampments	Number of women and children examined clinically	Number of interviewed women and children
1	10–15 Oct. 2005	Intoršawen Indiãrran Tin Timãyayãn In Ibrahim	N:17°23'80"/W:02°17'38" N:17°45'32"/W:01°59'55" N:17°54'36"/W:01°58'52" N:18°06'32"/W:02°51'34"	5	46	6
2	23–28 Oct. 2005	Buneyrub	N:18°04'36"/W:02°10'06"	5	45	7
3	6–11 Nov.2005	Inbagsa In Tešãq Inkomen Intikewen	N:17°54'44"/W:02°02'43" N:17°39'64"/W:02°21'05" N:17°05'54"/W:02°20'19" N:16°57'89"/W:02°15'76"	6	47	18
4	20–25 Nov. 2005	Intikewen Inkilla	N:16°57'89"/W:02°15'76" N:17°09'83"/W:01°46'58"	5	43	7
5	5–9 Dec. 2005	Iboggar Tinãhara	65 km south of Ber 30 km south of Rharous	5	46	0
6	20–24 Jan. 2006	Al Ma'mor In Ibrahim	N:18°00'58"/W:02°25'98" N:18°06'32"/W:02°51'34"	5	44	0
7	5–10 Feb. 2006	In Astilan W Tãbayãrt	N:17°05'46"/W:02°34'86" N:16°94'20"/W:02°51'94"	5	47	15
Total:				36	177 women 141 children	53

6.2. Clinical results among women

Sample

The selection of women for the study was largely determined by practical conditions and accessibility in the field and therefore, strongly influenced by, for example, impassable terrain, journey length and climatic conditions. During the seven missions, the medical team visited 36 different nomad encampments around 15 wells, examining between 19 and 25 women on each mission. Precise census data for the region are lacking, and so representative sampling among the women and children was not possible. Of the 177 women studied, 164 were approached at random and asked if they wished to participate, while 11 were selected by the doctor; one woman requested an auscultation, and for one woman the mode of selection is not known.

The analysis that follows is limited to the women who were selected randomly and were older than 14 years of age (n = 160). Of these women, 14 were single (8.7%), 118 married (73.7%), eight divorced (5%) and 20 widowed (12.5%).

The 53 women in the interview group were selected randomly from those in the clinical group during five missions to 26 encampments at 12 different wells.

The wells and encampments in the study area were selected to provide a cross-section of the entire nomadic range of the Kel Alhafra and to cover various geographic zones.

Data analysis

The data from completed questionnaires were entered in duplicate in a database (Access™, Microsoft Inc.), and double checked with Epi-Info™ (Centers for Disease Control, Atlanta, USA) to correct for input data errors. The data were analyzed statistically using SAS™ Version 9.1 (SAS Institute, Cary, USA).

Demographic data

Age distribution

The age distribution is based on the information given by the women themselves; however, many base this on events that took place in the year they were born rather than on knowing the actual year itself.

Figure 6.1. shows the age distribution of the women in the clinical and interview groups. The age structures of the two groups did not differ significantly (Mann-Whitney test: n = 213, Z = –0.32, p = 0.75).

Figure 6.1. *Age distribution*

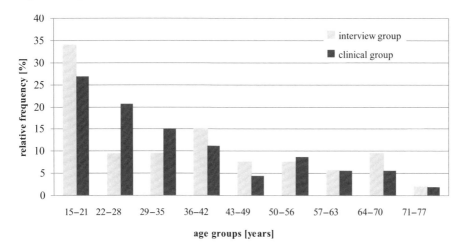

Fertility

The number of live births per woman varied between one and 12. In response to the medical questionnaire, 17% of the women reported they had never been pregnant, 80% had never had a miscarriage, and 95% had never had a stillbirth. In the interview group, these percentages were 8%, 70% and 83%, respectively.

Figure 6.2. illustrates the frequency distribution of pregnancies (black/dark grey) and live births (grey/light grey). The results obtained for the clinical and interview groups show only small differences.

The data in figure 6.3. for the frequency of miscarriages (black/dark grey)

Figure 6.2. *Frequency distribution of pregnancies and live births*

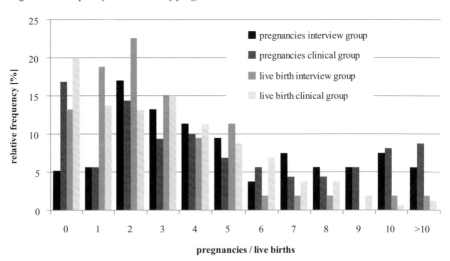

and stillbirths (grey/light grey) are for women who had been pregnant at least once: 133 in the clinical group and 49 in the interview group. In contrast to the pregnancy and live birth results, significantly more stillbirths were reported in the interview group compared to the clinical group (Mann-Whitney test: n = 182, Z = –2.65, p = 0.008).

The cohort fertility rate was calculated from the number of children borne by women now over 45 years of age in the clinical group. Forty-one women over 45 years of age had 335 pregnancies and 304 live births, to give an average of 7.4 live births per woman during her reproductive years.

Finally, the number of fertile years of all women between 15 and 45 was aggregated, giving 2,555 fertile years (n = 155) with a total of 771 pregnancies and 671 live births. The women in the clinical group therefore had on average one pregnancy resulting in a live birth every 3.8 years. However, because in the clinical study, miscarriages and stillbirths were mentioned less often than

Figure 6.3. *Relative frequency of miscarriages and stillbirths*

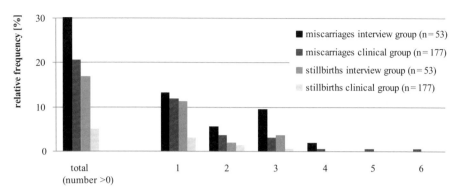

in the unstructured interviews, the interval between individual births is probably smaller, and women in the interview group reported that they became pregnant every two years.

Table 6.2. *Summary of the frequency of clinical diagnoses (including pregnancy) among 160 Tamasheq women between 15 and 75 years of age (n = 160). The relative frequency is given as prevalence with the upper and lower 95% confidence limits.*

Diagnosis	Number of women	Prevalence (%)	Lower 95% confidence limit (%)	Upper 95% confidence limit (%)
Joint and bone pain[1]	26	16.3	10.5	22.0
Pregnancy	18	11.3	6.4	16.1
Bronchitis	18	11.3	6.4	16.1
Endemic syphilis	8	5.0	1.6	8.4
High arterial blood pressure	5	3.1	0.4	5.8
Skin diseases[2]	5	3.1	0.4	5.8
Suspicion of tuberculosis	5	3.1	0.4	5.8
Ear, nose and throat[3]	5	3.1	0.4	5.8
Anemia[4]	4	2.5	0.1	4.9
Urinary tract disease[5]	4	2.5	0.1	4.9
Asthma	3	1.9	0	4.0
Stomach and intestinal tract disease[6]	3	1.9	0	4.0
Dental illness	3	1.9	0	4.0
Deafness	1	0.6	0	1.8
Obesity	1	0.6	0	1.8
Conjunctivitis	1	0.6	0	1.8

[1] *Knee, hip, post-traumatic (fall from an animal), loose pelvic symphysis, sciatica*
[2] *Including fungal skin infection ("Teigne")*
[3] *Colds, sore throat, otitis*

[4] *Sometimes postpartum*
[5] *Pyelonephritis, suspicion of bilharzia, urinary tract infection*
[6] *Dysentery*

Clinical status

The doctor made clinical diagnoses for 107 of the 160 women examined. Multiple diagnoses are listed separately in table 6.2.

Of the 160 women examined, the general condition of two was poor. Five were suffering from skin diseases and five more from pruritis (itching). Palpation identified one woman with an enlarged liver and two women with an enlarged spleen. During auscultation, a pathological cardiac murmur was found in one woman, and 14% had pathological lung findings. A body temperature greater than 37 °C was measured in 11% of the women, but 40% complained of an elevated temperature. At the time of the examination, 30% of the women had coughs; in one-fifth of these cases, the woman had been coughing for more than two weeks. Blood was found in the sputum (hemoptysis) of 4% of the women, while 6% complained of shortness of breath, with a suspicion of tuberculosis in 3% of all the women.

Nutritional status of the women

While children were weighed on a spring balance, scales were used for the women; the two instruments were not calibrated with each other. Nevertheless a general picture could be obtained, demonstrating a generally good nutritional status among the women. The women's weight rises between 15 and 20 years in age. This can be attributed on the one hand to pregnancy, on the other to a fat-rich diet (animal fat, butter and oil) and a lack of physical activity.

Figure 6.4. *Weight development in kilograms of children (white diamonds) and women (black dots) as a function of age in years*

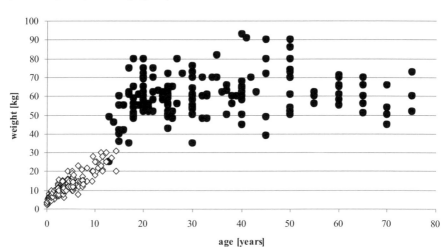

Relationship between blood pressure, weight and age

Systolic blood pressure greater than 130 mm HG was quite common between the ages of 15 and 30 years (figure 6.5.).

Multiple regressions showed that there was a significant correlation between

Figure 6.5. *Women's blood pressure (mm Hg) as a function of age*

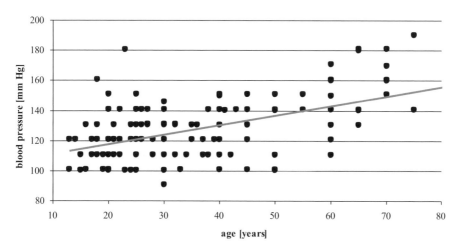

blood pressure and age (rate of increase 0.54 mm Hg/year, standard error 0.07 mm Hg/year, p < 0.0001) and between blood pressure and weight (figure 6.6.; rate of increase 0.38 mm Hg/kg, standard error 0.11 mm Hg/kg, p = 0.0011).

Figure 6.6. *Women's blood pressure (mm Hg) as a function of weight (kg)*

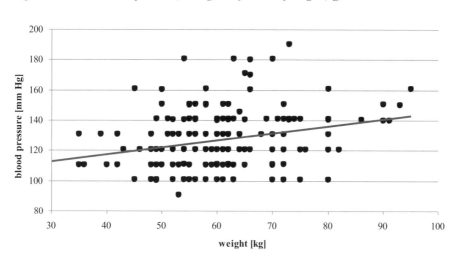

Seasonal influences on disease

Certain symptoms and diseases show a seasonal pattern. A distinction was made in this study between a phase after the rainy season, *γarat* (October–November: 53% of the probands), and the cold season, *tajrəst* (December–February: 47% of the probands).

There was a tendency for more women to be sick in the cold season (bronchitis, $p = 0.09$), with pathological lung findings in 29% of the women during this phase compared to only 14% after the rainy season. In contrast, during *γarat*, twice as many women complained of fever ($p < 0.001$) and hemoptysis ($p = 0.06$) than during the cold season of *tajrəst*.

Use of health care institutions

Of the examined women with medical complaints, 8% had sought treatment: 5% had treated themselves, one woman had gone to a marabout and three women had visited a health care center. One woman from an encampment near the CSCOM in Ber stated that she used the center regularly. Reasons given for not using the health care institutions included the large distances to the nearest CSCOM, lack of financial resources and dependence on male family kin without whose support and escort they could not visit a health care center.

Birth

Just one of the 160 women in the clinical group stated that she had had a prenatal examination in the health care center in Ber. Nearly all the women had given birth to their most recent child in their encampment, and the umbilical cord had been cut by female kin. Two women stated that they had given birth in an Algerian health care institution. There are no traditional midwives among this population group.

Vaccination

In the clinical group, 2% of the women stated they had an Algerian vaccination document. None of the women had a Malian vaccination document, and none had been vaccinated against tetanus (VAT).

Malaria

Among both the clinical and the interview groups, malaria appeared to be practically unknown, even though 85% of the women in the clinical group knew the substance chloroquine. About one-third of the women said that together with their family they used a mosquito net; the women were not aware of the existence of impregnated nets.

Nutritional practices

All the probands were asked what they had eaten in the last 24 hours. The responses are shown in table 6.3.

Table 6.3.
Food consumption

Food consumption per family
94% had eaten *cereals* such as millet and wheat (rice was less common)
93% had drunk *raw milk* from camels, goats and sheep (cow milk was also drunk, but with the lowest frequency)
76% had eaten *sugar*
58% had eaten *salt*
55% had eaten *meat*
None of the women had eaten *vegetables* or *fruit*

The average daily milk consumption was calculated from the total given for the family in *taɣəšut* (pl. *tiɣəšuten)* (= 2 liters) divided by the number of children plus 2 (parents), to give a value of 0.23 *taɣəšut* (standard deviation 0.16 *taɣəšut*). With an increasing number of children, this value leveled off at around 0.1 *taɣəšut* (200 ml) per person.

Work with animals

In response to the questionnaire, a quarter of the women in the clinical group stated that they tended goats and sheep, while only a few looked after camels. No woman herded cows. About half the women milked their goats and sheep themselves, 15% participated in milking camels, but no woman milked cows. Nearly all the women assisted when goats and sheep gave birth, fewer with camels, but, once again, the birth of calves is apparently a male affair. Most of the women slaughtered sheep and goats themselves, and also helped in the slaughter of camels and cattle.

Through the direct contact with animals in labor and during milking and slaughtering, the women are exposing themselves to various zoonoses, such as brucellosis, Q fever or bovine tuberculosis. However, more research is needed to determine the frequency and the significance of such diseases in the study area.

6.3. Clinical results among children

Sample

The mothers in the clinical group were often accompanied by their children and when the mothers requested it, the children were also given a clinical examination. The results reported below are for 141 children aged between 0 and 14 years. Over 75% of the children were less than 5 years old, and 57% were girls.

Clinical status

The most common diseases in both the children under five years as well as those between five and 15 years were acute respiratory diseases (bronchitis), conjunctivitis, skin diseases and gastrointestinal diseases. Fever and suspicion of malaria were much less common.

Table 6.4. *Summary of the frequency of clinical diagnosis among the children*

Clinical diagnosis	Number of children	Prevalence (%)	95% Confidence limits	Remarks
Children under 5 years (n = 72)				
Bronchitis	16	22.2	15.8–28.7	
Conjunctivitis	9	12.5	7.4–17.6	
Skin diseases	9	12.5	7.4–17.6	fungi, impetigo
Gastrointestinal diseases	7	9.7	5.1–14.3	dysentery, diarrhea
Malnutrition	5	6.9	3.0–10.9	
Ear, nose and throat	3	4.2	1.1–7.3	otitis, pharyngitis
Injuries	3	4.2	1.1–7.3	axe, shoulder dislocation
Lung infections	2	2.8	0.2–5.3	
Asthma	1	1.4	0.0–3.2	
Burns	1	1.4	0.0–3.2	
Hydrocephalus	1	1.4	0.0–3.2	
Leg paralysis	1	1.4	0.0–3.2	
Phimosis	1	1.4	0.0–3.2	
Premature birth	1	1.4	0.0–3.2	
Children between 5 and 15 years (n = 60)				
Bronchitis	15	25.0	18.3–31.7	
Skin diseases	6	10.0	5.4–14.6	fungi
Gastrointestinal diseases	5	8.3	4.1–12.6	
Conjunctivitis	3	5.0	1.6–8.4	
Lung infections	2	3.3	0.6–6.1	
Ear, nose and throat	2	3.3	0.6–6.1	Candida
Malaria	2	3.3	0.6–6.1	
Urinary stone	1	1.7	0.0–3.7	
Hydrocele	1	1.7	0.0–3.7	
Hearing loss	1	1.7	0.0–3.7	

Table 6.5. *Statistically significant seasonal differences for clinical findings in the children*

Disease	*γarat* October–November	*tajrast* December–February	Fisher exact test p
Dermatoses	1%	8%	0.06
Auscultation findings in the lung	15%	30%	< 0.05
Cornea changes	0%	4%	< 0.05
Conjunctivitis	4%	20%	< 0.01

The children suffer from more diseases of the skin, conjunctiva and respiratory tract during the cold season of *tajrɔst* than during the warm months of *ɣarat*.

Child mortality

Child mortality in this study was high. It was calculated from the information given in the 53 interviews in which were recorded precise details for the age of living and deceased children. Altogether 45 women who had given birth at least once knew the precise age at which their children had died. At the time of the interviews, of 199 births, 63 children had died, to give a mortality rate of 32%. Of these, 16 were stillbirths, 33 children had died at less than six years of age and 14 were older. Of the surviving children, 85 were more than five years old and 41 up to five years of age.

The Kaplan-Meier method was used for the survival function analysis. The 10 children under five years old whose age was not known exactly were excluded from the analysis.

Figure 6.7 shows the Kaplan-Meier curve for the survival in months of 198 children up to five years of age (including stillbirths). From this it can be seen that the probability for a newborn child to reach five years of age is 72%.

Figure 6.7. *Kaplan-Meier estimation for the age-dependent survival probability of the children (n = 198)*

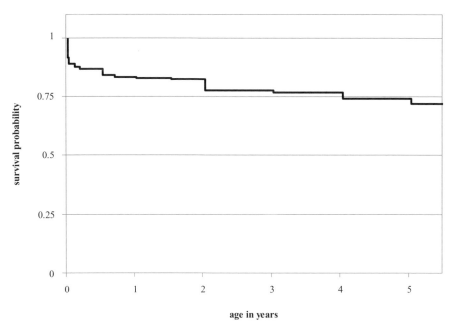

Malnutrition and undernourishment

Figure 6.8 shows the weight gain of girls and boys. Simultaneous measurement of the upper arm circumference (table 6.6.) confirmed low to medium undernourishment. (It should be mentioned here that April of the study year was marked by a serious food shortfall that led to the death of a number of children. Following a food aid campaign, the nutritional status of the children showed considerable improvement). Since the children rarely eat vegetables and fruit, milk is their only regular source of vitamin A. However, the estimated milk consumption (see above) is barely sufficient to cover their vitamin A needs, and hypovitaminosis A is likely. Further study is needed to examine the degree to which vitamin A may be lacking in the children's diet.

Most of the children were weaned on milk products and cereal porridge ("bouillie").

Figure 6.8. *Weight development of girls and boys*

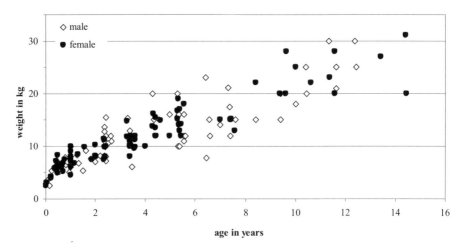

Table 6.6. *Upper arm circumference of children less than five years of age (n = 112)*

Upper arm circumference (cm)	Percentage of children
< 11	8.9%
< 12	14.0%
< 13	40.0%
< 14	65.0%

Access to health care services

Less than 3% of the children had received professional medical care for their complaints in the two weeks prior to the study. In most cases they were dependent on care and treatment by their parents.

Vaccination

Less than 3% of the children had received the standard child vaccinations provided by the state vaccination program PEV (Programme Elargi de Vaccination), and none had received vitamin A supplementation.

Table 6.7. *Immunization coverage by the standard child vaccinations among children under five years (BCG = Bacillus Calmette Guérin, tuberculosis; DTC3 = diphtheria/tetanus/pertussis).*

Vaccinations among children less than 5 years of age			
	vaccinated	not vaccinated	Percentage
BCG	3	113	< 3%
DTC3	2	109	< 2%
Polio	2	111	< 2%
Yellow fever	0	113	0
Measles	3	110	< 3%
Vitamin A	0	113	0

7. Interpretation and Perspectives

7.1. Correlation between clinical results and perceived health status

From the clinical study it is clear that Kel Alhafra women are highly unwilling to discuss topics such as pregnancy, miscarriages and stillbirths with a non-Kel Alhafra male. These are delicate matters concerning the subjective world of female intimacy and hidden internal processes, only discussed inside the protective environment of the tent with trusted peers of the same sex. Furthermore, because women are bonded to the natural world and to its creative powers, reproductive issues always bring into play the dreaded *kel tenere*, who are always implicated in such misfortunes as miscarriages and stillbirths. The Kel Alhafra take great pains in avoiding open reference to matters that involve the *kel tenere*, fearing that in naming them, they will draw the attention of the *kel tenere* or lure them into action. Stillbirths, *aratān immutnān*, are more likely to be mentioned, because after the seventh month of pregnancy, these children are fully developed and basically viable, although they are born dead, and thus have the right to a proper burial, which bestows on them a certain legitimacy. Early miscarriages, *išušəfān*, that take place during the first four months of a pregnancy are rarely mentioned by the Kel Alhafra women because the fetus at this stage is not recognized as a child with a divine soul, *iman*. According to the Kel Alhafra, this divine soul only enters the child after the fourth month, and from this point on, the women refer to a miscarriage, *eha*, as it is understood by western medicine. Strong emotions such as *tarəmmaq* (anxiety, shock, agitation), *tārha* or *derhan* (intense desire/passion) are held responsible as the primary causes of miscarriage. Since these feelings are always associated with *tašoṭṭ*, the evil eye, or with *terk mājārād*, bad speech, and thus with the pernicious powers of the *kel tenere*, a Kel Alhafra woman is very unlikely to lower her guard by mentioning her miscarriages to a foreign man during a clinical examination and thereby revealing her vulnerability.

The most frequently recorded diagnosis of joint and bone ailments in the clinical study corresponds to the perceived common image of the women interviewed. The Kel Alhafra in general complain of a steady rise in recent years of *tākmo n-iɣāssān*, internal, not easily localizable pains in the bones. These are attributed to the excessive consumption of foods classified as "hot", to malnutrition, to physically strenuous work and the privation of basic needs. *tākmo n-iɣāssān*, joint and bone pains, are also perceived by the Kel Alhafra as symptoms of *āmāɣras*, endemic syphilis, which was identified by the clinical study as the third most frequent disease. The women blame the lack of milk in particular for this ailment. There is overall agreement between the diseases identified by the doctor and the most common complaints mentioned and recognized by the women. High blood pressure, for example, which they refer to as *tākmo n-ulh*, "pain of the heart", is in their estimation a particular problem for women who have had several successive pregnancies closely following one another. Skin diseases, which they again claim are rapidly on the increase, are interpreted as a response to a change in diet, *āmāyrəs*, as well as the over-consumption of foods classified as "hot". The Kel Alhafra women do not perceive obesity as a pathology as such, more as a condition that can precipitate illnesses and suffering such as pains in the legs, *tākmo n-iḍarān, tāhafnent* or *tawār*. Especially noteworthy is that the clinical study identified no gynecological problems among the women. Four women were diagnosed with a urinary tract infection, *tijdil āwas*; this term though is used more vaguely by the Kel Alhafra women as a collective designation for genital tract problems. During auscultation, more precise information should be sought from a woman as to how she is specifically experiencing *tijdil āwas*, although out of modesty, the women are not likely to describe such troubles in great detail with a male doctor and/or his translator.

Although 40% of those examined complained of a raised body temperature, a temperature greater than 37° Celsius was measured in only 11%. This corresponds to the reported perception of excessive heat in the body, caused, according to the Kel Alhafra, by an imbalance in their current nutrition and their environment, dominated by elements classified as "hot". Since the clinical study was undertaken after the rainy season, *ɣarat*, and during the cold season of *tajrəst*, the seasonally typical "hot" diseases recognized by the Kel Alhafra, such as fever, *tenāde*, and respiratory complaints such as *iḍmārān* (bronchitis) and *tāsut* (coughing) predominate. More women reported feeling sick during the cold season of *tajrəst* than during the warmer season of *ɣarat*. At the end of this rainy season, the temperatures are still comfortable before they sink down to zero centigrade, and the poorly nourished nomads succumb to all forms of cold-associated diseases. Furthermore, during *ɣarat*, the nutritional situation is better: the animals have given birth, milk and meat are available, and Kel Alhafra families have recovered during the abundant months of the rainy season. *ɣarat*, however, is the season for the *Anopheles* mosquitoes, which breed during the rainy season in water pools as well as along the river and spread malaria particularly from September onward, as confirmed clinically by the increase in fever during this part of the year. This specific fever is referred to by the Kel Alhafra as *tenāde tamāssāɣarāt*, "the fever at the end of the rainy season". They are not aware that it is due to malaria. Both the questionnaire used for the clinical research as well as the unstructured interviews revealed that malaria is practically unknown among the Kel Alhafra. They attribute *tenāde tamāssāɣarāt* to milk drunk at the end of the rainy season, to excessive exposure to the sun, or to the dietary switch from milk to cereals. Although one-third of the women said they used mosquito nets, they made no association between "the fever at the end of the rainy season" and mosquitoes. The nets, rather, are used as protection from beetles, grasshoppers, spiders or small animals like scorpions and snakes when the temperatures are still too high to sleep inside the tents, when rains have ceased, and nights are spent under the open sky. The fact that 85% of the women know about the antimalarial drug chloroquine can be traced back to its prescription as an antifever medication at the health center and its widespread sale on the markets as an antipyretic.

The responses to questions about the use of health care institutions were similar in both arms of the study, the medical questionnaire and informal interviews: the women primarily make use of their own resources, and within two weeks of the study, only 8% had treatment for an illness, and for 5% this was in the form of self-medication. The reasons given in the medical questionnaire and in the informal conversations for the low usage rates of the health care center were similar. With regard to immunization, just 2% of the women had vaccination documents from Algeria, a strong indicator that the preventive medical efforts of the Malian government have not yet penetrated to the nomadic population in Azawad.

The nutritional data gathered by the medical questionnaire reflect the changes in dietary traditions described by the women in the more informal setting. At the time of the study, a woman was drinking on average just 200 ml milk per day, although a higher rate of milk consumption was expected. A study by Wagenaar-Brouwer on milk consumption by Tamasheq groups between June 1981 and December 1982 found that noble Tamasheq women in the Niger delta were drinking between 1.2 and 3 liters of milk per day during the cold season; only at the end of the dry season did this sink to 500 ml per adult.[222] This comparison clearly shows that today, the Kel Alhafra can only enjoy a milk-based diet from the end of June to the middle of September during the three-month season of *akāsa*. In the other months, cereals such as millet and white flour become the staple dietary components. Since the Kel Alhafra very rarely eat fruits and vegetables, deficiencies are likely. Malnutrition, *iba n-imənsiwān*, is viewed by the Kel Alhafra as a sickness in itself, a problem classified as "hot", which provokes other illnesses such as *āmāyras*, endemic syphilis, *āttaxma*, digestive problems, *aẓāndi*, hemorrhoids, *dāmbāraku*, night

---

222 See Martie Wagenaar-Brouwer, "Preliminary findings on the diet and nutritional status of some Tamasheq and Fulani groups in the Niger Delta of central Mali", in *Population, Health and Nutrition in the Sahel: Issues in the Welfare of Selected West African Communities*, ed. Allan G. Hill (London: Routledge & Kegan Paul, 1985) 226–253.

blindness, and *iba n-ašni*, anemia. Overall, though, what the Kel Alhafra perceive as the most troubling aspect of the dietary change is that it disturbs the internal thermal equilibrium: frequent consumption of cereals and other foods classified as "hot", like oil, sugar and salt, causes bodily overheating which in turn leads to the onset of diseases of a "hot" character.

In terms of body weight, the clinical study found relatively good nutritional status among the women – in contrast to the malnutrition identified in the children – but this finding must be treated with caution. Although the women are not very physically active, spend most of their time in and around the tent and tend to eat fat-rich foods and a lot of sugar, the ideals of beauty have changed, and the young women now wish to be well-nourished but not fat. The Kel Alhafra no longer force-feed girls with fat-rich foods, and indeed, it would be difficult to do so – there simply is not enough milk available any more to practice such a custom. The weight data, though, needs to be analyzed in more detail, taking into account pregnancy and post-pregnancy, since both obviously have an influence on body weight.

Among the Kel Alhafra, care and handling of animals is almost exclusively undertaken by the men. Women only help on a daily basis with the herds when male members of the family are absent. In contrast to their female Arab neighbors who sometimes tend flocks of goats or sheep and take them to the pastures, only Kel Alhafra men and boys move with the animals away from the protective environment of the tent and the encampment, while the women remain behind to take care of the girls and small children. The young women may help milk the small livestock in the mornings and evenings, but they never work with camels or cows, except in emergencies. The women are not aware that certain animal diseases can be transmitted to humans: they drink raw milk without hesitation, assist when animals are giving birth or are slaughtered, and also eat meat from animals that had clearly been sick. Further research is needed, however, to establish more clearly the meaning of animal health for the Kel Alhafra, the connections they perceive between animal and human health, and the actual incidence of zoonoses in the study area.

There was a substantial overlap between the clinically diagnosed pathologies among children and the sicknesses described by the mothers. Respiratory diseases, *iḍmārān*, eye inflammations, *ahənnəj*, mycoses, *ākorkor*, and diseases of the digestive tract (such as *tezzort n-tāsa*, abdominal pain, and diarrhea, *tufit*) are perceived by the Kel Alhafra as typical ailments for children up to 15 years of age. The clinical study, however, recorded none of the epidemic infectious diseases such chicken pox, *ubšej*, whooping cough, *sāqqārnen,* measles, *tassididet,* rubella, *šāggāɣ,* or meningitis, *eɣāf wa lābasān,* that the women also name as typical diseases of childhood. The high frequency of dermatoses and conjunctivitis might be attributable to the time of year, *tajrəst,* at which the study was undertaken. During this cold season, the Kel Alhafra wash infrequently in order not to cool the body down with water, a behavior that promotes the spread of mycoses and scabies. In addition, the lowered temperatures usher in flies that settle especially in the corners of the mouth and eyes of children and contribute to the development of eye infections. The women also acknowledge that because there is a shortage of clothing and children go around either naked or inadequately clothed, even when the temperatures are icy, they are much more susceptible to respiratory diseases during *tajrəst.* According to the Kel Alhafra women, it is between the ages of zero and five that their children are exposed to the most health risks, around two being seen as a particularly susceptible period, because the children may become quite weak while they are being weaned.

The clinically ascertained light to medium undernourishment among the children testifies to a generally inadequate diet. The Kel Alhafra point to the lack of milk and the necessity to feed the children cereals year round as the most significant factor contributing to this unsatisfactory situation. Faced with the shortage of fresh animal milk, some women have begun to give their children powdered milk. However, this is classified as "hot", and the women blame it for diarrhea, vomiting and pruritus and say that it weakens the young children's constitution. Although *tafəngora,* baobab powder, classified as "cold", used to be given to children as a milk substitute, it is now difficult to acquire in Azawad, the mothers say, because of the changes in the natural environment and the spread of the desert climate such that the tree can now only survive in the south.

Children are the weakest members of the Kel Alhafra society, and within the two weeks prior to the study, less than 3% of sick children had received medical treatment outside their family circle. Furthermore, less than 3% of the children had participated in the national vaccination program PEV (Programme Elargi de Vaccination). This suggests not only that the state health authorities do not reach the northern territories with this service, but that the nomadic population is unaware of and poorly informed about the effectiveness and value of immunization.

7.2. Health as a mirror of change and the turn to a reinterpreted Islam

The Kel Alhafra understand human health as a physical and psychic equilibrium dependent both on a balance in the natural surroundings as well the individual's relationship to the supernatural power. If this fragile balance in the interplay between the reciprocal energies in the daily lifeworld breaks down, or

if the believer errs from the righteous path and distances him- or herself from
the divine source of all life and death, the result for the individual is dishar-
mony and the onset of disease.

Confronted not only by climatic but also social changes, the Kel Alhafra
today are engaged in adapting themselves to unfamiliar living conditions and
an altered environment. Foreign occupying powers, drought, confusion caused
by war, refugee experience, breakdown of former social structures and loss
of assets and traditional values, have fundamentally disrupted what was perceived as a symbiotic relationship between the group and its lifeworld. This
disorder has carried over into all areas related to the nomads' health. The transformations and disbalances are experienced and reflected not only by the human body but are also seen in the medical system. With the dissection of the
large tribal fractions and the breakdown of earlier interdependencies between
individual groups, traditional families of healers in neighboring fractions have
moved to the cities. In doing so, they have become practically inaccessible to
the Kel Alhafra women who are rarely able to avail themselves of health services outside the tent and encampment. At the same time, the society's image
of its own health status has also changed: new and unfamiliar diseases have
appeared against which traditional healing knowledge and treatments are ineffective, ailments that were once specific to particular seasons are now oc-
curring year-round, and diseases that were restricted to a certain social group,
such as the elderly or children, are now found among the entire population.

Diseases that are novel for the Kel Alhafra and for which they have no
terms in their own language are usually given vague designations, such as "the
new fever", *tenāde tāšrayet,* or "the bad head", *eyāf wa lābasān,* that reflect
their lack of knowledge concerning these illnesses. Unable to explain these
strange ailments, they are often attributed to the noxious powers of the *kel tenere.* It needs to be emphasized that such diseases whose causal factor is explicitly ascribed to evil spirits need not necessarily be psychopathological in
nature, as previous research exploring medical understanding of the Tamasheq
has suggested, but express, rather, characteristics that the Kel Alhafra find inexplicable.

The decimation of their herds during the droughts, climatic change and
the failure of rains have had a dramatic impact on the dietary habits of the Kel
Alhafra. These changes in turn have made an impact on the body's equilibrium and the individual's health. Milk and milk products, once dietary staples,
are being increasingly replaced by cereals, primarily millet and refined white
flour from Algeria. Sunflower oil has replace butter, and children are given
powdered instead of fresh animal milk. The vast majority of these "new" and
strange foodstuffs are categorized as "hot" in the Kel Alhafra classification

system. In the nomads' view, skewed consumption in the form of too many and too much food classified as "hot" causes the body to accumulate excessive heat, leading to stagnation in the blood and hence to diseases that are likewise classified as "hot". Such diseases today vastly outnumber those of a "hybrid" or "cold" character. Whether this is a novel situation or whether such an imbalance has existed for some time would require further research comparing the past and contemporary disease repertoires. In addition, the change in traditional dietary behavior and the almost permanent shortage of milk result in a condition called *āmāγrəs*, "traversing a difficult situation", considered by the Kel Alhafra as one of the most serious disease pictures: it causes a general weakening of the entire organism and is regarded as a possible precursor for all other diseases, especially endemic syphilis, *āmāγras*.

During exile and while living in refugee camps, many Kel Alhafra women were exposed to a sedentary, different way of life. Comparing themselves with sedentary women who plant and tend gardens, have a school education and enjoy a certain degree of independence, the Kel Alhafra women have become conscious of their isolation and their dependence on male members of the group. The Kel Alhafra woman also feels, however, that as *wālāt ajāma*, as "daughter of the vast spaces/desert", she is labeled by the sedentary population as a "broussarde", as an "uncouth savage" who has no idea how to behave in the civilized world including state institutions like the health centers. Unable to access this strange world, and holding onto a sense of pride in her outsider status, the Kel Alhafra woman retreats into her familiar internal networks. Drawing on enormous reserves of self-control, a sick Kel Alhafra woman hides her suffering for as long as she can, discussing it only, if at all, with trusted female family members and friends. Only when the sickness is advanced and assistance must be sought outside the female networks will the (male) decision makers in the group be informed of her problem. The Kel Alhafra women say that it is during their reproductive years that they experience the most health problems, and as a first resort they help one another to alleviate and cure their ailments. Birth is perceived as an intimate, feminine experience that takes place in the protective environment of a familiar tent among, if possible, female kin. Only when a mother's life is in danger do the Kel Alhafra consider the services of the health care center, but by then she is often no longer in a state fit to be transported out of the encampment. If a woman dies during childbirth, however, the Kel Alhafra say her soul will go straight to paradise; such a death is not arbitrary and there is nothing that humans can do to avert it.

Following their belief in divine providence, the Kel Alhafra draw no distinction between natural and supernatural causes for disease: God alone is reality and nothing in nature happens independently of God. Solidarity with a sick person is, therefore, always more important than one's own fears of infection, because the occurrence of sickness lies in the hands of the creator alone: physical causality has no place in this worldview. Thus, many infectious diseases are misrecognized by the Kel Alhafra as hereditary diseases, imposed by the creator on certain families.

The Kel Alhafra are exceedingly mistrustful of the state health care services whose employees, the nomads believe, exploit their situation for their own benefit. In their illness behavior, the Kel Alhafra women remain withdrawn into their own networks until they are acutely ill, only then breaking out of their isolation to seek help elsewhere. It is especially difficult for women and children whose lives revolve around the tent and encampment to respond in any other way. When a healer from outside is consulted, he or she is almost invariably a practitioner from the folk sector who shares the cultural background of the Kel Alhafra. Because a marabout or *enāsāfar*, a traditional healer, is additionally endowed with *ālbarāka*, the divinely inspired power of blessing, and practices a holistic treatment which takes into account all aspects of the patient's circumstances, the Kel Alhafra feel much closer to such healers than to biomedically trained doctors or state-trained health personnel. Although the Kel Alhafra acknowledge the immediate effects of modern pharmaceuticals, in particular those that are given as injections or infusions, they nevertheless think that modern drugs only fight the symptoms and thereby superficially relieve the patient from his or her complaint but do not remove the disease out of the body. After treatment with modern medicines, the disease will reappear later in a different form or another part of the body. There is in every disease an element of divine wisdom, not always comprehensible to humans, and thus a total cure requires and comprises not only a physical healing but also an inner spiritual cleansing – both aspects are required to regain inner equilibrium and good health.

The recent past has brought political isolation and marginalization, expulsion and exile to the Kel Alhafra, and they perceive themselves as being excluded from the political development of the Malian state. In their remote nomadic range they have limited access to water, and their nomadic lifestyle makes it much more difficult for them to benefit from educational opportunities and preventive or curative health care provided by the state. The distant health care institutions in Ber and Timbuktu are not adapted to the needs of this population group. During famines, the nomads are turned into political pawns, their health becomes a discourse of power and once again it is the weakest members of the society who suffer the consequences.

In this contemporary situation where the Kel Alhafra are torn between rebellion and capitulation, between an idealized past and an uncertain future, be-

tween a nomadic lifestyle and settlement in villages or cities, and not least between traditional and modern medicine, religious values are being reassessed
as a source of greater stability in such precarious times. The identificatory role,
once played by the now disbanded tribal associations and discredited traditions, is being transferred to a nascent religiosity. A general return to and reinterpretation of religious values is apparent, in which coreligionists are forming a social network set within the context of a shared Islamic origin, history
and culture. During the struggles for emancipation, especially in the rebellion years of 1991–1996 and not least in the recent political unrest, an idealized Islamic prototype began to take shape among the Kel Alhafra, bestowing
on them a new sense of community and security in times of change. Since de-
velopments in Malian politics either rarely penetrate or benefit the remote areas of Azawad or meet with general indifference among the nomads, religious
structures internal to Kel Alhafra society are gaining in importance. Because
virtues such as piety and godliness now win both recognition and respect, the
role of the marabout within the nomadic society is gaining in significance and
influence. This revived piety has two important consequences for health concepts and behavior among the Kel Alhafra. On one hand, it brings with it a religious fatalism in certain circles that smothers any personal responsibility
and action; children in particular suffer in such cases because they are absolutely dependent on their parents. The second effect is the rejection of secular influences, including modern medicine. The effectiveness of modern medicine is placed in doubt not only because it does not offer a holistic approach
to the patient's suffering and treatment, but also because it is perceived as
the product of profit- and power-greedy western industrialized nations and
their sidekicks in the local health care sector. *"āṣṣexāt ašəkrəš n-alxer"*, they
say in Tamasheq, "health is a garden of good fortune". *"mušan torhənna
tojarāt āṣṣahāt-nanāy"*, the Kel Alhafra add, "however, sickness surpasses our
means", because they are subject to the divine power, and recovery is a decided by God alone.

7.3. Critical reflections

It is hoped that this study will provide a deeper understanding of disease
concepts among the Kel Alhafra, their representations of illness and disease,
their social practices and norms, and the risks to which they are exposed in
their specific cultural context. As the medical investigation shows, standardized epidemiological questionnaires are not entirely adequate to capture a target group's thinking about sickness and health. Local interpretation strategies have a high explanatory value, and biomedical diagnostics and therapies

will receive greater recognition if they can be translated into the local context. However, in order to perform such a translation, the cultural context of the Kel Alhafra has to be recognized first and then be translated to the biomedical perspective.

In a patriarchal society like that of the Kel Alhafra, where quite strict divisions between the sexes prevail, only female researchers will be allowed access to the feminine milieu. Such researchers from outside must know the group's language if they are seeking real and nuanced insights into the women's world. This study is distinctive among research on the health of the Tamasheq in that conversations and interviews were conducted directly with Kel Alhafra women without using an interpreter. Their statements have been translated as literally as possible for incorporation into this book. All my interpretations and reflections were also discussed with the Kel Alhafra women for their endorsement before I included them in the text.

This is the first study that has been undertaken in the remote nomadic range of the Kel Alhafra, and it shows that the mode of life and the medical resources of this nomadic group in Azawad are significantly different from those of other Tamasheq groups, such as those based in the southern and western Niger delta, and also from those living in Algeria and Niger. However, this study makes no claims to completeness, and the clinical investigation alone highlights medical issues that require more extensive and more comprehensive investigation. For a representative and accurate analysis of the nutritional status of the Kel Alhafra, it will be necessary to study and follow a target group for at least one entire year. The same goes for the pathologies, which in this study were only diagnosed during a limited phase of two seasons. Detailed investigations are also required to confirm or dispel the suspicion of tuberculosis, hypovitaminois A and various zoonoses. The efficacy of traditional therapies (phytotherapies) remains an open question, as does the use and impact of the various pharmaceutical products that are sold at the local markets or are smuggled in from Algeria. In addition, it appears that veterinary products, such as ivermectin, are being used to treat humans. Differentiations also need to be made between the population's self-medication with modern medicines and their prescription and use by the "Agents de Santé". Finally, this study has only been able to provide an initial picture of the various healer types to which the Kel Alhafra have recourse, and their circles of influence. How and where healers establish their networks and a more precise understanding of their practices requires a separate study to detail the outlines that have been provided here.

This study was by no means a straightforward undertaking. Officially Azawad is still defined by the government as a "zone d'insécurité", and "le grand Nord", the far north of Mali, is associated with the perpetual flare up of conflicts and conspiracies. State authorities initially viewed interest in a population group that had in recent years become a politically intractable topic with some mistrust. When the local Malian health authorities received a report from a foreign academic in April 2005 of a developing food crisis in the research area, they reacted with indignation and questioned the veracity of my observations, although facts, confirmed later by Médicins sans Frontières from a medical point of view, spoke another language. At the same time, a developing food shortage was observed by international organizations in neighboring Niger. In several locations, conditions were on the verge of famine, but the authorities there continued to deny its existence. Corruption, mismanagement and favoritism prevail in northern Mali, severely impeding any development efforts to assist the marginalized nomadic groups. To undertake research in an area like Azawad requires not only permission and support by the state institutions, one must also gain the trust of the nomads, not always an easy task.

At the end of my fieldwork, it was possible to organize a conference in the study area on the theme "The Well-Being of the Nomadic Populations". There, representatives of the state authorities, the nomadic population and international organizations discussed together, for the first time, appropriate health care interventions and possible development measures for this region of Mali and its people. Surprisingly, women of the Kel Alhafra, in particular, came forward to speak. They called first and foremost for the installation of a solar pump at the relatively centrally located well of Tin Timāγayān. *"aman iman"*, they say in Tamasheq, "water is life, is the soul". The women stated that without water, no local markets will grow, and development interventions can only be implemented if basic human needs are guaranteed. When asked about healthcare, the Kel Alhafra women do not talk about how they hope for a health center, access to medicine or doctors. Instead, they say: *"tafāja dat iləktan"* – "a tree must have a trunk before it can grow branches", but before the trunk itself can grow, three things are needed: peace, *ālγafγāt*, water, *aman,* and education, *tāmusne.*

"We don't want to be afraid any more", said one woman at the conference, "peace and security should be guaranteed in the region", she continued, because *"akənnəs wār itəmmādrāy"* – "a conflict is never minor". When families have to flee, pastures that are already barren suddenly become overpopulated, leading to further conflicts over scarce natural resources, food shortages and hunger. Further, in their search for pastures, Tamasheq families are often separated by enormous distances, and the men are away with the herds while the women remain at the camp near a well. Drawing water from a well is seen as men's work, however, and a Tamasheq woman will not go to the well by herself. If the men of the family are away, the water that has already been drawn must be used very carefully. "Simple access to water would not only end our isolation", the women say, "we could also plant vegetable gardens, as we have seen in refugee camps in Algeria and Mauritania". Growing vegetables would not only allow the women to supplement their one-sided diet but would also give them the opportunity to improve their financial situation. "If access to water were easier, we could settle with the children for longer periods while the men are away with the animals. The children would have the chance of going to school, and we women could also be trained in what to do against disease. The girls could marry later than they do now". However, the Tamasheq women emphasize, "we women will not go to a health center to have our children – that is not a matter for doctors, and it is not in our tradition, but we want to learn how we can better support our sisters and daughters when they are giving birth".[223]

223 The Tamasheq women attending the Tin Timāɣayān conference on March 11ᵗʰ – 12ᵗʰ 2006: Tiyāyya Wālāt Muttalāmin, Taitini Wālāt Hammoutāfa, Matou Wālāt Maḥmoud, Aicha Wālāt Alḥajj, Tiyāyya Wālāt Tāhamāt, Tafakou Wālāt Tāhamāt, Taima Wālāt Muḥammad Aṣṣaliḥ, Tismakout Wālāt Muḥammad, Bouba Wālāt Ḥāmmāta, Mansola Wālāt Ḥāmmāta.

8. Annex

8.1. List of figures

Chapter 4: Cultural Interpretations of Illnesses

Chapter 5: Therapeutic Networks

Chapter 6: The Clinical Status of Women and Children

8.2. List of plants

Plants used as medicines		
Tamasheq term	Latin name	Plant part used
akāmen	Zornia glochidiata	timəttāwt (pl. timəttwen) seeds
ahārjəjəm	Cassia italica	tabsāyt (pl. tibsāyen) bush
ahəjjar	Acacia adansonii/Acacia nilotica	timəttāwt (pl. timəttwen) seeds, āla – leaves
akārkāra	?	efārket (pl. ifārkitān) n-emāyt leaves of the tree
al'anbar	Jasminum floribundum	eki (pl. ikiwān) roots
ālyānfar (aḍutān)	Syzygium aromaticum	cloves
ālḥālba	Trigonella foenum graecum	timəttāwt (pl. timəttwen) fenugreek seeds
ālišwaḍ	Cymbopogon schoenanthus	āla- fine leaves of the tebāremt plant
ālmuxāynes	Cleome bradycarpa	tabsāyt (pl. tibsāyen) bush
balāssa	Commelina forskalei	timəttāwt (pl. timəttwen) seeds
boylām	Quercus suber	cork of the cork oak
əššāyḥ	Artemisia santonica	tabsāyt (pl. tibsāyen) bush, wormwood
hālla	Lawsonia inermis	tabsāyt (pl. tibsāyen) bush, henna
ižəkimba	Xylopia aethiopica	alkāḍ (pl. ilkaḍān) fruit, pepper
tāborāyt	Balanites aegyptiaca	āla, iləktān, issənnanān, ikiwān leaves, twigs, thorns, roots of tree
tadhānt	Boscia senegalensis	efārket (pl. ifārkitān) leaves of the tree
tāhahist	Cadaba glandulosa	tabsāyt (pl. tibsāyen) bush
tājārt	Maerua crassifolia	āla n-emāyt leaves of the tree
tajəllət	Citrullus colocynthis	alkāḍ (pl. ilkaḍān) colocynth
tafəngora	Adansonia digitata	alkāḍ (pl. ilkaḍān) pulverized fruit of the baobab tree
tānafyāk	?	timəttāwt (pl. timəttwen) seeds
tanust n-āwārwār	Gummi arabicum	
tebāremt	Andropogon nadus	tešše (pl. taššiwen) herb

Plants used as medicines		
Tamasheq term	Latin name	Plant part used
tešāɣt	Salvadora persica	efārket (pl. ifārkitān) leaves of the tree
təlšušād	?	alkāḍ (pl. ilkaḍān) fruit
təsuya	Picris asplenioides	tabsāɣt (pl. tibsāɣen) bush
torša	Calotropis procera	(tiẓuẓamn-torša) carbonized pieces of the plant

Edible plants		
Tamasheq term	Latin name	Plant part used
abāka (pl. ibakatān)	Zizyphus saharae	alkāḍ (pl. ilkaḍān) fruit
abədebəd	Boerhavia coccinea	timəttāwt (pl. timəttwen) seeds
āborāɣ (pl. iborāɣen)	Balanites aegyptiaca	alkāḍ (pl. ilkaḍān) fruit, wild date
afāẓo	Panicum turgidum	timəttāwt (pl. timəttwen) seeds
asɣāl	Panicum laetum	timəttāwt (pl. timəttwen) seeds, fonio
ajəruf	Tribulus terrestris	timəttāwt (pl. timəttwen) seeds, fenugreek
bərjut	Echnochloa stagnina	timəttāwt (pl. timəttwen) seeds (only near the river)
emeitāɣtāɣ	Agama colonorum	timəttāwt (pl. timəttwen) seeds
idumumān	Diospyros mespiliformis	alkāḍ (pl. ilkaḍān) fruits of the tādumut tree
infin	Grewia villosa	timəttāwt (pl. timəttwen) seeds
tamāssālt	Limeum indicum	timəttāwt (pl. timəttwen) seeds
tarākaḍt	Grewia tenax	alkāḍ (pl. ilkaḍān) fruits
tašit	Eragrostis pilosa	timəttāwt (pl. timəttwen) seeds
teɣrāggāɣen	Leptadenia pyrotechnica	alkāḍ (pl. ilkaḍān) fruits of the ana plant
tejābārt	Echinochloa colona	timəttāwt (pl. timəttwen) seeds
telājāṣt	Citrullus lanatus	alkāḍ (pl. ilkaḍān) fruit, wild melon
titanɣen	Balanites aegyptiaca	alkāḍ (pl. ilkaḍān) fruit, nuts of the wild date
waẓẓāj also aɣālas/tākane	Cenchrus biflorus	timəttāwt (pl. timəttwen) seeds, cram-cram

Plants used as animal feed	
Tamasheq term	Latin name
afāẓo	Panicum turgidum
ajāsāy	Gynandropsis gynandra
ana	Leptadenia pyrotechnica
aləmmoẓ	Eragrostis tremula
efāyād	Blepharis linariifolia
iləs n-tas	Polygala arenaria
tāfādofādot	Tragus berteronianus
tāfaytok	?
taləggid	Cyperus jeminicus

Plants used as animal feed	
Tamasheq term	Latin name
tasəskārt	Dactyloctenium aegyptium
əššāyḥ	Artemisia santonica
hālla (anhālla)	Lawsonia inermis
iẓəkimba	Xylopia aethiopica
tāhahist	Cadaba glandulosa
tafəngora	Adansonia digitata
tebāremt	Cymbopogon schoenanthus
təsuya	Picris asplenioides

Trees	
Tamasheq term	Latin name
ādārās	Commifora africana
āhākš	Acacia raddiana
ājār	Maerua crassifolia
tāborāyt	Balanites aegyptiaca
tadhānt	Boscia senegalensis only found near the river

Trees	
Tamasheq term	Latin name
tādumut	Diospyros mespiliformis
tājārt	Maerua crassifolia
temewt	Acacia flawa
tešāyt	Salvodora persica
torša	Calotropis procera

Most of the Latin names for the identified Tamasheq plants are taken from the dissertation by El Mehdi Ag Hamahady: *Nosographie tamachèque des gastro-enterites dans la région de Tombouctou*. Thèse de Doctorat à l'Ecole Nationale de Médecine et de Pharmacie du Mali. Bamako: 1988.

The sources for all plant names whose Latin designations are not in Ag Hamahady's catalogue are:

– Anne-Catherine Benchelah, Hildegard Bouziane and Marie Maka, *Arbres du Sahara. Voyage au coeur de leurs usages*. Paris: Ibis Press, 2006;

– Anne-Catherine Benchelah, Hildegard Bouziane, Marie Maka, Colette Ouahès, *Fleurs du Sahara. Voyage ethnobotanique avec les Touaregs du Tassili*. Paris: Ibis Press, 2000;

– Marceau Gast, *Moissons du désert. Utilisation des ressources naturelles au Sahara central*. Paris: Ibis Press, 2000.

8.3. Bibliography

Aghali-Zakara, Mohamed. Psycholinguistique touarègue. Interférences culturelles. Paris: Inalco, 1992.

Ag Hama, Ahmed Ismail. "Consommation et commercialisation des produits pastoraux chez les Kel Tamasheq de la boucle du Niger (Mali)". L'avenir des peuples pasteurs. Eds. Galaty, John G., Dan Aronson, and Philip C. Salzman. Ottawa : Centre de recherches pour le développement international: 1983. 270–276.

Ag Hamahady, El Mehdi. Nosographie tamachèque des gastro-enterites dans la région de Tombouctou. Doctoral thesis, Ecole Nationale de Médecine et de Pharmacie du Mali. Bamako: 1988.

Al Wardi, Ali. Soziologie des Nomadentums. Neuwied and Darmstadt: Luchterhand, 1972.

ʿArīb Ibn Saʿīd al-Kātib al-Qurṭubī. Kitāb Ḫalq al-ǧanīn wa -tadbīr al-ḥabālā wa-l-maulūdīn. Le livre de la génération du foetus et le traitement des femmes enceintes et des nouveau-nés. Eds. Jahier, Henri, and Abdelkader Noureddine. Algiers: Publications de la faculté mixte de médecine et de pharmacie d'Alger, 1975/1956.

Assmann, Jan. Das kulturelle Gedächtnis. Schrift, Erinnerung und politische Identität in frühen Hochkulturen. Munich: Beck, 2002.

Azarya, Victor, Nomads and the State in Africa: The Political Roots of Marginality. Leiden: African Studies Centre, 1996.

Basso, Keith H. "Western Apache Witchcraft." Anthropological Papers of the University of Arizona No. 15. Tucson: University of Arizona Press, 1969.

Bastien, Joseph W. "Qollahuaya-Andean Body Concepts: A Topographical-Hydraulic Model of Physiology." American Anthropologist 87.3 (1985): 595–611.

Benchelah, Anne-Catherine, Hildegard Bouziane, and Marie Maka. Arbres du Sahara. Voyage au cœur de leurs usages. Paris: Ibis Press, 2006.

Benchelah, Anne-Catherine, Hildegard Bouziane, Marie Maka, and Colette Ouahès. Fleurs du Sahara. Voyage ethnobotanique avec les Touaregs du Tassili. Paris: Ibis Press, 2000.

Bernus, Edmond. "Laits touaregs. Usages et symboles". Ressources vivrières et choix alimentaires dans le bassin du lac Tchad. Eds. Raimond, Christine, Eric Garine, and Olivier Langlois. Paris: IRD Editions / Prodig Editions, 2005. 399–412.

– "Colporteurs de charmes magiques: les Ikadammatan." Journal des Africanistes 55.1–2 (1985): 16–27.

– Touaregs nigériens. Unité culturelle et diversité régionale d'un peuple pasteur. Paris: L'Harmattan, 1981.

– "Maladies humaines et animales chez les Touaregs sahéliens." Journal de la Société des Africanistes 39.1 (1969): 111–137.

– "Cueillette et exploitation des ressources spontanées du Sahel nigérien par les Kel Tamasheq." Cahiers d'ORSTOM, Série Sciences humaines 4.1 (1967): 31–49.

Bernus, Edmond, Pierre Boilley, Jean Clauzel, and Jean-Louis Triaud. Nomades et commandants. Administration et sociétés nomades dans l'ancienne AOF. Paris: Karthala, 1993.

Boilley, Pierre. Les Touaregs Kel Adagh. Dépendances et révoltes: du Soudan français au Mali contemporain. Paris: Karthala, 1999.

Boisbouvier, Christophe. "ATT entre en guerre." Jeune Afrique, 27 January 2009.

Boll, Franz. "Die Lebensalter. Ein Beitrag zur antiken Ethologie und zur Geschichte der Zahlen." Neue Jahrbücher für das klassische Altertum 16.31 (1913): 89–145.

Bonnier, Gaetan. L'occupation de Tombouctou. Paris: Monde moderne, 1926.

Bourdieu, Pierre. Esquisse d'une théorie de la pratique (précédé de trois études d'ethnologie kabyle). Paris: Editions du Seuil, 2000.

Brunet-Jailly, Joseph. Se soigner au Mali: une contribution des sciences sociales. Paris: Karthala/ ORSTOM, 1993.

al-Buḫārī, Muḥammad Ibn Ismaʿīl. Ṣaḥīḥ al-Buḫārī. al-ǧamiʿ aṣ-ṣaḥīḥ. Liechtenstein: Thesaurus Islamicus Foundation, 2000.

Byl, Simon. Le dualisme ou les couples d'opposées. Recherches sur les grands traités biologiques d'Aristote: sources écrites et préjuges. Brussels: Académie Royale Belgique, 1980. 210–237.

Casajus, Dominique. La Tente dans la solitude. La société et les morts chez les Touaregs Kel Ferwan. Paris: Fondation de la Maison des Sciences de l'Homme, 1987.

Chelhod, Joseph. "La baraka chez les Arabes ou l'influence bienfaisante du sacré." Revue de l'histoire des religions 148 (1955): 68–88.

Claudot-Hawad, Hélène. "Neither Segmentary, nor Centralized. The Sociopolitical Organization of a Nomadic Society (Tuaregs) beyond Categories." Orientwissenschaftliche Hefte 14 (2004): 57–69.

– Les Touaregs. Portrait en fragments. Aix-en Provence: Edisud, 1993.

Comte, Auguste. Cours de philosophie positive. Paris: Hermann, 1975.

"Corruption Perception Index." Transparency International. 6 November 2006. http://www.transparency.org (accessed 11 Nov. 2006).

Cunningham, Clark. "Order in the Atoni House." Right and Left: Essays on Dual Symbolic Classification. Ed. Needham, Rodney. Chicago: Chicago University Press, 1973. 204–238

Daou, Ousmane. "Insécurité au nord: L'Etat entretien le conflit ethnique." Le Républicain, 16 January 2009.

Decraene, Philippe. "Une arme politique contre les Touaregs du Mali." Le Monde, 6 February 1974. 1 and 3–4.

Defo, Barthelemy Kuate. "Areal and Socioeconomic Differential in Infant and Child Mortality in Cameroon." Social Science and Medicine 4.32 (1996): 399–420.

Deichgräber, Karl, ed. Hippokrates: Über Entstehung und Aufbau des menschlichen Körpers. Περί σαρκών. Leipzig, Berlin: Teubner, 1935.

Diakité, Birama Djan. "Problèmes de nomades au Gourma." Se soigner au Mali: une contribution des sciences sociales. Ed. Brunet-Jailly, Joseph. Paris: Karthala ORSTOM, 1993. 189–209.

Diallo, Birama. Rapport de la mission médicale, aire d'Oudéika, région de Tombouctou-Mali, 07 au 09 avril 2005. Programme santé nomade de Médecins Sans Frontières Luxembourg (MSF-L). Timbuktu (Mali): MSF-L, 2005.

Douglas, Mary. Ritual, Tabu und Körpersymbolik. Frankfurt am Main: Fischer, 2004.

Ebin, Victoria. "Interpretations of Infertility: the Aowin People of Southeast Ghana." Ethnography of Fertility and Birth. Ed. McCormack, Carol. London: Academic Press, 1982. 131–149.

ECHO. Rapport d'évaluation des actions humanitaires financées par ECHO dans le Nord-Mali et le Nord-Niger, 1998–1999. April 2000.

El Moctar, Mohamed. "Logiques de production et utilisation des services de santé en milieu nomade au Mali: Cas de la commune de Ber (Tombouctou)." Doctoral thesis, Faculté de Médecine de Pharmacie et d'Odonto-Stomatologie. Bamako: Université du Mali, 2006.

Encyclopedia of Islam. Vol. 2. Leiden: Brill, 2000.

Fabrega, Horacio. Disease and Social Behavior: An Interdisciplinary Perspective. Cambridge MA: MIT Press 1974.

Feachem, Richard G, Dean T. Jamison. Disease and Mortality in Sub-Saharan Africa. Oxford: Oxford University Press, 1991.

Ferro-Luzzi, Gabriella. "Women's Pollution Periods in Tamilnadu (India)." Anthropos 69 (1974): 113–161.

Figueiredo-Biton, Cristina. "Initiation sentimentale et sexuelle chez les Touaregs du Mali." L'autre 4.2 (2003): 225–237.

Fiore, Barbara. "La maladie 'naturelle' et soins chez les Touaregs." Isefran. Maladies et soins en milieu Touareg. Walett Faqqi, Fadi. Bandiagara (Mali), Perugia (Italy): Editions CRMT/PSMTM, 1993. 53–62.

Foley, Henri. Moeurs et médecine des Touareg de l'Ahaggar. Calvisson: Jacques Gandini, 1995.

Foster, Stanley O., Gadir H. El Sid, and Abdullahi Deria. "Spread of Smallpox among a Somali Nomadic Group." Lancet 2.8094 (1978): 831–833.

Foucauld, Charles de. Dictionnaire Touareg-Français. Dialecte de l'Ahaggar. 4 vols. Paris: Imprimerie nationale, 1951–1952.

Foucauld, Charles de, and Adolphe de Calassanti-Motylinski. Textes Touaregs en prose (dialecte de l'Ahaggar). Critical edition by Salem Chaker, Hélène Claudot, and Marceau Gast. Aix-en Provence: Edisud, 1984.

Gast, Marceau. Moissons du désert. Utilisation des ressources naturelles au Sahara central. Paris: Ibis Press, 2000.

Geertz, Clifford: Die künstlichen Wilden. Frankfurt am Main: Fischer, 1993.

– Observer l'Islam: Changement religieux au Maroc et en Indonésie. Paris: la Découverte, 1992.

– Works and Lives: The Anthropologist as Author. Cambridge: Polity Press, 1988.

– Dichte Beschreibung. Beiträge zum Verstehen kultureller Systeme. Frankfurt am Main: Suhrkamp, 1983.

Giuffrida, Alessandra. "Clerics, Rebels and Refugees: Mobility Strategies and Networks among the Kel Antessar." The Journal of North African Studies 10.3–4 (2005): 529–543.

Goldziher, Ignaz. Gesammelte Schriften. Vol. 5. Hildesheim: Olms, 1970.

Good, Byron J. Medicine, Rationality, and Experience. An Anthropological Perspective. New York: Cambridge University Press, 1994.

Good, Byron J., and Mary J. Del Vecchio Good. "The Comparative Study of Greco-Islamic Medicine: The Integration of Medical Knowledge into Local Symbolic Contexts." Paths to Asian Medical Knowledge. Eds. Leslie, Charles, and Allan Young. Berkeley: University of California Press, 1992. 257–271.

– "The Semantics of Medical Discourse." Sciences and Cultures. Eds. Mendelsohn, Everett, and Yehuda Elkana. Dordrecht: Reidel, 1981. 177–212.

– "The Meaning of Symptoms: A Cultural Hermeneutic Model for Clinical Practice." The Relevance of Social Science for Medicine. Eds. Eisenberg, Leon, and Arthur Kleinman. Dordrecht: Reidel, 1980. 165–196.

Good, Byron J., Mary J. Del Vecchio Good, and Robert Moradi. "The Interpretation of Dysphoric Affect and Depressive Illness in Iranian Culture." Culture and Depression: Studies in the Anthropology and Cross-Cultural Psychiatry of Affect and Disorder. Eds. Kleinman, Arthur, and Byron J. Good. Berkeley: University of California Press, 1985. 369–428.

Greifeld, Katarina, ed. Ritual und Heilung: Eine Einführung in die Ethnomedizin. Berlin: Dietrich Reimer 2003.

Grémont, Charles, André Marty, Rhissa ag Mossa, and Younoussa H. Touré. Les liens sociaux au Nord-Mali. Entre fleuve et dunes. Paris: IRAM/Karthala, 2004.

Griaule, Marcel. Conversations with Ogotemmeli. Oxford: Oxford University Press, 1965.

Guide de Transcription du Tamasheq: Anāsbərij n-tanəktubt n-Tāmašāγt. Ministère de l'Education de Base DNAFLA/AEN-Mali. Bamako: Imprimerie DNAFLA, Edition 1995.

Guthrie, William K.C. A History of Greek Philosophy. 2 vols. Cambridge: University Press, 1962–1965.

Hahn, Robert: Sickness and Healing: An Anthropological Perspective. New Haven: Yale University Press, 1995.

Hall, Edward T. The Dance of Life: The Other Dimensions of Time. Garden City NY: Anchor Press, 1984.

Hampshire, Kate. "Networks of Nomads Negotiating Access to Health Resources among Pastoralist Women in Chad." Social Science and Medicine 54.7 (2002): 1025–1037.

Harwood, Alan. "The Hot-Cold Theory of Disease. Implications for Treatment of Puerto Rican Patients." Journal of the American Medical Association 216.7 (1971): 1153–1158.

Heath, Jeffrey. Dictionnaire Touareg du Mali. Tamachek-Anglais-Français. Paris: Karthala, 2006.

Helman, Cecil G. Culture, Health and Illness. New York: Oxford University Press, 2001.

Hertz, Robert. "La prééminence de la main droite: étude sur la polarité religieuse." Revue philosophique de la France et de l'étranger 11 (1909): 553–580.

Hill, Allan G. Population, Health and Nutrition in the Sahel. London: Routledge & Kegan Paul, 1985.

Hilton-Simpson, Melville W. Arab Medicine & Surgery: A Study of the Healing Art in Algeria. London: Oxford University Press, 1992.

Hörbst, Viola. Heilungslandschaften. Umgangsweisen mit Erkrankungen und Heilung bei den Cora in Jesus Maria, Mexiko. Münster: Lit, 2006.

Hoffman, Lawrence A. "Healing the Sick as an Exercise in Religious Metaphor." Metaphor Canon, and Community: Jewish, Christian, and Islamic Approaches. Eds. Bisschops, Ralph, and James Francis. Bern, New York: Lang, 1999.

Hugh-Jones, Christine. From the Milk River. Cambridge: Cambridge University Press, 1979.

Hunwick, John O., ed. The Writings of Western Sudanic Africa. Leiden: Brill, 2003.

Hureiki, Jacques. Tuareg. Heilkunst und spirituelles Gleichgewicht. Schwülper/Hülperode: Cargo Verlag, 2004.

– Essai sur les origines des Touaregs. Paris: Karthala, 2003.

– Les médecines touarègues traditionnelles. Approche ethnologique. Paris: Karthala, 2000.

Hureiki, Jacques, and Xavier Laqueille. "The Tuareg Addiction to Tea, to Smokeless Tobacco and to Milk: Ethnological and Clinical Approach." Encéphale, le Journal de Neurologie de Psychiatrie et de Médecine Psychosomatique 29.1 (2003): 42–48.

http://english.aljazeera.net

http://globalsecurity.org/military/ops/pan-sahel.htm

http://globalsecurity.org/military/ops/tscti.htm

http://www.temoust.org/mali-les-rebelles-touaregs-fuient,7632

Ibn Ḥanbal, Aḥmad Ibn Muḥammad. Musnād al-imām Aḥmad Ibn Ḥanbal / ḥaqqaqalu wa-ḫarraǧa aḥādīṯahu wa-'allaqa 'alayhi. Šu'ayb al-Arna'ūṭ, 'Adil Muršid al-Musnad. Bayrūt: Mu'assasat ar-risāla, 1999–2001.

Imperato, Pascal J. "Problems in Providing Health Services to Desert Nomads in West Africa." Tropical Doctor 5 (1974): 116–117.

Izutsu, Toshihiko. God and Man in the Koran: Semantics of the Koranic Weltanschauung. North Stratford: Ayer, 1998.

Jachimowicz, Edith: "Islamic Cosmology." Ancient Cosmologies. Eds. Blacker, Carmen, and Michael Loewe. London: George Allen & Unwin, 1975. 143–171.

Joffre, Maréchal J. "Rapport sur les opérations de la colonne Joffre avant et après l'occupation de Tombouctou." Rapport de M.J. Joffre, lieutnant-colonel du Génie. Revue du Génie militaire. Paris: Berger-Levrault, 1895.

Khuri, Fuad I. The Body in Islamic Culture. London: Saqi Books, 2001.

Klein, Thamar. Globale und lokale Medizinen in Benin. Münster: Lit, 2006.

Klein-Franke, Felix. Vorlesung über die Medizin im Islam. Wiesbaden: Franz Steiner, 1982.

Kleinman, Arthur. Patients and Healers in the Context of Culture. An Exploration of the Borderland between Anthropology, Medicine, and Psychiatry. Berkeley: University of California Press, 1980.

Klute, Georg. "Die Rebellionen der Tuareg in Mali und Niger." Habil.-Schrift Univ. Siegen 2001/2. Cologne: Köppe Verlag [in print].

– Die schwerste Arbeit der Welt. Alltag von Tuareg-Nomaden. München: Trickster, 1992.

Knipper, Michael. Krankheit, Kultur und medizinische Praxis. Eine medizinethnologische Untersuchung zu "mal aire" im Amazonastiefland von Ecuador. Münster: Lit, 2001.

Koch, Lars-Christian. Die ethnischen Varianten des "Krankseins": Krankheitsvorstellungen und Krankheitsverhalten in Stammeskulturen. Bonn: Holos, 1987.

Kriss, Rudolf and Hubert Kriss-Heinrich. Volksglaube im Bereich des Islam. 2 vols. Wiesbaden: Harrassowitz, 1960–1962.

Krönke, Frank. "Perception of Ill-Health in a Fulbe Pastoralist Community and Its Implications on Health Interventions in Chad." Doctoral thesis, University of Basel, 2001.

Laderman, Carol. "Symbolic and Empirical Reality: A New Approach to the Analysis of Food Avoidances." Amercian Ethnologist 8.3 (1981): 468–493.

Le Jean, Yannick. "Médecine traditionnelle en milieu nomade dans la région de Tombouctou." Doctoral thesis in medicine, Faculté de Médecine de Paris-Sud, 1986.

Leslie, Charles ed. Asian Medical Systems: A Comparative Study. Berkley: University of California Press, 1977.

L'Essor. No. 15740, 7. October 2006.

Lexiques Spécialisés: Français-Tamasheq. tālqamust: təfransist-tāmašāɣt. Ministère de l'Education de Base DNAFLA/AEN-Mali. Bamako: Imprimerie DNAFLA, 1995.

Lhote, Henri. Comment campent les Touaregs. Paris: Susse, 1947.

L'Indépendant. 13 July 2006, and 17 July 2006.

Lloyd, Geoffrey. Polarity and Analogy. Two Types of Argumentation in Early Greek Thought. Bristol: Bristol Classical Press, 1987.

Loustaunau, Martha O., and Elisa J. Sobo. The Cultural Context of Health, Illness, and Medicine. Westport: Bergin & Garvey, 1997.

Loutan, Louis. "Les problèmes de santé dans les zones nomades." La santé en pays tropicaux. Eds. Rougement, André, and Joseph Brunet-Jailly. Paris: Doin, 1989. 219–253.

– "Seasonal Variations in Nutrition among a Group of Nomadic Pastoralists in Niger." Lancet 8383 (1984): 945–947.

Lux, Thomas, ed. Kulturelle Dimensionen von Medizin. Ethnomedizin – Medizinethnologie – Medical Anthropology. Berlin: Reimer, 2003.

Maïga, Mohamed Tiessa-Farma. Le Mali: de la sécheresse à la rébellion nomade. Chronique et analyse d'un double phénomène du contre-développement en Afrique sahélienne. Paris: L'Harmattan, 1997.

Mali, République. Commissariat à la Sécurité Alimentaire (CSA). "Plan de sécurité alimentaire commune rurale de Ber, 2006–2010." Bamako: 2006.

Mali, République. "Loi N° 02–049 du 22 Juillet 2002." Portant loi d'orientation sur la santé. Assemblée Nationale. Bamako: 20 July 2002.

Mali, République. Ministère de l'Administration Territoriale et des Collectivités Locales. "Commune rurale de Ber. Présentation générale." Bamako: 2006.

Mali, République. Ministère de la Santé. "SLIS (Système Local d'Information Sanitaire): Annuaire statistique sanitaire du système locale d'informations sanitaires." Bamako: 2002.

Marty, Paul. Etudes sur l'islam et les tribus du Soudan. Vol. 1: Les Kounta de l'Est, les Bérabiches, les Iguellad. Paris: Leroux, 1920.

McGilvray, Dennis. Symbolic Heat: Gender, Health & Worship among the Tamils of South India and Sri Lanka. Ahmedabad: Mapin, 1995.

McLuhan, Marshall. Understanding Media: The Extensions of Man. Corte Madra: Gingko, 2003.

Macpherson, Calum N. "Epidemiology and Control of Parasites in Nomadic Situations." Veterinary Parasitology 54. 1–3 (1994): 87–102.

Meyerhof, Max. Ḥunain ibn Isḥāq. Cairo: Government Press, 1928.

Murphy, Robert F. "Social Distance and the Veil." American Anthropologist 66 (1964): 1257–1274.

Muslim, Ibn al-Ḥaǧǧāǧ al-Qušayrī. Ṣaḥīḥ Muslim. Liechtenstein: Thesaurus Islamicus Foundation, 2000.

Musnāt i-efes. āssexāt 1&2. Bamako : Ministère de l'Education de Base de la République du Mali (DNAFLA) / UNICEF, 1989.

Nesselrath, Heinz-Günther. "Mythos-Logos – Mytho-Logos: Zum Mythos-Begriff der Griechen und ihrem Umgang mit ihm." Form und Funktion des Mythos in archaischen und modernen Gesellschaften. Eds. Rusterholz, Peter, and Ruppert Moser. Bern: Haupt, 1999. 1–26.

Nicolaisen, Johannes. "Essai sur la religion et la magie touarègues." Folk 3 (1961): 113–162.

Norris, Harry. The Tuaregs: Their Islamic Legacy and Its Diffusion in the Sahel. Warminster, Aris & Phillips, 1975.

Ouazani, Cherif. "Les dessous d'une attaque." Jeune Afrique, 20 May 2007.

Ousmane, Mohamed. "La médecine traditionnelle tamachèque en milieu malien." Doctoral thesis, Ecole Nationale de Médecine et de Pharmacie du Mali. Bamako: 1981.

Pandolfi, Paul. Les Touaregs de l'Ahaggar, Sahara algérien. Parenté et résidence chez les Dag-Ghâli. Paris: Karthala, 1998.

Paret, Rudi: Der Koran. Translated by Rudi Paret. Stuttgart, Berlin, Cologne: Kohlhammer, 1996.

Pfleiderer, Beatrix, and Wolfgang Bichmann. Krankheit und Kultur. Eine Einführung in die Ethnomedizin. Berlin: Dietrich Reimer, 1985.

Poulton, Robin E. "Après cinq ans de guerre: vers la réintégration des Touaregs au Mali." Le Monde Diplomatique. November 1996.

Prasse, Karl-G. Dictionnaire Touareg-Français (Niger). 2 vols. Copenhagen: Museum Tusculanum, 2003.

Prinz, Armin. "Die Lyme-Borreliose als 'Culture-bound Syndrome' bei den Azande Zentralafrikas: Beispiel einer ethnozentrischen Fehlinterpretation." Special reproduction Curare 14 (1991).

Prudhon, Claudine. La malnutrition en situation de crise. Manuel de prise en charge thérapeutique et de planification d'un programme nutritionnel. Paris: Action contre la Faim, Karthala, 1995.

Raimond, Christine, Eric Garine, and Olivier Langlois, eds. Ressources vivrières et choix alimentaires dans le bassin du lac Tchad. XI Colloquium International Mega-Tchad, 20–22 November 2002. University of Paris X-Nanterre. Paris: IRD, 2005.

Randall, Sara. "The Demographic Consequences of Conflict, Exile and Repatriation: A Case Study of Malian Tuareg." European Journal of Population – Revue Européenne de Démographie 21.2–3 (2005): 291–320.

– Fertility of Malian Tamasheq Repatriated Refugees. The Impact of Forced Migration. Washington, DC: The National Academic Press, 2004.

– "Enquête au Gourma en vue d'une intervention sanitaire appropriée." Se soigner au Mali. Ed. Brunet-Jailly, Joseph. Paris: Karthala, 1993.

– "Différences géographiques et sociales dans la mortalité infantile et juvénile au Mali." Population 6 (1984): 921–946.

Randall, Sara, and Alessandra Giuffrida. "Mariage et ménages chez les Kel Tamasheq du Mali: bouleversements socio-économiques et continuité démographique." Communication préparée pour les Cinquième Journées Scientifiques du Réseau Démographique de l'AUF, London, 2004.

– "Forced Migration, Sedentarisation and Social Change: Malian Kel Tamasheq." Nomadic Societies in the Middle East and North Africa: Entering the 21st century. Ed. Chatty, Dawn. Leiden: Brill, 2005. 431–462.

"Rapports de missions sur l'action d'urgence à Inagouzmi (Commune de Ber, Cercle de Tombouctou, Région de Tombouctou)." Implementation: Vétérinaires Sans Frontières, Centre de Référence de Tombouctou, Financing: Swiss Development Cooperation SDC, Programme Alimentaire Mondiale PAM. July 2005.

Rasmussen, Susan J. "From Childbearers to Culture-Bearers: Transition to Postchildbearing among Tuareg Women." Medical Anthropology 19.1 (2000): 91–116.

– "Parallel and Divergent Landscapes: Cultural Encounters in the Ethnographic Space of Tuareg Medicine." Medical Anthropology Quarterly 14 (2000): 242–270.

– "Ritual Powers and Social Tensions as Moral Discourse among the Tuareg." American Anthropologist 100.2 (1998): 458–468.

– "Female Sexuality, Social Reproduction, and the Politics of Medical Intervention in Niger: Kel Ewey Tuareg Perspectives." Culture, Medicine and Psychiatry 18.4 (1994): 433–462.

– "Lack of Prayer: Ritual Restrictions, Social Experience, and the Anthropology of Menstruation among the Tuareg." American Ethnology 18.4 (1991): 751–769.

– "Accounting for Belief: Causation, Misfortune and Evil in Tuareg Systems of Thought." Man 24.1 (1989): 124–144.

– "Interpreting Androgynous Woman: Female Aging and Personhood among the Kel Ewey Tuareg." Ethnology 26 (1987): 17–30.

Reichel-Dolmatoff, Gerardo. Amazonian Cosmos: The Sexual and Religious Symbolism of the Tukanao Indians. Chicago: Chicago University of Chicago, 1971.

R.N. "Ag Bahanga demande à réintégrer l'Accord d'Alger. El-Watan (Algeria), 2 April 2009.

Roche Lexikon Medizin. Hoffmann La Roche AG. 4th edition. Munich: Urban & Fischer, 1999.

Roussel, M. "Ether et chaleur dans l'embryologie aristotélicienne: influences archaïques." Mélanges d'études anciennes offerts à Maurice Lebel. Quebec: 1980. 157–160.

Rusterholz, Peter, and Rupert Moser. Form und Funktion des Mythos in archaischen und modernen Gesellschaften. Bern: Haupt, 1999.

Ṣaḥīḥ al-Buḫārī. Nachrichten von Taten und Aussprüchen des Propheten Muhammad. Edited and translated by Dieter Ferchl. Stuttgart: Reclam, 1991.

Schelling, Esther. "Human and Animal Health in Nomadic Pastoralist Communities of Chad: Zoonoses, Morbidity and Health Services." Doctoral thesis, University of Basel, 2002.

Schopen, Armin: Traditionelle Heilmittel in Jemen. Wiesbaden: Franz Steiner, 1983.

Schreiber, Wolfgang. Das Kriegsgeschehen 2008. Wiesbaden: VS Verlag für Sozialwissenschaften, 2010.

Sheper-Hughes, Nancy, and Margaret Lock. "The Mindful Body: A Prolegomenon to Future Work in Medical Anthropology." Medical Anthropology Quarterly 1.1 (1987): 6–41.

Siebert von, Silke. Traditionelle Medizin, Körper- und Krankheitsverständnis in Boca do Acre, Brasisilien. Dissertation der Universität Düsseldorf, 2000.

Spittler, Gerd. Les Touaregs face aux sécheresses et aux famines. Les Kel Ewey de l'Aïr (Niger). Paris: Karthala, 1993.

Spitz Georges. Le Soudan français. Paris: Editions Maritimes et Coloniales, 1955.

Staiano-Ross, Kathryn. Interpreting Signs of Illness: A Case Study in Medical Semiotics. Berlin; New York: Mouton de Gruyter, 1986

Stolz, Fred: Nomadismus. Theorie und Wandel einer sozio-ökologischen Kulturweise. Stuttgart: Franz Steiner, 1995.

Sudlow, David. The Tamasehq of North-East Burkina Faso. Vol. 1. Cologne: Rüdiger Köppe, 2001.

Swift, Jeremy. "Sahelian Pastoralists: Underdevelopment, Desertification, and Famine." Annual Review of Anthropology 6 (1977): 457–478.

Swift, Jeremy, C. Toulmin, and S. Chatting. "Providing Services for Nomadic People." UNICEF Staff Working Papers No. 8. New York: UNICEF, 1990.

Synnott, Anthony. The Body Social. Symbolism, Self and Society. London, New York: Routledge, 1993.

Ṭabarī, Abū l-Ḥasan ʿAli Ibn Sahl Rabban. Firdausu-l-Ḥikmat. Die propädeutischen Kapitel aus dem Paradies der Weisheit über die Medizin des ʿAli Ibn Sahl Rabban aṭ-Ṭabarī. Translated and commented by Alfred Siggel. Mainz: Akademie der Wissenschaften und der Literatur, Abhandlungen der geistes- und sozialwissenschaftlichen Klasse 14, 1953.

Touré, Laurence. "Une innovation sanitaire: l'appropriation des médicaments par les populations touaregs du Mali." Panser le monde, penser les médecines. Traditions médicales et développement sanitaire. Ed. Pordié, Laurent. Paris: Karthala, 2005. 269–286.

True, William R. "Epidemiology and Medical Anthropology." Medical Anthropology: A Handbook of Theory and Method. Eds. Johnson, Thomas M., and Carolyn F. Sargent. New York: Greenwood Press, 1990.

UNICEF. Enfants et femmes au Mali. Une analyse de situation. Paris: L'Harmattan, 1989.

Vogt, Evon. The Zinacantecos of Mexico: A Modern Mayan Way of Life. Belmont: Wadsworth, Thomson Learning, 2002.

Wagenaar-Brouwer, Martie. "Preliminary findings on the diet and nutritional status of some Tamasheq and Fulani groups in the Niger Delta of central Mali." Population, Health and Nutrition in the Sahel: Issues in the Welfare of Selected West African Communities. Ed. Hill, Allan G. London: Routledge & Kegan Paul, 1985. 226–253.

Walentowitz, Saskia. "Enfant de soi, enfant de l'autre. La construction symbolique et sociale des identités à travers une étude anthropologique de la naissance chez les Touaregs (Kel Eghlal et Ayttawari de l'Azawagh, Niger)." Paris: Thèse de doctorat, Ecole des Hautes Etudes en Sciences Sociales, 2003.

– "L'enfant qui n'a pas atteint son lieu. Représentations et soins autour des prématurés chez les Touaregs de l'Azawagh (Niger)." L'autre, cliniques, cultures et sociétés 5.2 (2004) : 227–242.

Walett Faqqi, Fadi. Isefran. Maladies et soins en milieu Touareg. Ed. Fiore, Barbara. Bandiagara (Mali), Perugia (Italy): Editions CRMT/PSMTM, 1993.

Werner, David. Là où il n'y a pas de docteur. Dakar: Enda Tiers-Monde, 2004.

Westermarck, Eduard. Ritual and Belief in Morocco. Vol. 1. London: McMillan, 1926.

Wiese, Martin. The Context of Vulnerability to Ill-Health as Experienced by Nomadic Pastoralists. A Case Study from Dazagada and Arab Pastoral Communities in Chad. Freiburg: University of Freiburg and the Swiss Tropical Institute, 2002.

Winter, Michael. "Slavery and the Pastoral Twareg of Mali." Cambridge Anthropology 9 (1984): 4–30.

Zahan, Dominique. The Religion, Spirituality, and Thought of Traditional Africa. Chicago: Chicago University Press, 1979.

Zbinden, Ernst. Die Djinn des Islam und der altorientalische Geisterglaube. Bern: Haupt, 1953.

8.4. Clinical study questionnaires

Sélection par: code d'identification|__|__|__|__|__|__|__|__|__|__|

Choix Aléatoire |__| Médecin |__| Présentation |__| **1** Femmes; **3** Hommes: **2** Garçons; **4** Filles; **5** enfants

Santé des nomades au Mali
Questionnaire Individuel ADULTE et Consultation médicale

Informations générales (à remplir par le médecin)

Date de l'entretien : |__|__| jours |__|__| mois **2005**

1) Nom et Prénom de l'enquêté et consulté

Nom_____ Prénom _____

2) Ethnie?

     1. Arabe |__|
     2. Tamasheq |__|
     3. Songhay |__|

Autre → *Préciser* _____   code|____|

3) Sexe?

     1. Féminin |__|
     2. Masculin |__| code|____|

4) Age?   ans |__|__|

5) Quel est votre statut matrimonial?

     1. célibataire |__|
     2. marié (e)/ monogame |__|
     3. marié (e)/polygame (co-épouses) |__| → *si oui:*   Nbre|__|__|
     4. divorcé (e) |__|
     5. veuf (ve) |__| code|____|

6) Nombre d'enfants vivants?   Nbre|__|__|

7) Nombre total d'accouchements?   Nbre|__|__|

8) Nombre d'enfants de moins de 5 ans?   Nbre|__|

8) Nombre d'avortements?   Nbre|__|

8) Causes des avortements?   1|_____|
                                     2|_____|
                                     3|_____|

Sélection par:	code d'identification |__|__|__:__|__|__|__|__|__:__|
Choix Aléatoire |__| Médecin |__| Présentation |__|	1 Femmes; 3 Hommes: 2 Garçons; 4 Filles; 5 enfants

Pathologie générale (à remplir par le médecin)

9) Etat général

1. Bon |__|
2. Mauvais |__|
3. Très mauvais |__| code|____|

10) Etat de la peau

1. Normal	|__|	5. Ulcère de buruli	|__|
2. Dartre	|__|	6. Gale	|__|
3. Lèpre	|__|	7. Autre _____
4.Charbon cutané (Anthrax)	|__|	_____
5.Teigne (Trichophytie)	|__|	code|____|

11) Conjonctives (Vitamine A)

1. Normal |____| 1: oui; 0: non
2. Conjonctivite |____| 1: oui; 0: non
3. Pâles |____| 1: oui; 0: non
4. Ictériques |____| 1: oui; 0: non
5. Xérose |____| 1: oui; 0: non
6. Bitot |____| 1: oui; 0: non
7. Cicatrice |____| 1: oui; 0: non

12) Cornée (Vitamine A)

1. Xérose |____| 1: oui; 0: non
2. Erosion |____| 1: oui; 0: non
3. Ulcère |____| 1: oui; 0: non
4. Autres : _____

13) Palpation FOIE

1. Normal |__|
2. Augmenté |__| code|____|

14) Palpation RATE

1. Non palpable |__|
2. Palpable |__| code|____|

15) Palpation GANGLIONS

1. Ganglions cervicales |____| 1: augmenté; 0: normal
2. Ganglions inguinales |____| 1: augmenté; 0: normal
3. Ganglions généralisés |____| 1: augmenté; 0: normal

Auscultation (Sans valeur analytique mais médicalement nécessaire)

Sélection par: code d'identification|__|__|__!__|__|__|__|__!__|
Choix Aléatoire |__| Médecin |__| Présentation |__| **1** Femmes; **3** Hommes: **2** Garçons; **4** Filles; **5** enfants

16) Auscultation CŒUR

    1. Normal |__|
    2. Pathologique |__| code|____|

17) Auscultation POUMONS

    1. Normal |__|
    2. Pathologique |__| code|____|

18) Tension artérielle / Poids / Température

       Tension artérielle |__!__| mmHg   Poids |__!__| kg   Température |__!__| C

19) Etes-vous malades ces derniers 14 jours?

    0. Non |__| → *Question 21)*
    1. Oui |__| code|____|

20) *Si oui*, quelle maladie?

→ *donner le nom local* _____

Maladie	Nom local	Code
Paludisme		1 |__|
Bronchite		2 |__|
TBC		3 |__|
Brucellose		4 |__|
IRA		5 |__|
Diarrhée		6 |__|
Ulcère de Buruli		7 |__|
Avitainose A		8 |__|
Blessure par un animal		9 |__|
Autre Blessure (accident)		10 |__|
Brûlure		11 |__|
Fracture		12 |__|
Anémie		13 |__|
		14 |__|
		15 |__|
		16 |__|

Sélection par: code d'identification |__|__|__|__|__|__|__|__|__|__|

Choix Aléatoire |__| Médecin |__| Présentation |__| **1** Femmes; **3** Hommes: **2** Garçons; **4** Filles; **5** enfants

Soins et utilisation des services de santé (à remplir par le médecin)

21) Aviez-vous reçu de traitement pour cette maladie

0. Non |__| → *Question 23)*

1. Oui |__| code |____|

22) *Si oui*, de qui?

1) Automédication |____| *(Numéroter selon l'ordre cité par l'enquêté*

2) Marabout |____|

3) Structure sanitaire |____|

4) Guérisseur |____|

23) Quand vous êtes malades, fréquentez-vous une structure sanitaire?

0. Non |__|

1. Oui |__| → *Question 25)*   code |____|

24) *Si non*, pourquoi?

1. Pas de temps |__|	6. N'est pas dans nos habitudes |__|
2. Chère |__|	7. _____ |__|
3. Loin |__|	8. _____ |__|
4. Mauvais accueil |__|	9. _____ |__|
5. Mauvaise qualité de soins |__|	

codes |____|;|____|;|____|;|____|;|____|

Examen clinique pour les zoonoses (à remplir par le médécin)
Symptomatologie cardinale Tuberculose, Brucellose, Coxiellose

25) Avez-vous la toux?

0. Non |__| → *Question 28)*

1. Oui |__| code |____|

26) *Si oui*, depuis combien de temps?   jours |__|__| mois |__|__| années |__|__|

27) Votre crachat contient-il du sang?

0. Non |__|

1. Oui |__| code |____|

28) Avez-vous de la fièvre?

0. Non |__|

1. Oui |__| code |____|

29) De quels autres symptômes souffrez vous
(La symptomatologie suivante est d'abord demandée sans spécification (réponse ouverte), ensuite les symptomes non mentionnés sont explorés en les spécifiant)

Sélection par: code d'identification |__|__|__|¦|__|__|__|__|__|¦|__|

Choix Aléatoire |__| Médecin |__| Présentation |__| **1** Femmes; **3** Hommes: **2** Garçons; **4** Filles; **5** enfants

Complexe TBC, Brucellose, Coxiellose	Réponse ouverte	1=oui 0=non		Réponse fermée	1=oui 0=non
Dyspnée	1)			14)	
Perte de poids	2)			15)	
Douleurs dans la poitrine	3)			16)	
Fatigue	4)			17)	
Perte d'appetit	5)			18)	
Fièvre ondulé prolongée	6)			19)	
Transpiration nocturne	7)			20)	
Myalgie isolé ou diffuse	8)			21)	
Arthralgie	9)			22)	
Maux de tête	10)			23)	
Frontale	11)			24)	
Latérale	12)			25)	
Nuque	13)			26)	

Soins prénatales et couverture vaccinale des mères (à remplir par le médecin)

30) Nombre total de grossesses?   *(à comparer avec réponse 6 - 8)*   Nbre|__|__|

31) Nombre de décès périnatal?   Nbre|__|__|

32) Date de naissance dernier enfant?   jours |__|__| mois |__|__| année |__|__|__|__|

33) Avez vous une carte de vaccination ou un carnet?

      0. Non |__|

      1. Oui |__| → *Vérifier* : _____   code|__|

34) Nombre de consultations prénatales durant la dernière grossesse?   Nbre|__|

35) Accouchement du dernier enfant

      1. Hôpital |__|
      2. Férik |__|
      3. Autres:_____   code|__|

36) Qui a coupé le cordon ombilicale?

      1. Sage femme |__|
      2. Accoucheuse |__|
      3. Parent |__|
      4. Voisine |__|
      5. Autres: _____   code|__|

37) Etes-vous vacciné au moins une fois pendant votre dernière grossesse?

Sélection par: code d'identification |__|__|__|__|__|__|__|__|__|__|

Choix Aléatoire |__| Médecin |__| Présentation |__| 1 Femmes; 3 Hommes: 2 Garçons; 4 Filles; 5 enfants

    0. Non |__| → *Question 39)*

    1. Oui |__| → *Question 38)*   code|__|

38) Vous avez reçu quelles vaccinations pendant votre grossesse et quand?

  1. VAT1   jour |__|__| mois |__|__| année |__|__|__|__|

  2. VAT2   jour |__|__| mois |__|__| année |__|__|__|__|

  3. VAT3   jour |__|__| mois |__|__| année |__|__|__|__|

  4. VAT4   jour |__|__| mois |__|__| année |__|__|__|__|

  5. VAT5   jour |__|__| mois |__|__| année |__|__|__|__|

  6. VitA   jour |__|__| mois |__|__| année |__|__|__|__|

                  jour |__|__| mois |__|__| année |__|__|__|__|

  7. Prévention contre le paludisme jour |__|__| mois |__|__| année |__|__|__|__|

                  jour |__|__| mois |__|__| année |__|__|__|__|

Facteurs d'exposition aux zoonoses et questions nutritionnelles (Vitamine A) et paludisme (à remplir par un assistant)

39) Connaissez vous la chloroquine?

42) ← 0. Non |__| 1. Oui |__| →   code|__|

   40) *Si oui*: Vous la prenez quand vous avez le paludisme

   42) ← 0. Non |__| 1. Oui |__| →   code|__|

      41) *Si non*: Pourquoi?

        1. Vomissement |__|

        2. Prurits |__|

        3. Ne soigne pas |__|

        4. Autres:_____ code|__|

42) Utilisez vous une moustiquaire pour dormir?

44) ← 0. Non |__| 1. Oui |__| →   code|__|

   43) *Si oui*: Quand l'utilisez vous?

      1. Toute l'année |__|

      2. Pendant la saison des pluies |__|

      3. Quand il fait chaud |__|

      4. Autres:_____ code|__|

Sélection par: code d'identification |__|__|__|__:__|__|__|__|__:__|
Choix Aléatoire |__| Médecin |__| Présentation |__| **1** Femmes; **3** Hommes: **2** Garçons; **4** Filles; **5** enfants

---

44) Qui dors sous la moustiquaire?

    1.   Toute la famille |__|
    2.   Seulement les enfants |__|
    3.   Seulement les parents |__|
    4.   Seulement le père |__|
    5.   Autres:_____ code|____|

45) Avez vous entendu parler des moustiquaires imprégnées

47) ← 0. Non |__| 1. Oui |__| →   code|____|

      46) Si oui: Où?

Aliments les plus consommés (Rappel de 24 h qualitatif en relation avec la vitamine A).

47) Qu'est-ce que vous avez mangé hier et quelle en était la quantité?

    1. Lait |__| 1=oui 0=non   ¼ coro |__| ½ coro |__| ¾ coro |__| 1 coro |__|
    2. Céréales |__| 1=oui 0=non
    3. Légumes frais |__| 1=oui 0=non
    4. Fruits |__| 1=oui 0=non
        Si oui: spécifier _____
    5. Viande |__| 1=oui 0=non
    6. Poisson |__| 1=oui 0=non
    7. Sucre |__| 1=oui 0=non
    8. Sel |__| 1=oui 0=non

48) Est-ce que vous gardez un troupeau?

50) ← 0. Non |__| 1. Oui |__| →   code|____|

      49) Si oui: de quelles espèces?

        Espèce
        1. Bovins → |__|
        2. Chèvres → |__|
        3. Moutons → |__|
        4. Chameaux → |__|

50) Est-ce que vous traitez les cuirs?

52) ← 0. Non |__| 1. Oui |__| →   code|____|

Sélection par: code d'identification |__|__|__¦__|__|__|__|__¦__|__|

Choix Aléatoire |__| Médecin |__| Présentation |__| **1** Femmes; **3** Hommes: **2** Garçons; **4** Filles; **5** enfants

---

51) *Si oui:* de quelles espèces?

Espèce
1. Bovins → |__|
2. Chèvres → |__|
3. Moutons → |__|
4. Chameaux → |__|

---

52) Est-ce que vous faites la traite du bétail, même si c'est plus exceptionnellement?

54) ← 0. Non |__| 1. Oui |__| →   code|__|

53) *Si oui*: a) quelles espèces et b) avec quelle fréquence?

	Fréquence				
Espèce	1. Chaque **jour** ↓	2. Au moins une fois par **semaine** ↓	3. Au moins une fois par **mois** ↓	4. moins qu'une fois par mois ↓	5. Autres:
1. Bovins →	|__|	|__|	|__|	|__|	
2. Chèvres →	|__|	|__|	|__|	|__|	
3. Moutons →	|__|	|__|	|__|	|__|	
4. Chameaux →	|__|	|__|	|__|	|__|	

---

54) Est-ce que vous consommez le lait cru, c-à-d non bouilli?

56) ← 0. Non |__| 1. Oui |__| →   code|__|

55) *Si oui:* a) de quelles espèces et b) avec quelle fréquence

	Fréquence			
Espèce	1. Chaque **jour** ↓	2. Au moins une fois par **semaine** ↓	3. Au moins une fois par **mois** ↓	4. Autres: ↓
1. Bovins →	|__|	|__|	|__|	
2. Chèvres →	|__|	|__|	|__|	
3. Moutons →	|__|	|__|	|__|	
4. Chameaux →	|__|	|__|	|__|	

---

56) Est-ce que vous assistez aux mises bas (vêlages, agnelages)?

58) ← 0. Non |__| 1. Oui |__| →   code|__|

57) *Si oui:* 1) chez quelles espèces et 2) avec quelle fréquence environ.?

	Fréquence			
Espèce	1. Au moins une fois par **mois** ↓	2. Au moins une fois les **six mois** ↓	3. Au moins une fois par **an** ↓	4. Moins qu'une fois par an ↓
1. Bovins →	|__|	|__|	|__|	|__|
2. Chèvres →	|__|	|__|	|__|	|__|
3. Moutons →	|__|	|__|	|__|	|__|
4. Chameaux →	|__|	|__|	|__|	|__|

---

58) Est-ce que vous avez jamais eu un contact direct avec un placenta animal ou un avorton animal?

60) ← 0. Non |__| 1. Oui |__| →   code|____|

59) *Si oui*: a) de quelles espèce et b) placenta et/ou avorton?

Espèce	1. Placenta	2. Avortons
1. Bovins →	|__|	|__|
2. Chèvres →	|__|	|__|
3. Moutons →	|__|	|__|
4. Chameaux →	|__|	|__|

60) Quand un animal est abattu, est-ce que vous assistez à l'égorgement et/ou au découpage?

62) ← 0. Non |__| 1. Oui |__| →   code|____|

61) *Si oui*: a) quelles espèces et b) l'égorgement et/ou découpage?

Espèce	1. Egorgement	2. Découpage
1. Bovins →	|__|	|__|
2. Chèvres →	|__|	|__|
3. Moutons →	|__|	|__|
4. Chameaux →	|__|	|__|

62) Est-ce qu'il y a des parties de la carcasse qui sont consommez cru?

0. Non |__| 1. Oui |__| →   code|____|

63) *Si oui*: Quelles pièces?

---

64) Diagnostic préliminaire

---

65) Prescription

---

66) Prélèvements pris du patient et traitement des échantillons sur le terrain

1. Prélèvement Sang |__| 1=oui 0=non	5. Urines |__| 1=oui 0=non	Hématocrite:
2. Goutte épaisse |__| 1=oui 0=non	6. Hématocrite |__| 1=oui 0=non	
3. Crachat	__	1=oui 0=non	7. Inoculation du sang complet	
4. Selles |__| 1=oui 0=non	|__| 1=oui 0=non	

Sélection par: code d'identification|__|__|__|__|__|__|__|__|__|__|
Choix Aléatoire |__| Médecin |__| Présentation |__| 1 Femmes; 3 Hommes: 2 Garçons; 4 Filles; 5 enfants

Santé des nomades au Mali
Questionnaire Individuel MERE-ENFANTS et Consultation médicale

Informations générales (à remplir par le médecin)

Date de l'entretien : |__|__| jours |__|__| mois **2005**

1) Nom et prénoms de l'enfant

Nom_____Prénom_____

2) Nom du père

_____

3) Nom de la mère

_____

4) Sexe?

    1. Féminin |__|

    2. Masculin |__| code|____|

5) Age?   ans |__|__| mois |__|__|

6) Date de naissance   jour |__|__| mois |__|__| ans |__|__|

7) A t-il été vu au moins une fois dans une structure sanitaire?

9) ← 0. Non |__| 1. Oui |__| →   code|____|

    8) *Si oui*: y a-t-il un document prouvant?

    0. Non |__|

    1. Oui |__| → *demander à voir le document*

9) A t-il été vacciné une fois dans sa vie?

11) ← 0. Non |__| 1. Oui |__| →   code|____|

    10) *Si oui*, y a-t-il un document prouvant?

    0. Non |__|

    1. Oui |__| → *demander à voir le document*

B.C.G	jour |__|__|	mois |__|__|	année |__|__|__|__|	Cicatrice 1: Oui |__| 0: Non |__|
DTC 1	jour |__|__|	mois |__|__|	année |__|__|__|__|	
DTC 2	jour |__|__|	mois |__|__|	année |__|__|__|__|	
DTC 3	jour |__|__|	mois |__|__|	année |__|__|__|__|	
Polio 1	jour |__|__|	mois |__|__|	année |__|__|__|__|	
Polio 2	jour |__|__|	mois |__|__|	année |__|__|__|__|	
Polio 3	jour |__|__|	mois |__|__|	année |__|__|__|__|	
F. jaune jour |__|__|	mois |__|__|	année |__|__|__|__|		
Rougeole	jour |__|__|	mois |__|__|	année |__|__|__|__|	
Vit. A	jour |__|__|	mois |__|__|	année |__|__|__|__|	

11) A t-il été malade ces 14 derniers jours?

    0. Non |__| → *Question 15)*

    1. Oui |__| code|____|

12) *Si oui*, quelle maladie?

→ *donner le nom local* _____

Maladie	Nom local	Code
Paludisme		1 |__|
Bronchite		2 |__|
Otite		3 |__|
Pharyngite		4 |__|
Malnutrition		5 |__|
Diarrhée		6 |__|
Anémie		7 |__|
TBC		8 |__|
Brucellose		9 |__|
Ulcère de Buruli		10 |__|
Avitainose A		11 |__|
Blessure par un animal		12 |__|
Autre Blessure (accident)		13 |__|
Brûlure		14 |__|
Fracture		15 |__|
Fièvre		16 |__|
Rougeole		17 |__|
		18 |__|
		19 |__|
		20 |__|

13) A t-il été traité pour cette maladie?

    0. Non |__| → *Question 15)*

    1. Oui |__| code|____|

14) *Si oui*, de qui?

    5) Automédication |____| *(Numéroter selon l'ordre cité par l'enquêté)*

    6) Marabout |____|

    7) Structure sanitaire |____|

    8) Guérisseur |____|

15) Votre enfant a t-il fait la rougeole?

    0. Non |__|

    1. Oui |__| code|____|

Sélection par: code d'identification|__|__|__'__|__|__|__|__'__|__|
Choix Aléatoire |__| Médecin |__| Présentation |__| **1** Femmes; **3** Hommes: **2** Garçons; **4** Filles; **5** enfants

---

16) Quel est le principal aliment de sevrage de vos enfants ?

1) Lait |__|
2) Bouillie |__|
3) Boule |__|
4) Autres → *préciser, nom local* _____ code|____|

17) Etat général

4. Bon |__|
5. Mauvais |__|
6. Très mauvais |__| code|____|

18) Etat de la peau

1. Normal |__| 5. Ulcère de buruli |__|
2. Dartre |__| 6. Gale |__|
3. Lèpre |__| 7. Autres _____
4. Charbon cutané (Anthrax) |__| _____
5. Teigne (Trichophytie) |__| code|____|

19) Conjonctives (Vitamine A)

8. Normal |____|1: oui; 0: non
9. Conjonctivite |____|1: oui; 0: non
10. Pâles |____|1: oui; 0: non
11. Ictériques |____|1: oui; 0: non
12. Xérose |____|1: oui; 0: non
13. Bitot |____|1: oui; 0: non
14. Cicatrice |____|1: oui; 0: non

20) Cornée (Vitamine A)

5. Xérose |____|1: oui; 0: non
6. Erosion |____|1: oui; 0: non
7. Ulcère |____|1: oui; 0: non
8. Autres : _____

21) Oreilles

1. Normales |____|1: oui; 0: non
2. Pathologiques → *Préciser* _____ code|____|

22) Palpation FOIE

3. Normal |__|
4. Augmenté |__| code|____|

23) Palpation RATE

3. Non palpable |__|
4. Palpable |__| code|____|

24) Palpation GANGLIONS

4. Ganglions cervicales |____|1: augmenté; 0: normal
5. Ganglions inguinales |____|1: augmenté; 0: normal
6. Ganglions généralisés|____|1: augmenté; 0: normal

Sélection par: code d'identification |__|__|__|'|__|__|__|__|'|__|
Choix Aléatoire |__| Médecin |__| Présentation |__| 1 Femmes; 3 Hommes: 2 Garçons; 4 Filles; 5 enfants

25) Auscultation CŒUR

    3. Normal |__|

    4. Pathologique |__| code|____|

26) Auscultation POUMONS

    3. Normal |__|

    4. Pathologique |__| code|____|

27) Périmètre brachiale / Poids / Température

Périmètre brachiale |__|__| cm |__|__| mm   Poids |__|'|__| kg   Température |__|'|__| C

28) Diagnostic préliminaire

29) Prescription

Laboratoire

30) Prélèvements pris du patient et traitement des échantillons sur le terrain

    8. Prélèvement Sang |__| 1=oui 0=non
    9. Goutte épaisse |__| 1=oui 0=non
    10. Crachat |__| 1=oui 0=non
    11. Selles |__| 1=oui 0=non
    12. Urines |__| 1=oui 0=non
    13. Hématocrite |__| 1=oui 0=non   →   Hématocrite:
    14. Inoculation du sang complet |__| 1=oui 0=non

8.5. *Index*